Caring for Patients with Mesothelioma: Principles and Guidelines

W0106329

Mary Hesdorffer • Gleneara E. Bates-Pappas
Editors

Caring for Patients with Mesothelioma: Principles and Guidelines

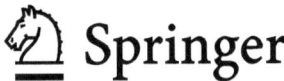 Springer

Editors
Mary Hesdorffer
Mesothelioma Applied Research
Foundation
Alexandria, VA
USA

Gleneara E. Bates-Pappas
City University of New York,
Graduate Center
New York, NY
USA

ISBN 978-3-319-96243-6   ISBN 978-3-319-96244-3   (eBook)
https://doi.org/10.1007/978-3-319-96244-3

This Springer imprint is published by the registered company Springer Nature Switzerland AG
The registered company address is: Gewerbestrasse 11, 6330 Cham, Switzerland

Foreword

Mesothelioma remains a lethal cancer with increasing global incidence. While there have been modest incremental advances, there is no clear optimal surgical approach, and presently, only one standard systemic treatment option, cisplatin and pemetrexed, is widely approved. Median overall survival remains, even with aggressive multimodality treatment, poor. Many attempts over the past decade to improve upon the established chemotherapy regimen and surgical treatment paradigm have been unsuccessful. While there has been an influx of new systemic treatments over the past 10 years for patients with molecularly characterized malignancies, no such progress has been made for patients with malignant mesothelioma. Similarly, the advent of immunotherapy with checkpoint inhibitors is under investigation in mesothelioma. These agents do appear active but, as in other diseases, only in a subset of patients. Consequently, a tremendous unmet need remains for mesothelioma treatments, and much research is ongoing.

Within this book, Mary Hesdorffer and Gleneara E. Bates-Pappas have gathered key experts across a variety of domains related to surgical treatment, systemic therapies, supportive care, public health, future mesothelioma research, and patient perspectives. Each chapter adds perspective and insight into current standards of care and potential future developments. The inclusion and emphasis on supportive care is an important differentiator for this book. Addressing the many adjunctive treatment domains such as nutrition, physical therapy, occupational therapy, pulmonary rehab, palliative care, survivorship, and end-of-life care is a unique element of this text and ensures that it will be useful to those providing care to patients with mesothelioma. Furthermore, the section on the public health impact of asbestos is vital for understanding the complex socioeconomic and psychosocial elements of this disease for patients, caregivers, families, colleagues, and other global citizens.

Caring for Patients with Mesothelioma thoughtfully touches upon basic science, clinical research, and the future of mesothelioma care, treatment, and research. Connecting all of these domains is a key component of facilitating preventative approaches and treatment advances. Only through better understandings of the molecular mechanisms of mesothelioma will we be able to bring more rational and effective therapies to this devastating disease so that we can overcome the current therapeutic plateau. Additionally, given the substantial environmental contribution of asbestos to mesothelioma and other health conditions, advocacy and public health endeavors are essential to stem the growing burden of this disease and direct necessary resources toward environmental protections, prevention, and research funding. Mesothelioma remains a disease where all involved in caring for patients, whether professionally or personally, can have a tremendous impact and many opportunities exist for researchers to advance the field in meaningful ways.

Marjorie G. Zauderer
Assistant Attending, Thoracic Oncology Service, Division of Solid Tumor Oncology, Department of Medicine, Memorial Sloan Kettering Cancer Center, Co-Director MSK Mesothelioma Program, Assistant Professor of Medicine
Weill Cornell Medical College
New York, NY, USA

Contents

Part III   Supportive Health Care for Treatment

Part IV   Public Health Impact of Asbestos Worldwide

Part V   The Future of Mesothelioma Research

Part VI   Patient's Perspective

Mary Hesdorffer Received her undergraduate degree at the College of New Rochelle in New York and went on to receive her Master of Science at the same institution. She is a Nurse Practitioner and spent nearly 20 years actively treating patients with mesothelioma. Ms. Hesdorffer has an expertise in the development and implementation of clinical trials. Her work has been published in peer-reviewed scientific journals, and she has lectured both nationally and internationally on the topics pertaining to mesothelioma with particular emphasis on clinical trials as well as symptom and disease management.

Ms. Hesdorffer has been a strong voice in urging increased transparency to the medical and legal issues surrounding mesothelioma with a strong emphasis on ethics. She is passionate in her commitment to the treatment and management of this disease and hopes to increase awareness of the need to advance the science that will lead to a cure. Mary is the Executive Director of the Mesothelioma Applied Research Foundation.

Gleneara E. Bates-Pappas LMSW, is currently a doctoral candidate at CUNY Graduate Center; an adjunct lecturer at Columbia University School of Social Work, Silberman School of Social Work at Hunter College, and New York University Silver School of Social Work; and a psychological counselor at CUNY School of Labor and Urban Studies. She received her bachelor's degree from the University of Arizona in political science and economics minoring in Africana studies and went on to receive her master's, basic science and legal training from Columbia University.

Her doctoral research explores the environmental risk factors for lung cancer mortality among racially ethnic minorities living in New York. Her current research projects aim to elucidate the biophysiological aspects of tumor resistance in response to chemotherapy and the use of telemedicine to improve quality of life and cognitive function in post-treatment cancer survivors. In addition to exploring ways to use virtual and augmented reality to reduce anxiety during treatment in pediatric oncology patients.

As a cancer researcher, she managed a translational research laboratory at Columbia University Medical Center where she conceptualized and conducted research on heat shock proteins and their role in tumor resistance in response to chemotherapy and the role of platinum agents in inducing checkpoint inhibitors related to tumor progression on the quality of life of patients and their primary care-givers during and post-treatment. In addition, she serves on the American Society of Clinical Oncology Cancer Survivorship Committee and the International Association for the Study of Lung Cancer Smoking Cessation Committee.

Part I

Mesothelioma Treatment

Dharmaraj Chauhan and Wickii T. Vigneswaran

Surgery for malignant pleural mesothelioma has had an interesting history and in selected patients remains vital for best outcome. Malignant pleural mesothelioma is a diffuse neoplasm that renders it difficult to obtain surgical resection margins free of disease. In order to achieve surgical oncologic resection (R0 resection), it would be necessary to remove all the structures that are in contact with the pleura. As there are many structure that are vital in the chest cavity that are in continuity with the parietal and mediastinal pleura, complete resection with clear margins is not achievable. Therefore, the best resection that is possible with "curative intent" is a macroscopic complete resection (MCR), a R1 resection (microscopic residual tumor). The operative procedures that are used for MCR were developed in the past to treat *Mycobacterium tuberculosis* infection. The surgery with "curative intent" is extensive surgeries and at its onset was a radical pleural pneumonectomy. This surgical procedure was fraught with very high surgical morbidity and mortality which overshadowed any potential benefit that was gained (Butchart et al. 1976). With improvement in surgical technique, anesthetic, and critical care management, the morbidity and mortality reduced significantly to appreciate the benefits. In a multimodality setting, the median survival of 21, 19, 14, and 10 months has been observed in patients with stage I, II, III, and IV MPM (Rusch et al. 2016). The optimal surgical procedure and various multimodal protocols are in flux, but the principles that are important include a complete MCR either by pleurectomy and decortication or extrapleural pneumonectomy. A uniform nomenclature was developed by the International Society for Study of Lung Cancer and International Mesothelioma Interest Group to describe various pleural surgical procedures that

D. Chauhan · W. T. Vigneswaran (✉)
Department of Thoracic and Cardiovascular Surgery, Loyola University Health System, Maywood, IL, USA
e-mail: Wickii.vigneswaran@lumc.edu

© Springer Nature Switzerland AG 2019
M. Hesdorffer, G. E. Bates-Pappas (eds.), *Caring for Patients with Mesothelioma: Principles and Guidelines*,
https://doi.org/10.1007/978-3-319-96244-3_1

are performed for MPM (Rice et al. 2011). Additionally surgical procedures are also performed for symptom relief, particularly controlling the pleural effusion and rarely for pain, or to establish diagnosis or both. These are often considered in patients who are not suitable for extensive surgical procedures but to relieve symptoms as definitive procedures or while working up for MCR.

1   Macroscopic Complete Resection (MCR) Surgery

1.1   Pleurectomy and Decortication

Pleurectomy and decortication was introduced in the 1950s for treatment of trapped lung associated with tuberculous empyema. The treatment was later adopted for malignant pleural mesothelioma. The surgery is reserved for patients that are elderly, with comorbidities, and not suitable for a pneumonectomy.Two thin layers of the pleura envelop the pleural space: (1) the visceral pleura that covers the surface of the lung and (2) parietal pleura that lines the inside of the chest wall. The former is attached to the lung surface firmly and the latter is attached to the chest wall somewhat loosely. The space between the pleurae is the pleural space where malignant cells can be found with mesothelioma.The surgical procedure of pleurectomy and decortication entails two different components. Decortication is defined as separation of visceral pleura from underlying lung parenchyma. An incision is made in the tumor, and a plane is established between the visceral pleura and lung parenchyma. Tumor invasion in visceral pleura extends into different fissure planes and can cause loss of lung expansion. Therefore, decortication should separate the fissures to allow the lung re-expansion (Fig. 1.1). The challenge of this procedure is to remove as much of the tumor

Fig. 1.1 Dissection of the visceral and parietal pleura including in the fissures

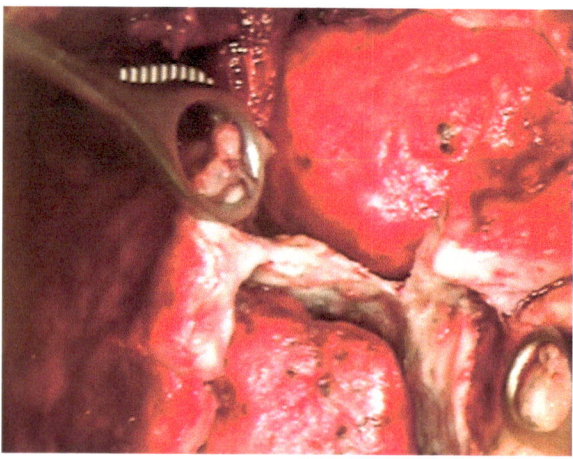

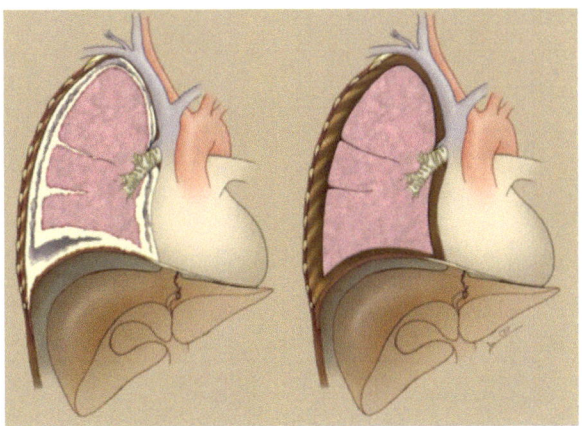

as possible without causing injury to underlying lung. Pleurectomy involves dis-section of the parietal pleura off the chest wall, pericardium, and diaphragm. This is usually achieved with blunt and sharp dissection. Extreme care is taken when dissecting at the apex and around the pericardium to avoid injury to vascu-lar structures. Inferiorly, the pleurectomy may involve peeling or removing the tumor off the diaphragm (Fig. 1.2) (Rice 2012).

Peeling of the pleura leaves raw surface on the chest wall and lung parenchyma that can lead to significant blood loss. Hemostasis can be achieved with high power electrocautery and packing. The removal of visceral pleura leaves lung parenchyma exposed, which can cause an air leak. A majority of air leaks seal within 72 hours with good drainage and full lung expansion. Drainage tubes are left behind to allow blood and air to evacuate. In the process of healing, the lung will scar and form adhesions to the chest wall which will eliminate the space where fluid normally accumulates. At times chemical agents such as talc or povidone-iodine are used to assist the scarring process.It is not unusual that the tumor involves the diaphrag-matic surface which cannot be peeled off and requires either partial or total removal. Diaphragm reconstruction may be necessary if a large portion of the diaphragm is removed. Additionally, in some patients, the pericardium that is involved is resected. Both the diaphragm and often the pericardium require reconstruction. If the diaphragm is resected and reconstructed, this is termed extended pleurectomy/decortication (EPD) (Fig. 1.3). Most surgeons use Gore-Tex prosthesis for this purposes, but a bioprosthesis can be used particularly if there is concern for infection or in patient who had a long-standing drainage tube to control pleural effusion before definitive surgery.

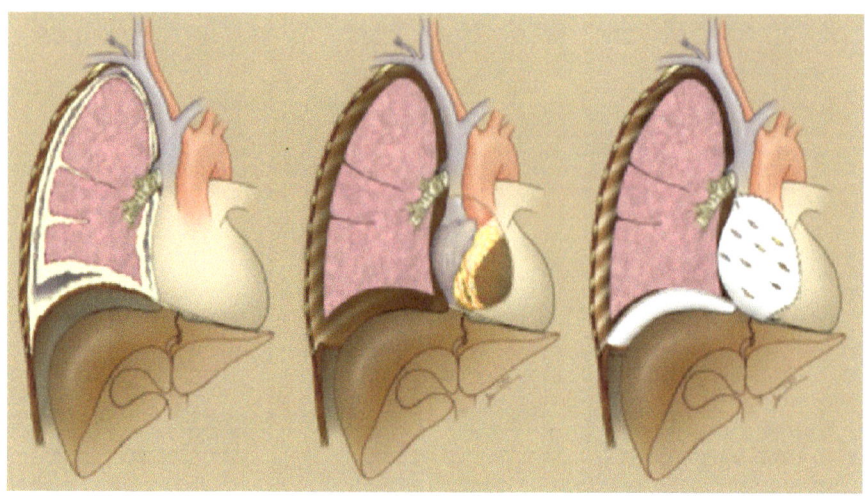

Fig. 1.3 Extended pleurectomy/decortication (EPD). (Copyrights from AME History of PleuralPublishing Company. All rights reserved. www.annalscts.com. Rice D, Ann Cardiothorac Surg 2012;1(4):497–501)

1.2　Extrapleural Pneumonectomy

Extrapleural pneumonectomy (EPP) is the removal of the entire diseased lung, part of the pericardium, diaphragm, and parietal pleura off the chest wall. In 1949, Dr. Irving Sarot performed the first extrapleural pneumonectomy for tuberculous empyema. Since then, EPP is primarily reserved for malignant pleural mesothelioma.

Patient selection is critical for surgery in order to have best outcomes. The considered patient should have optimal lung capacity in order to survive with a single lung; this is assessed via pulmonary function tests. The disease has to be of non-sarcomatoid cell subtype, preferably epithelioid cell subtype, which has the best prognosis. Since the goal of surgery is to remove all malignant cells, the patient must not have any extension of disease in the mediastinum. As part of the staging workup, CT and PET scans are obtained which can provide information regarding disease outside of the chest or in the lymph nodes. Some programs perform additional procedures such as mediastinoscopy or thoracoscopy to identify enlarged lymph nodes in the mediastinum that are not identified on the PET scan. Talc pleurodesis can provide symptomatic relief during a thoracoscopic evaluation, if malignant pleural effusion is identified while patient is worked up for EPP. The pleural adhesion can also assist in extrapleural dissection if patient is selected to undergo EPP.

EPP is performed via posterolateral thoracotomy or a lateral thoracotomy although the technique used can vary. If a previous invasive procedure was performed on the same side, the goal is then to incorporate the incision as part of the thoracotomy site. To begin the dissection, a plane is developed between the chest

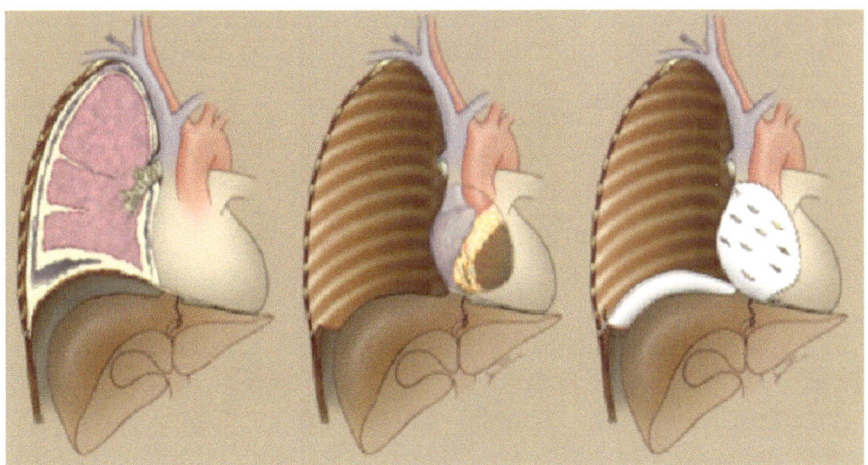

Fig. 1.4 Extrapleural pneumonectomy (EPP). (Copyrights from AME Publishing Company. All rights reserved. www.annalscts.com. Rice D, Ann Cardiothorac Surg 2012;1(4):497–501)

wall and parietal pleura. Care is taken not to enter the pleural cavity as to prevent spillage of malignant cells. Blunt and sharp dissection is used to stay in the extrapleural space inferiorly and superiorly. Medially, the dissection at the hilum is carried in the pericardium, and it is removed as part of the specimen. This is later reconstructed with patch to prevent the heart from herniating into the chest. Inferiorly, the diaphragm is excised in its entirety and reconstructed with a Gore-Tex patch (Fig. 1.4).

Managing these patients postoperatively is just as important as performing the operation. Adequate pain control is necessary to allow patients to participate in physical therapy and to prevent atelectasis of the contralateral lung caused by splinting. During and after the surgery, patients are given intravenous fluid that is managed very carefully in order to prevent fluid shift and development of post-pneumonectomy pulmonary edema.

2 Palliative Surgical Procedures

2.1 Parietal Pleurectomy

As the disease progresses, many patients will develop malignant pleural effusions. One method of treating the pleural effusion is by removing the parietal pleura. This procedure is performed in the presence of minimal disease in the pleura and to remove pleural effusion and encourage pleural adhesion to chest wall. Generally parietal pleurectomy is partial removal of parietal and/or visceral pleura for diagnostic or palliative purposes but leaving gross tumor behind (Fig. 1.5). It is a palliative procedure and is less extensive than the MCR. For the procedure to be effective, the lung should be able to completely expand following the removal of the pleural

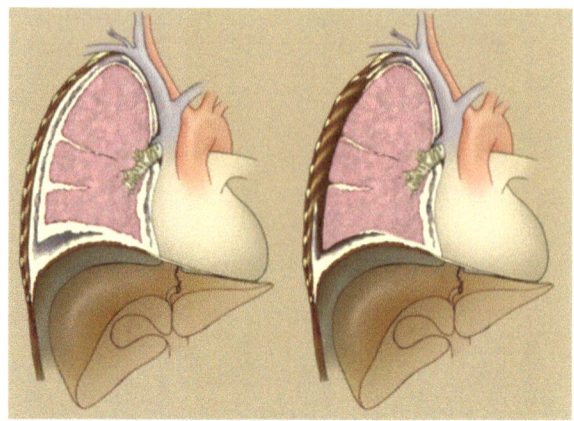

effusion to fill the chest cavity. This is often performed using video-assisted thora-coscopic approach or small thoracotomy. The procedure offers symptomatic relief in patients with pleural effusion.

2.2 Pleurodesis/PleurX Catheter

For patients who have advanced disease or those that cannot tolerate surgery, there are less invasive procedures that can be performed for symptomatic relief. Pleurodesis is a less aggressive form of treating pleural effusion. The goal is to eliminate the pleural space between the two separate pleurae where fluid accumulation can occur by instilling a caustic agent that causes scarring. The most commonly used agent currently is sterile talc powder. In order for talc pleurodesis to work successfully, the lung has to re-expand and fill the chest to allow adhesion of pleura.

In cases where there is persistent pleural effusion despite multiple interventions, or the lung will not expand to fill the chest cavity, an indwelling cuffed tunneled catheter can be placed. The procedure can be performed under local anesthesia for patients that are too sick to tolerate general anesthesia. After the procedure, patients can attach the catheter to a vacuum canister periodically and drain the fluid to help relieve their symptoms.

3 Outcomes

Despite multiple surgical options, no current consensus exists on which procedure offers the best long-term survival. Each surgical option has its own postoperative complications that need to be considered (Batirel et al. 2016). Complications common to both procedures and MCR resections include arrhythmia (atrial fibrillation, supraventricular tachycardia), bleeding requiring reoperation, and prolonged ventilation. For EPP, common complications are bronchopleural fistula and chylothorax and significantly increased morbidity and mortality (Table 1.1). Pleurectomy and

Table 1.1 Comparison of the early results of EPP and P/D

Author (year)	Total number (n)	EPP (n)	PD (n)	Major morbidity % EPP/PD	Mortality % EPP/PD
Flores et al. (2008)	663	385	278	10/6.4	7/4
Burt et al. (2014)	225	95	130	24.2/3.8	10.5/3.1
Batirel et al. (2016)	130	42	66	20/5	7/2
Sharkey et al. (2016)	362	133	229	15/6.2	6/3.5

decortication complications are prolonged air leak and mucus plugging with atelectasis. A focused systematic review on trimodality therapy involving neoadjuvant or adjuvant chemotherapy, EPP, and adjuvant radiotherapy reported a perioperative mortality rate of 0–12.5%, a morbidity rate of 50–83%, and a median overall survival of 12.8–46.9 months (Cao et al. 2012).

Overall median survival favors pleurectomy and decortication over EPP with ranges from 12 to 23 months for EPP and 19 to 32 months for pleurectomy and decortication (Flores et al. 2008; Taioli et al. 2015; Kostron et al. 2017). Quality of life is generally better for patients undergoing PD compared to EPP, for an extended period following surgery (Ploenes et al. 2013). Given the need for multimodality therapy and the aggressive nature of MPM, quality of life outcomes should be strongly considered when recommending type of surgery (Vigneswaran et al. 2017). Considering the overall survival and quality of life following surgery, pleurectomy and decortication is the preferred approach for MCR in majority of patients with MPM (Schwartz et al. 2017). Both surgical procedures are combined with multimodality treatment either neoadjuvant or adjuvant therapy for maximal benefit. In the patient in whom the comorbidities preclude MCR, palliative procedures to improve symptoms should be considered, which will allow nonsurgical treatment or best supportive care.

4 Multimodality Treatment

Surgery is not expected to achieve a complete resection without any residual disease. Therefore, chemotherapy and/or radiotherapy is added as part of multimodality treatment either in the neoadjuvant or adjuvant setting. Currently cisplatin-pemetrexed chemotherapy regimen is the first-line therapy. Bevacizumab in combination with cisplatin-pemetrexed may provide an additional benefit of 2.7 months in select patients (Wu and de Perrot 2017). Radiotherapy using intensity-modulated radiation therapy (IMRT) has been used for palliation of pain, for reduction of the risk of local metastasis at intervention sites, or as part of a multimodality approach. IMPRINT and SMART trials looked at radiation therapy with pleurectomy/decortication and EPP, respectively, and found that IMRT is a safe and feasible option (Rimner et al. 2016). There are numerous ongoing studies that will shed light into the best treatment combination modality. Current standard of care for this deadly disease remains suboptimal which has prompted researchers to explore innovative treatment alternatives. Immunotherapy is an emerging therapeutic modality that harnesses the power of the human immune system. Immune checkpoint blockade, immunotoxin therapy, anticancer vaccines, oncolytic viral therapy, and adoptive cell therapy are currently being assessed in clinical trials. Although some dramatic responses have been observed with these approaches, there are many limitations that remain, and these need to be overcome to improve the efficacy of these new therapies (Dozier et al. 2017).

References

Batirel HF, Metintas M, Caglar HB, Ak G, Yumuk PF, Yildizeli B, Yuksel M. Adoption of pleurectomy and decortication for malignant mesothelioma leads to similar survival as extrapleural pneumonectomy. J Thorac Cardiovasc Surg. 2016;151:478–84. https://doi.org/10.1016/j.jtcvs.2015.09.12.

Burt BM, Cameron RB, Mollberg NM, Kosinski AS, Schipper PH, Shrager JB, et al. Malignant pleural mesothelioma and the society of thoracic surgeons database: an analysis of surgical morbidity and mortality. J Thorac Cardiovasc Surg. 2014;148:30–5. https://doi.org/10.1016/j.jtcvs.2014.03.011.

Butchart EG, Ashcroft T, Barnsley WC, Holden MP. Pleuropneumonectomy in the management of diffuse malignant mesothelioma of the pleura. Experience with 29 patients. Thorax. 1976;31:15.

Cao C, Tian D, Manganas C, Matthews P, Yan TD. Systematic review of trimodality therapy for patients with malignant pleural mesothelioma. Ann Cardiothorac Surg. 2012;1:428–37.

Dozier J, Zheng H, Adusumilli PS. Immunotherapy for malignant pleural mesothelioma: current status and future directions. Transl Lung Cancer Res. 2017;6(3):315–24. https://doi.org/10.21037/tlcr.2017.05.02.

Flores RM, Pass HI, Seshan VE, Dycoco J, Zakowski M, et al. Extrapleural pneumonectomy versus pleurectomy/decortication in the surgical management of malignant pleural mesothelioma: results in 663 patients. J Thorac Cardiovasc Surg. 2008;135:620–6.

Kostron A, Friess M, Inci I, Hillinger S, Schneiter D, Gelpke H, et al. Propensity matched comparison of extrapleural pneumonectomy and pleurectomy/decortication for mesothelioma patients. Interact Cardiovasc Thorac Surg. 2017;24(5):740–6. https://doi.org/10.1093/icvts/ivw422.

Ploenes T, Osei-Agyemang T, Krohn A, et al. Changes in lung function after surgery for mesothelioma. Asian Cardiovasc Thorac Ann. 2013;21:48–55. https://doi.org/10.1177/0218492312454017.

Rice D. Standardizing surgical treatment in malignant pleural mesothelioma. Ann Cardiothorac Surg. 2012;1(4):497–501. https://doi.org/10.3978/j.issn.2225-319X.2012.11.05.

Rice D, Rusch V, Pass H, Asamura H, Nakano T, Edwards J, et al. Recommendations for uniform definitions of surgical techniques for malignant pleural mesothelioma: a consensus report of the international association for the study of lung cancer international staging committee and the international mesothelioma interest group. J Thorac Oncol. 2011;6(8):1304–12.

Rimner A, Zauderer MG, Gomez DR, Adusumilli PS, Parhar PK, et al. Phase II study of hemithoracic intensity-modulated pleural radiation therapy (IMPRINT) as part of lung-sparing multimodality therapy in patients with malignant pleural mesothelioma. J Clin Oncol. 2016;34(23):2761–8.

Rusch VW, Chansky K, Kindler HL, et al. The IASLC mesothelioma staging project: proposals for the M descriptors and for revisions of the TNM stage groupings. J Thorac Oncol. 2016;11:2112–9.

Schwartz RM, Watson A, Wolf A, Flores R, Taioli E. The impact of surgical approach on quality of life for pleural malignant mesothelioma. Ann Transl Med. 2017;5(11):230. https://doi.org/10.21037/atm.2017.03.41.

Sharkey AJ, Tenconi S, Nakas A, Waller DA. The effects of an intentional transition from extrapleural pneumonectomy to extended pleurectomy/decortication. Eur J Cardiothorac Surg. 2016;49:1632–41.

Taioli E, Wolf AS, Flores RM. Meta-analysis of survival after pleurectomy decortication versus extrapleural pneumonectomy in mesothelioma. Ann Thorac Surg. 2015;99(2):472–80. https://doi.org/10.1016/j.athoracsur.2014.09.056. Epub 2014 Dec 20.

Vigneswaran WT, Kircheva DY, Rodrigues AE, Watson S, Celauro AD, et al. Influence of pleurectomy and decortication in health-related quality of life among patients with malignant pleural mesothelioma. World J Surg. 2017. https://doi.org/10.1007/s00268-017-4264-4. [Epub ahead of print].

Wu L, de Perrot M. Radio-immunotherapy and chemo-immunotherapy as a novel treatment paradigm in malignant pleural mesothelioma. Transl Lung Cancer Res. 2017;6(3):325–34. https://doi.org/10.21037/tlcr.2017.06.03.

History Cytoreductive Surgery and Hyperthermic Intraperitoneal Chemotherapy for Peritoneal Metastasis and Evolution and Contemporary Application in Peritoneal Mesothelioma

Gautham Malhortra, Ashish Patel, and Jason M. Foster

1   History of Cytoreductive Surgery

Mesothelioma is a rare tumor that develops from the cells that line the pleural space (chest cavity) and abdominal cavity (peritoneal space) and rarely can present as a soft tissue mass or growth. Malignant peritoneal mesothelioma (MPM) similar to pleural mesothelioma presents with disseminated cancer that spreads on the surfaces of abdominal organ such as the intestine, liver, spleen, omentum, and lining surfaces on the inner abdomen that cover the muscle. Other malignancies that similarly grow and metastasize in the peritoneal cavity with high frequency include tumors of the appendix, colon, and ovary. Peritoneal metastasis is a different type of cancer spread than hematogenous metastasis, which occurs due to cancer cells traveling through the blood stream to distant organ such as the liver, lung, bone, or brain and will be discussed further in this chapter. Patients with peritoneal metastasis frequently experience symptoms related to their cancer metastasis, and common symptoms include abdominal distention, ascites, pain, appetite loss, early satiety, fistula, and infection. Untreated peritoneal metastatic disease has a poor prognosis with a mean and median overall survival of 6 and 3 months, respectively (Sadeghi et al. 2000). During this short survival time, patients often endure poor quality life from tumor symptoms and malnutrition that accompanies the progression of peritoneal disease. In an effort to palliate symptoms and improve quality of life, surgery was identified as the treatment with most utility to address this problem.

The use of surgery to remove bulky, symptomatic tumor dates back to the early twentieth century in the 1930s (Meigs 1934). It was initially labeled debulking

G. Malhortra · A. Patel
Division of Surgery, University of Nebraska Medical Center, Omaha, NE, USA
e-mail: gmalhotra@unmc.edu; asish.patel@unmc.edu

J. M. Foster (✉)
Division of Surgical Oncology,
Nebraska Medical Center, University of Nebraska Medical Center, Omaha, NE, USA
e-mail: jfosterm@unmc.edu

© Springer Nature Switzerland AG 2019   13
M. Hesdorffer, G. E. Bates-Pappas (eds.), *Caring for Patients with Mesothelioma: Principles and Guidelines*,
https://doi.org/10.1007/978-3-319-96244-3_2

surgery, and the first tumor type for which surgery was conducted was ovarian cancer. The rationale for considering surgery started with the rudimentary understanding of peritoneal metastasis. Conceptually, peritoneal metastasis is similarly to the process of the shedding of skin cells, which is part of the life cycle of all cells in the human body. Microscopically cancer cells (and normal cells) shed in abdominal cavity; however, cancer cells develop molecular and biological changes that allow cancer cells to grow on other abdominal organs such as the omentum, bowel, liver, or spleen surfaces. Normal cells die after they shed in the abdominal cavity and the immune system eliminates these cells. Cancer cells, either through mutations or through cellular pathway perturbations, develop mechanisms to survive in the abdominal cavity and avoid immune detection. The cancer cells that become peritoneal metastasis must have the ability to grow on the surface of another organ as microscopic cells and once established grow eventually become visible tumor implants. The tumors continue this cycle of cancer spread and can disseminate throughout the abdominal cavity as well as grow/invade the organs where the microscopic cells implant. The lining surface where these cells attach is called the peritoneal layer (lining) and it composed of mesothelial cells. This peritoneal lining surface wraps around all of the abdominal muscles, diaphragm, and pelvic walls housing the organs called the parietal peritoneal layer, while the peritoneal lining on the organs such as the liver, intestine, spleen, etc. is called the visceral peritoneal layer. Peritoneal metastasis (PM) has also been called peritoneal carcinomatosis (PC).

The first reported experiences with debulking surgery was in the 1930s with the goal of palliation to relieve symptoms of ascites, bowel obstructions, pain, and bowel fistulas. While patients did experience some symptom relief, this was transient as tumor (and symptoms) recurrence was frequent with only a minority of patients experiencing long-term survival benefit. Groups continued to explore how surgery might benefit more patients with peritoneal metastasis, and it was not until the late 1960s when published reports began to emerge demonstrating survival benefits for patients with advanced ovarian cancer who underwent a more aggressive and comprehensive resection of their peritoneal disease. This surgical approach, called cytoreductive surgery (CRS), has the primary goal of surgery to maximally remove the abdominal tumor burden (ideally to remove all visible disease). This is different from classic debulking for palliation as the goal of CRS is to remove all the tumor, not just the tumor causing symptoms.

In quick succession, independent investigators began to confirm the survival benefit of aggressive CRS in patients with advanced staged ovarian cancer. As experience expanded, these groups began to demonstrate that the size of residual disease after CRS was the most important factor that predicted survival benefit (Griffiths et al. 1979; Munnell 1968). Specifically, patients with either no visible disease or minimal residual disease were observed to experience the longest survival benefit. This renewed the medical communities' interest in surgery for peritoneal metastasis with a change in the intent of surgery from a palliative procedure to a therapeutic procedure. Given the benefits observed with ovarian cancer, interest in using CRS for other cancer types with peritoneal metastasis as appendix, mesothelioma, and gastric – the most common being mucinous appendiceal neoplasms (MAN) that present as pseudomyxoma peritonei (PMP) – was also being explored (Ghosh et al. 1972).

Although aggressive CRS improved survival from 2 to 6 months without therapy to a 40% 5-year survival (Munnell 1968), long-term survival was observed in a minority of patients. Demonstrably survival time was 2–3 times longer; the majority of patients were still relapsing in the peritoneal cavity (local recurrence), while distant (hematogenous) metastatic events were rare. Around this time in the 1970s, laboratory research and clinical efforts began understanding what contributed to peritoneal recurrence. Both the lab and clinical evidence revealed residual disease, both microscopic and gross tumor, that remained after CRS was responsible for peritoneal cancer recurrence. Further investigation showed a clear inverse relationship between residual tumor size and long-term survival (Griffiths 1975).

Efforts to identify adjuvant treatments that could be given after CRS to prevent disease relapse, extend the time to relapse, or further improve patient survival were pursued. Early success of adjuvant radiation in other tumors prompted attempt at radiation therapy after CRS, but this was fraught with many side effects and no clinical benefit. Importantly, chemotherapeutic drug development was gaining momentum in the late 1970s, and trials for many cancers with these drugs being administered intravenously (IV) were being investigated. Some early favorable responses to IV chemotherapy were observed in ovarian cancer when given following CRS surgery (Griffiths et al. 1979). Currently the mainstay of contemporary advanced ovarian cancer management is the combination of maximal CRS surgery combined with chemotherapy, specifically a patinum and taxane agent.

During the 1970s, the same time as the first interest in IV chemotherapy, investigators began developing the tools necessary for delivery of intraperitoneal (IP) chemotherapy (Palta 1977). This was of particular interest to surgeons performing CRS procedures for cancers arising from the appendix, stomach, and mesothelioma. Although IV chemotherapy was benefiting ovarian cancer, PC from other tumor types did not achieve the same benefit. Many of the same researchers were also exploring the effects of hyperthermia in humans and specifically investigating its cytotoxic effects on cancer cells (Shingleton and Parker 1964). The work ultimately revealed that the combination of IP chemotherapy with hyperthermia yields the most robust cytotoxic effects to cancer cells in preclinical experimental models and the first clinical application of combined CRS followed by hyperthermic intraperitoneal chemotherapy (HIPEC) was performed on a patient with extensive pseudomyxoma peritonei arising from the appendix in 1979 by JS Spratt with success (Spratt et al. 1980). At this time IV chemotherapy provided no benefit for patients with appendix and mesothelioma tumors in the 1970s–1980s, and with this benefit being observed increasing interest in administering chemotherapy directly in peritoneal cavity with or without hyperthermia, CRS with HIPEC (or IP) became the major treatment paradigm for treating these types of tumors with PC.

It is important to understand some of the peritoneal space biology to appreciate the rationale for utilizing HIPEC after CRS surgery. Key to the concept of CRS surgery is the understanding that the peritoneal cavity, where the abdominal organs are "housed," provides an environment to maintain the organs and allow them to function normally. The mesothelial cellular lining on the surface of the peritoneum is responsible for this homeostasis. Therefore, the peritoneal cavity should be considered an organ that houses and protects the abdominal organs. Tumors, like mesothelioma, grow on the surface and establish a metastatic tumor on this perito-neal lining layer. As the tumor spreads and grows, sites of metastasis can involve several organs establishing disease on the peritoneal surface disease as previously described in this chapter. When the tumor burden in the abdomen is limited (low tumor burden), the CRS surgery may only require removal of the primary tumor and an organ called the omentum. When the tumor burden is more extensive, the CRS may include removal of several organs such as the spleen, portions of the colon, small bowel, pancreas, liver, peritoneum, and in woman ovaries and uterus. Again, the goal of CRS is to remove all visible disease or remove the disease down to small tumor lesions. The risk and benefits of the CRS are discussed with each patient, and the surgical selection section below addresses the patient selection decision-making in more detail for mesothelioma. When CRS can achieve removal of all visible dis-ease or minimal tumor burden (nodules 2–5 mm), HIPEC which is performed at the time of surgery will treat the remaining disease within the peritoneal cavity.

HIPEC research has determined the safest temperature range for hypethermia is 40–42.5 °C (or 104–108.5 °F) for a duration of 90–120 minutes. The drugs that are most commonly use in the peritoneal cavity are drugs with a high molecular weight and have demonstrable activity against the tumor cells. The most common drug is mitomycin C; however, other drugs used include cisplatin, carboplatin, and oxali-platin. A unique feature of the peritoneal cavity, similar to the "blood-brain barrier concept," is that drugs with high molecular weight remain contained in the abdomi-nal cavity where the drug is needed most with limited drug entry in the bloodstream. This allows medications to be given at significantly higher doses directly to the organ (peritoneal cavity) where the tumor resides. Specifically, the peritoneal-cavity-partition pharmacologically will limit the amount of drug absorbed in the blood stream, and the highest concentration of the drug is peritoneal lining, organ surfaces where either small volume or microscopic cancer cells remain. HIPEC therapy penetrates the surface to depth of 5–8 mm with maximal drug dose. This concept is central to the utilization of not only HIPEC but IP chemotherapy in general.

Persistent research in this field during the 1970–1990s has culminated in the expanded utilization of CRS/HIPEC, which has now become the primary therapy for mesothelioma and appendix tumors with PC. Both of these tumor types histori-cally, and currently, share a common problem with limited response to our best chemotherapy and no survival benefit with chemotherapy alone in patients where CRS/HIPEC is not an option. Worldwide many groups and hospitals have estab-lished CRS/HIPEC programs, and all continue to focus on refining the surgery to reduce surgical complications and improving patient selection. Two early adopters and pioneers in CRS/HIPEC are Dr. Sugarbaker in the USA and Dr. Gilly in France (Sadeghi et al. 2000; Sugarbaker 1995). Both championed the use of CRS/HIPEC, and their persistence began to shift in the oncological communities' perception of peritoneal disease from a "systemic" problem to a "locoregional" problem best treated with a surgical approach. This concept is rooted in the surgical approach to cancer of single organ such as the colon, stomach, or pancreas that are amenable to complete surgical resection and are resected after a proper cancer workup. The surgical removal of a primary colon cancer or gastric cancer yields the best outcome for patients but does not necessarily guarantee that all patients will get the best same benefit and survival. Similarly, when colon cancer metastasizes to the liver, complete resection of the metastatic foci yields the best survival outcome for patients. Conceptually CRS, when the peritoneum is viewed as an organ that can have metastatic disease that may involve multiple sites, is a similar philosophy or approach when optimal tumor resection can be achieved, and HIPEC is the second therapy to address minimal or micrometastatic disease. In 1995 one of the first comprehensive reports outlining methods for approaching a cytoreductive surgery with a focus on techniques for performing peritonectomy procedures was published and provided a foundation upon which to build (Sugarbaker 1995). As surgical technique and patient selection continue to improve, the use of CRS/HIPEC has been applied to a variety of tumor types that spread in the peritoneal cavity, expanding from mesothelioma and appendix to now include colon, stomach, as well as a renewed interest in ovarian cancer.

2   Mesothelioma Patient Selection for CRS/HIPEC

Mesothelioma is a rare but aggressive malignancy. While the majority of cases present in the pleural space, malignant peritoneal mesothelioma (MPM) accounts for approximately 30% of all mesothelioma with an annual US incidence of only 300–500 cases (Yan et al. 2007). Unfortunately, the non-specific clinical symptoms associated with MPM result in the majority of patients presenting with advanced peritoneal disease. Untreated mesothelioma has a very poor prognosis and a life expectancy between 4 and 12 months. Even though there have been many advancements in chemotherapy, use of IV systemic chemotherapy only provides a modest survival benefit, ranging between 7 and 13 months. However, with the success of CRS/HIPEC on a variety of peritoneal malignancies, investigators starting in the 1980s began utilizing CRS/HIPEC in the management of MPM with significant improvements in overall survival rates ranging from 34 to 100 months (Helm et al. 2015). Currently, CRS/HIPEC is the primary treatment for patients with optimally resectable disease and appropriate histology (Table 2.1) and confers significant survival benefit in comparison to other treatment modalities.

As discussed above, CRS is effective because it leads to locoregional control of the diseases in peritoneal cavity and surface. Consequently, when selecting patients who may be candidates for this procedure, it is essential to rule out patients with

Table 2.1 Overall survival of MPM by varying treatments

Treatment	Median overall survival (months)
No treatment	4–12 months Chua et al. (2009)
Chemotherapy	7–13 months Janne et al. (2005)
CRS/HIPEC	34–100 months Helm et al. (2015)

hematogenous metastases outside of the abdominal compartment. All patients require extensive radiologic testing utilizing computed tomography (CT) of the chest, abdomen, and pelvis with contrast and whole body with F-fluorodeoxyglucose (FDG) positron emission tomography (PET)/CT. This imaging evaluates the chest for pleural disease, chest and abdomen for nodal disease, and liver metastasis. Once extra-abdominal disease has been excluded, qualitative and quantitative assessment of the tumor burden is necessary and will determine the extent of resection necessary to achieve complete cytoreduction. The tools to determine peritoneal disease burden again are CT and magnetic resonance imaging (MRI). Blood tests for cancer markers usually CEA, CA 19-9, and CA-125 which are all types of glycoproteins are obtained primarily because these tests can be used after surgery and in follow-up to help monitor for disease recurrence/progression.

CT is often the initial imaging modality used when patients are diagnosed with PC due to its availability, ease of use, and cost. The most common finding on CT imaging includes involvement of the greater omentum seen as reticular retraction, nodular appearance, and occasionally large plaques, and in some cases, the omentum is diffusely involved and appears as a large heterogeneous density referred to as "omental caking." In addition, we commonly see focal or diffuse thickening of the peritoneal folds, or large tumor deposits depending on the underlying pathology. There are limitations to imaging, and small tumor deposits (<5 mm) are difficult to appreciate unless deposited on the surface of the liver or spleen. Finally, ascites (abdominal fluid) is a common radiographic finding. This may be seen as free intra-abdominal ascites or loculated collections and can be easily identified on CT if 50 ml of fluid is present.

MRI has emerged as another imaging option and its utility has increased over the last decade primarily due improvements in MRI access, technology, and protocols. The use of fat suppression and delayed contrast sequences has allowed MR imaging to achieve greater resolution, and some view it as a tool that might be better than CT for detecting smaller tumor deposits. There is limited comparative data of MRI and CT, and both are acceptable modalities to evaluate patients. MRI is limited because of availability and the duration of the test compared to CT is significant.

The goal of preoperative imaging after determining the absence of metastatic disease is to estimate peritoneal disease burden. Unfortunately, MRI and CT both have difficulty with smaller tumor nodules, and imaging alone is fraught with underestimating disease burden particularly small lesions on the small intestine, which is an organ that comprises a large surface area in the abdomen. Majority of surgeons who treat mesothelioma also perform a diagnostic laparoscopy to explore and directly visualize the abdominal cavity and organs. This is an invasive procedure performed in the OR, but the value is not only in determining the disease extent, but also tumor biopsies can be performed to provide adequate tissue to confirm the diagnosis. In addition, for patients with ascites, this can temporarily relieve symptoms, and it can be performed safely with the patient being discharged either the same day or the next. A staging system for peritoneal metastasis was established in the 1990s to help standardize how preoperative tumor burden was measured, and this system is called the peritoneal cancer index (PCI). It was not only useful in quantifying disease burden, but it also has value in determining the risk of relapse and survival outcomes (Harmon and Sugarbaker 2005). With this system, the abdomen is divided into nine sections, and the small bowel is further divided into four sections. For each section, a lesion size (LS) score is assigned related to the disease burden:

- LS 0: no macroscopic evidence
- LS 1: maximum diameter of the lesion up to 0.5 cm
- LS 2: maximum diameter of the lesion up to 5 cm
- LS 3: maximum diameter of the lesion greater than 5 cm or confluent nodules

The total score of all sectors yields the PCI.

The PCI provides a composite objective measurement of disease burden based upon which recommendations can be made regarding the value of cytoreduction for each patients and the timing of the surgery as well. The PCI threshold for surgery varies based on the tumor of origin as each tumor has its own inherent biological potential for relapse in both the peritoneal cavity and hematogenous metastasis. This suggests that the underlying tumor biology is another key determinant in patient outcomes. In general, a PCI score of 15–20 has been the threshold for proceeding with CRS/HIPEC in mesothelioma, but other factors also can influence this decision as well.

Achieving optimal tumor removal at the time of CRS is the most important factor in patient outcomes. In part the PCI is an estimation of our ability to achieve complete cytoreduction and important in selection particularly when surfaces such as the small intestine are involved and cannot be cleared of disease. Scoring systems to measure the volume of residual disease have also been established which are useful in determining risk of recurrence and survival. The scoring systems are based in the general principles that guide resection of many cancers in general defined by the R-stage classification system part of the internationally accepted TNM staging system (Wittekind et al. 2002) (Table 2.2). The R score has been modified for peritoneal metastasis and reflects the categories of tumor debulking based on the size of the residual disease of the largest lesion (Table 2.3). In this system, optimal CRS is defined as R0-R2a (Foster et al. 2009, 2016). Since limited benefit was observed outside of the R2a, other groups explored further defining stratifying the residual lesion size, and this is called the completeness of cytoreduction (CC) score (Glehen and Gilly 2003) (Table 2.4).

Table 2.2 R-Classification system used for oncologic resection

Resection margin (R score)	Definition
R0	Complete resection with microscopically free margins
R1	Macroscopically complete resection with microscopic residual disease
R2	Macroscopically incomplete resection

Table 2.3 R score for cytoreduction

Resection margin (R score)	Definition
R0	Complete resection with negative cytology of peritoneal fluid
R1	Complete resection with positive cytology of peritoneal fluid
R2a	Macroscopically incomplete resection with lesions ≤5 mm
R2b	Macroscopically incomplete resection with lesions >5 mm≤ 2 cm
R2c	Macroscopically incomplete resection with lesions >2 cm

Table 2.4 Completeness of cytoreduction (CC) classification system widely accepted for PC

Definition	CC score	Description
Complete	0	No visible tumor remaining
	1	Tumor implants <0.25 cm remaining
Incomplete	2	Tumor implants between 0.25 cm and 2.5 cm remaining
	3	Tumor implants >2.5 cm or layered disease remaining

These tools help to establish patient selection criteria for surgery and design treatment strategies for patients with mesothelioma. In 2004 and 2006, international consensus meetings for MPM were held, and treatment guidelines were published (Hassan et al. 2006). Patients are initially evaluated with extensive laboratory and imaging workup. Staging laparoscopy was recommended to (1) obtain tissue diagnosis (if this has not yet been done), (2) accurately determine disease burden, (3) calculate their PCI, and (4) estimate the completeness of cytoreduction that is achievable. If the patient's histological diagnosis is responsive to CRS/HIPEC (epithelioid histology), and the patient can achieve a CC0, CC1, or CC2 cytoreduction, then proceed with CRS/HIPEC followed by adjuvant systemic chemotherapy. If these conditions are not met, the patient starts systemic chemotherapy initially and is reevaluated for surgical resection (Sugarbaker et al. 2016).

3 Factors in Outcome and Survival in MPM and CRS/HIPEC

A small subset of patients with MPM will have advanced unresectable disease and will not be surgical candidates, while a few other patients may have medical comorbidities that increase surgical risk and preclude safe conduct of CRS/HIPEC. For these patients' chemotherapy is the primary treatment. Unfortunately, this subset of patient has the worst prognosis.

The majority of mesothelioma patients are candidates for CRS/HIPEC, and several prognostic factors have been identified to determine risk of recurrence and survival. These factors can be divided into patient factors, tumor factors, and surgical factors. The two primary patient factors are age and sex. Older patients (>60 years) at diagnosis experience a shorter survival, while female patients have been found to have a favorable survival after CRS/HIPEC (Alexander et al. 2013). More important, tumor histology and subtype have a major impact on both patient selection and survival. Patients with sarcomatoid or biphasic tumors have the worst prognosis but represent a small minority of MPM patients. Most patients are epithelioid subtype, 90–95% which overall has favorable prognosis.

Surgical factors can be divided into the burden of disease at the time of surgery and the amount of residual disease at the conclusion of surgery. The scoring systems were discussed earlier, but to briefly recap, peritoneal carcinoma index (PCI) is the burden of disease before surgery, and the cytoreduction score (CC) or R score measures the residual disease at the conclusion of CRS (Tables 2.2, 2.3, and 2.4). The more bulky disease at diagnosis is associated with a worse prognosis, and not surprisingly, patients with bulky disease are less likely to undergo optimal tumor debulking. Optimal tumor debulking as defined by the CC or R score is when all visible disease can be removed, labeled either CC-0,1 or R0-R2a. The higher the CC or R score, the bulkier the residual disease following surgery, and the higher the risk of recurrence and worse survival. Other surgical poor prognostic factors include nodal metastasis and exclusion of HIPEC administration following optimal CRS (Chua et al. 2009).

CRS/HIPEC has emerged as the most effective therapy for peritoneal mesothelioma, with reported 5-year overall survival (OS) around 41–67%, and in general, adjuvant chemotherapy is given to these patients (Kepenekian et al. 2016). Yan et al. reported a median OS of 53 months in a multi-institutional retrospective study of 405 patients with improved survival dependent upon epithelioid subtype, absent lymph node metastasis, and complete cytoreduction (CCR-0 or CCR-1) (Yan et al. 2009). Helm et al. reported improved 5-year survival with intraperitoneal chemotherapy (Helm et al. 2015). A second multi-institutional retrospective study of 211 mesothelioma patients treated with CRS/HIPEC reported by Alexander et al. demonstrated overall median survival of 38.4 months, with 5- and 10-year survivals of 41% and 26% (Alexander et al. 2013). In Alexander et al. multivariate analysis demonstrated significantly worse prognosis for age greater than 60 (HR 2.05, CI 1.24–3.39), CCR-2-CCR-3 resection (HR 1.81, CI 1.11–2.95), and high-grade histology (HR 2.14, CI 1.17–3.91). Thirty percent of patients experienced a postoperative complication and operative mortality was 2.3%. In both studies (Yan and Alexander et al.), there was some evidence that platinum-based chemotherapy (cisplatin) was associated with improve survival compared to mitomycin C, but this will require further investigation.

4 Emerging Therapies and Future Direction

Repeated application of intraperitoneal therapy (HIPEC and/or IP) has been the area of interest and may be a simple but impactful strategy to help improve outcomes in MPM. Specifically, patients with bulky disease determined by a high PCI (>20–25) remain a high-risk group, and efforts to improve outcomes with this strategy have been explored. One strategy is a two-staged procedure where patients undergo limited debulked with omentum resection and large bulky tumor but avoid major resection (incomplete debulking) combine with HIPEC. Next patients receive adjuvant chemotherapy and return to the OR for a second CRS/HIPEC. Heller et al. demonstrated a median recurrence-free survival of 38.5 months for optimally treated patients with MPM undergoing two-stage CRS/HIPEC. Their study found that completeness of cytoreduction score ≤CC1 at the first and second operations resulted in a median OS of 6.65 years (95% CI 5.03–14.41). Tumor histology was not a significant factor in recurrence, but biphasic and sarcomatoid tumors were a minority of the patients. In this study, only lesions greater than 0.5 cm were resected, providing evidence of the efficacy of HIPEC for small and microscopic disease (Heller et al. 2017).

The concept of repeat intraperitoneal chemotherapy has also been explored with normothermic intraperitoneal chemotherapy (NIPEC) after definitive CRS/HIPEC in 29 patients. This is conceptually similar to the use of IP chemotherapy following CRS in ovarian cancer (Armstrong et al. 2006). This early experience reported by Sugarbaker et al. demonstrated that CRS/HIPEC with NIPEC improved survival despite high preoperative PCI and reported a 5-year survival was 75%. Similarly, in this treatment model, CC score was relevant as survival benefit was only observed in optimally debulked CC0, CC-1 patients (Sugarbaker and Chang 2017).

Laboratory research focus on identifying the biological mechanisms involved in peritoneal mesothelioma will lead to novel therapies that help improve survival outcomes (Esquivel et al. 2007). Additionally, efforts to develop clinical trial to help identify the best combination and sequencing of these therapies are being designed. In a subset of patients, CRS/HIPEC and systemic chemotherapy have significantly improved outcomes and prolonged survival, but continued research is necessary to improve patient selection and improve outcome for all patients with MPM.

In conclusion, significant progress has been achieved through a robust understanding of the biology of peritoneal metastasis and peritoneal base therapy. This work has yielded improved outcomes for patients with peritoneal mesothelioma patients, and for a subset, long-term survival can be achieved. CRS/HIPEC is currently the most effective therapy in the management of peritoneal mesothelioma. Majority of patients will also receive chemotherapy as part of their treatment. Further progress is still necessary in optimizing outcomes, patients' selection, and the development of new therapies effective in mesothelioma.

References

Alexander HR Jr, et al. Treatment factors associated with long-term survival after cytoreductive surgery and regional chemotherapy for patients with malignant peritoneal mesothelioma. Surgery. 2013;153(6):779–86.

Armstrong DK, et al. Intraperitoneal cisplatin and paclitaxel in ovarian cancer. N Engl J Med. 2006;354(1):34–43.

Chua TC, Yan TD, Morris DL. Outcomes of cytoreductive surgery and hyperthermic intraperitoneal chemotherapy for peritoneal mesothelioma: the Australian experience. J Surg Oncol. 2009;99(2):109–13.

Esquivel J, et al. Cytoreductive surgery and hyperthermic intraperitoneal chemotherapy in the management of peritoneal surface malignancies of colonic origin: a consensus statement. Society of Surgical Oncology. Ann Surg Oncol. 2007;14(1):128–33.

Foster JM, Gatalica Z, Lilleberg S, Haynatzki G, Loggie BW. Novel and existing mutations in the tyrosine kinase domain of the epidermal growth factor receptor are predictors of optimal resectability in malignant peritoneal mesothelioma. Ann Surg Oncol. 2009;16(1):152–8.

Foster JM, et al. Early identification of DPAM in at-risk low-grade appendiceal mucinous neoplasm patients: a new approach to surveillance for peritoneal metastasis. World J Surg Oncol. 2016;14(1):243.

Ghosh BC, Huvos AG, Whiteley HW. Pseudomyxoma peritonei. Dis Colon Rectum. 1972;15(6):420–5.

Glehen O, Gilly FN. Quantitative prognostic indicators of peritoneal surface malignancy: carcinomatosis, sarcomatosis, and peritoneal mesothelioma. Surg Oncol Clin N Am. 2003;12(3):649–71.

Griffiths CT. Surgical resection of tumor bulk in the primary treatment of ovarian carcinoma. Natl Cancer Inst Monogr. 1975;42:101–4.

Griffiths CT, Parker LM, Fuller AF Jr. Role of cytoreductive surgical treatment in the management of advanced ovarian cancer. Cancer Treat Rep. 1979;63(2):235–40.

Harmon RL, Sugarbaker PH. Prognostic indicators in peritoneal carcinomatosis from gastrointestinal cancer. Int Semin Surg Oncol. 2005;2(1):3.

Hassan R, et al. Current treatment options and biology of peritoneal mesothelioma: meeting summary of the first NIH peritoneal mesothelioma conference. Ann Oncol. 2006;17(11):1615–9.

Heller DR, et al. Recurrence of Optimally Treated Malignant Peritoneal Mesothelioma with Cytoreduction and Heated Intraperitoneal Chemotherapy. Ann Surg Oncol. 2017;24(13):3818–24.

Helm JH, et al. Cytoreductive surgery and hyperthermic intraperitoneal chemotherapy for malignant peritoneal mesothelioma: a systematic review and meta-analysis. Ann Surg Oncol. 2015;22(5):1686–93.

Jacquet P, Sugarbaker PH. Clinical research methodologies in diagnosis and staging of patients with peritoneal carcinomatosis. Cancer Treat Res. 1996;82:359–74. Review

Janne PA, et al. Open-label study of pemetrexed alone or in combination with cisplatin for the treatment of patients with peritoneal mesothelioma: outcomes of an expanded access program. Clin Lung Cancer. 2005;7(1):40–6.

Kepenekian V, et al. Diffuse malignant peritoneal mesothelioma: Evaluation of systemic chemotherapy with comprehensive treatment through the RENAPE Database: Multi-Institutional Retrospective Study. Eur J Cancer. 2016;65:69–79.

Meigs JV. Tumors of the female pelvic organs. New York: The Macmillan Company; 1934. p. xxxiv. p. 1 l., 533 p.

Munnell EW. The changing prognosis and treatment in cancer of the ovary. A report of 235 patients with primary ovarian carcinoma 1952-1961. Am J Obstet Gynecol. 1968;100(6):790–805.

Palta JR. Design and testing of a therapeutic infusion filtration system. M.S. thesis, University of Missouri, Columbia; 1977.

Sadeghi B, et al. Peritoneal carcinomatosis from non-gynecologic malignancies: results of the EVOCAPE 1 multicentric prospective study. Cancer. 2000;88(2):358–63.

Shingleton WW, Parker RT. Abdominal Perfusion for Cancer Chemotherapy Using Hypothermia and Hyperthermia. Acta Unio Int Contra Cancrum. 1964;20:465–8.

Spratt JS, Adcock RA, Muskovin M, Sherrill W, McKeown J. Clinical delivery system for intraperitoneal hyperthermic chemotherapy. Cancer Res. 1980;40(2):256–60.

Sugarbaker PH. Peritonectomy procedures. Ann Surg. 1995;221(1):29–42.

Sugarbaker PH, Chang D. Long-term regional chemotherapy for patients with epithelial malignant peritoneal mesothelioma results in improved survival. Eur J Surg Oncol. 2017;43(7):1228–35.

Sugarbaker PH, Turaga KK, Alexander HR Jr, Deraco M, Hesdorffer M. Management of malignant peritoneal mesothelioma using cytoreductive surgery and perioperative chemotherapy. J Oncol Pract. 2016;12(10):928–35.

Wittekind C, Compton CC, Greene FL, Sobin LH. TNM residual tumor classification revisited. Cancer. 2002;94(9):2511–6.

Yan TD, Welch L, Black D, Sugarbaker PH. A systematic review on the efficacy of cytoreductive surgery combined with perioperative intraperitoneal chemotherapy for diffuse malignancy peritoneal mesothelioma. Ann Oncol. 2007;18(5):827–34.

Yan TD, et al. Cytoreductive surgery and hyperthermic intraperitoneal chemotherapy for malignant peritoneal mesothelioma: multi-institutional experience. J Clin Oncol. 2009;27(36):6237–42.

Cytoreductive Surgery and Intraperitoneal Chemotherapy for Treatment of Malignant Peritoneal Mesothelioma

3

Paul H. Sugarbaker

1 The Natural History of Malignant Peritoneal Mesothelioma

In 1972, Charles Meortel at the Mayo Clinic, Rochester, Minnesota, reviewed the information available to that point in time concerning malignant peritoneal mesothelioma (Moertel 1972). He noted that death occurs as a result of abdominal involvement alone before there is any detectable metastatic disease. He finishes the review by stating that "Death has uniformly been reported to occur in less than 12 months after the diagnosis is established." Brenner and coworkers in 1981 at Memorial Sloan Kettering Cancer Center reviewed their experience with 25 patients with malignant peritoneal mesothelioma over a 30-year time span (Brenner et al. 1981). Surgery and chemotherapy treatments were not effective. There were 4 long-term survivors treated with radiation therapy and 32 p instillation. They observed that most patients died of extensive intra-abdominal disease with a median survival of only 12 months. Chahinian and coworkers in 1982 reporting from Mount Sinai School of Medicine, New York, presented their experience with 12 patients with malignant peritoneal mesothelioma (Chahinian et al. 1982). Median survival was 10 months from the first symptom and 7 months from the initiation of treatment with doxorubicin and radiation therapy. Clearly, the treatments with systemic chemotherapy or radiation therapy did little or nothing to improve survival with MPM patients. In the review of 514 patients reported in 2000 from the Surveillance, Epidemiology, and End Results (SEER) database, Verschraegen et al. concluded that there had been no therapeutic progress with this disease in the last 30 years (Verschraegen et al. 2005).

P. H. Sugarbaker (✉)
Center for Gastrointestinal Malignancies, MedStar Washington Hospital Center, Washington, DC, USA
e-mail: Paul.Sugarbaker@medstar.net

© Springer Nature Switzerland AG 2019
M. Hesdorffer, G. E. Bates-Pappas (eds.), *Caring for Patients with Mesothelioma: Principles and Guidelines*,
https://doi.org/10.1007/978-3-319-96244-3_3

2   Intraperitoneal Chemotherapy Alone for Malignant Peritoneal Mesothelioma

The use of intraperitoneal chemotherapy for this disease that exclusively involves the abdominal and pelvic space has been slow to develop. The initial use of intraperitoneal chemotherapy for this disease is difficult to determine because it occurred as a result of case reports and small series of patients. The early reports of limited benefit of intraperitoneal (IP) chemotherapy as compared to an absence of benefit from IV chemotherapy were reviewed by Averbach and Sugarbaker in 1996 (Averbach et al. 1996). Plaus in 1988 from the University of Colorado reported a single 38-year-old patient who by second-look surgery had a documented complete pathological response (Plaus 1998). Treatment was by IP cisplatin and IV doxorubicin. Long-term follow-up on this patient is not available, and the chemotherapy doses and schedules were not provided. Several other small series of benefit from IP chemotherapy for MPM have been published (Piccigallo et al. 1988; Vidal-Jove et al. 1991; Moore et al. 1992; Sugarbaker and Fernandez-Trigo 1996).

Three groups from the United States reported a more extensive experience with this treatment modality. Treatment strategies developed by Antman and colleagues (Antman et al. 1985) and Lagerman and coworkers (Lederman et al. 1987, 1988) combined tumor debulking, intraperitoneal administration of doxorubicin and cisplatin, and whole abdominal radiation. To decrease the incidence of chemical peritonitis from doxorubicin, corticosteroids were used. The results of these studies from the Dana-Farber Cancer Institute did produce a moderately prolonged survival estimated at 16 months. The role of abdominal irradiation in prolonged survival was not clear, and these results were achieved in a highly selected group of patients (Markman 1993).

Another group from the University of California, San Diego, applied high-dose intraperitoneal cisplatin with systemic thiosulfate protection in an unselected group of patients with peritoneal mesothelioma (Pfeifle et al. 1985; Markman et al. 1986). The objective response was recorded in 57% of patients, including a complete response in 28.5% of patients. The median survival of all patients was 14 months with that of responders being 18 months.

The combination of intraperitoneal cisplatin and mitomycin C was evaluated by Markman and Kelsen (Markman and Kelsen 1989, 1992). This treatment was based on the synergy of these drugs in experimental systems and their known activity in peritoneal mesothelioma. Treatment was reasonably well tolerated although most patients had therapy discontinued due to failure of the catheter to maintain access to the peritoneal space. In 47% of patients, control of ascites reaccumulation was achieved for a median of 8 months. The median survival of all patients was 9 months, and it was 17.8 months among responders. Twenty-one percent of patients survived 3 years, and 10.5% of patients survived 5 years.

It should be mentioned that in studies from the University of California and from the Memorial Sloan Kettering Cancer Center, debulking surgery was not an important part of the treatment protocol. A possible role of debulking was emphasized by Lederman and coworkers (Lederman et al. 1987).

3 Results of Treatment Combining Cytoreductive Surgery with Intraperitoneal Chemotherapy

In 1988, Antman and colleagues stated that complete surgical removal of MPM was rarely feasible and did not show survival benefit (Antman et al. 1988). Only as the combination of complete cytoreductive surgery plus perioperative chemotherapy that was developed for the treatment of appendiceal and colorectal peritoneal metastases was applied to MPM did results of treatment improve (Sugarbaker and Jablonski 1995; Sebbag et al. 2000). Vidal-Jove and coworkers in 1991 reported favorable results with a curative approach to MPM using cytoreductive surgery including peritonectomy combined with perioperative intraperitoneal chemotherapy (Vidal-Jove et al. 1991). In this report, two cycles of intraperitoneal doxorubicin were used prior to the cytoreductive surgery. Histologic assessment of the tumor prior to treatment and at the time of second-look showed a marked response of the disease to the effects of the intraperitoneal chemotherapy. Pharmacologic studies of the potential benefit of intraperitoneal as compared to systemic doxorubicin in peritoneal mesothelioma patients were presented. In 1996, Fernandez-Trigo and Sugarbaker reported an evolution of treatments in seven patients with malignant peritoneal mesothelioma (Sugarbaker and Fernandez-Trigo 1996). The management plan recommended was cytoreductive surgery followed by hyperthermic intraperitoneal chemotherapy with cisplatin and then early postoperative intraperitoneal chemotherapy (EPIC) with doxorubicin. Long-term survival was reported in four of the seven patients. A complete cytoreduction was emphasized in this report if long-term benefit was to be achieved. In 2000 at ASCO, Sebbag and colleagues reported on 33 patients treated between 1989 and 1999 at the Washington Cancer Institute who had cytoreductive surgery and perioperative chemotherapy as a new and definite treatment strategy (Sebbag et al. 2000). The mean survival since diagnosis in these patients was 31 months with a 33% and 26% overall survival at 3 and 5 years, respectively. The most significant positive predictive factors of survival were complete cytoreduction ($p = 0.0002$), low prior surgical score ($p = 0.0025$), female gender ($p = 0.0031$), and patients able to undergo a second-look surgery ($p = 0.0191$). Twenty-two of the 33 patients had long-term relief of their ascites. The morbidity rate was 33.5%, and perioperative mortality was 3%. They concluded that although MPM is a rare disease, progress in its management had occurred. Their survival had been extended, and ascites was successfully palliated. Some long-term survivors were seen, and the selection factors by which these long-term survivors might be selected for aggressive treatment strategies were defined. They conclude that MPM is a disease that can be treated with long-term benefits.

In 1997, Ma and coworkers from the National Cancer Institute, Bethesda, Maryland, reported nine patients treated between 1993 and 1996 with debulking surgery followed by chemohyperthermic peritoneal perfusion. The intraoperative treatments were heated cisplatin (Ma et al. 1997). Eight of nine patients were optimally debulked and had no evidence of disease with a median follow-up of 10 months.

In 1999, Mongero and coworkers from Columbia Presbyterian Medical Center, New York City, reported on three patients who had induction IP chemotherapy, CRS, and then HIPEC (Mongero et al. 1999). They concluded that intraoperative hyperthermic peritoneal chemotherapy may play a role in novel approaches to the treatment of peritoneal malignancies previously unresponsive to traditional systemic chemotherapy regimens.

Also in 1999, Park and colleagues from the National Cancer Institute, Bethesda, Maryland, reported on 18 patients from 3 consecutive phase I trials (Park et al. 1999). All patients had tumor debulking followed by escalating doses of hyperthermic intraperitoneal cisplatin. Median follow-up after treatment was 19 months (range 2–56) with no operative- or treatment-related mortality. Overall, morbidity was 24%. Nine of ten patients had resolution of ascites, and the three who developed recurrent ascites were retreated with resolution of their ascites. The median progression-free survival was 26 months, and the overall 2-year survival was 80%. The median overall survival was not reached. These authors conclude that hyperthermic intraperitoneal chemotherapy with cisplatin can be added to aggressive surgical debulking with no mortality and a minimal morbidity. Compared to historical controls, their patients showed a prolonged survival.

The Washington Cancer Institute, National Cancer Institute, and Columbia Presbyterian Hospital mesothelioma treatment centers continued their work over the next two decades. Due to their continued clinical investigations and those of many other institutions, in 2006 Yan and colleagues performed a systematic review on the efficacy of cytoreductive surgery combined with perioperative intraperitoneal chemotherapy for the treatment of MPM (Yan et al. 2007). They found seven prospective observational studies available allowing for the assessment of 240 MPM patients. The median survival ranged from 34 to 92 months. The 1-, 3-, and 5-year survival was 60–88%, 43–65%, and 29–59%, respectively. The perioperative morbidity varied from 25% to 40% and the mortality from 0% to 8%. In 2009, Yan and colleagues performed a multi-institutional study of 405 patients with MPM treated with CRS plus HIPEC (Yan et al. 2010). The median overall survival in this large group of patients was 53 months, and 3- and 5-year survival rates were 60% and 47%, respectively. Four prognostic variables were independently associated with improved survival in the multivariate analysis. They were epithelial subtype ($p < 0.001$), absence of lymph node metastases ($p < 0.001$), completeness of cytoreduction ($p < 0.001$), and the use of HIPEC ($p = 0.002$).

Helm and colleagues in 2015 performed another systematic review and meta-analysis (Helm et al. 2015). They were able to collect 20 articles reporting on 1047 patients. The median peritoneal cancer index was 19 (range 16–23), and complete cytoreduction was performed in 67% of patients. The estimates of survival at 1, 3, and 5 years were 84%, 59%, and 42%, respectively. Perioperative chemotherapy was associated with prolonged survival. Both HIPEC and EPIC were recognized as effective, but no inferences regarding a preferred perioperative chemotherapy were possible.

4   Current Standard of Care for Treatment of MPM

In 2016, Sugarbaker and colleagues summarized the current management strategies for peritoneal mesothelioma (Sugarbaker et al. 2016). They cite numerous single-institution studies as well as systematic reviews reporting median survival of 3–5 years with a combined treatment using cytoreductive surgery and hyperthermic perioperative chemotherapy. At experienced centers, these markedly improved survival statistics were achieved with a 1% mortality and 20% morbidity. Data had shown that knowledgeable patient selection is required to prevent patients unlikely to benefit from undergoing these interventions. Their publication in the *Journal of Oncology Practice* concluded that patients with MPM can experience long-term progression-free survival or significant palliation with CRS plus HIPEC. This management plan should be considered the standard of care for properly selected patients with MPM at experienced centers around the globe.

5   Recent Results with Cytoreductive Surgery, HIPEC, and NIPEC

Several reports of intraperitoneal chemotherapy followed by surgery show marked histopathologic regression of the disease from the regional chemotherapy. Also, a majority of patients treated with long-term normothermic intraperitoneal chemotherapy show a response. It is a treatment recommended for patients who have debilitating ascites. Sugarbaker and Chang reported on the treatments of long-term normothermic intraperitoneal chemotherapy that followed cytoreductive surgery and HIPEC (Sugarbaker and Chang 2017). This long-term chemotherapy was administered via an intraperitoneal port. For 100 patients treated with CRS plus HIPEC and/or EPIC, the 5-year survival was 52%. In 29 patients who received 6 cycles of normothermic intraperitoneal chemotherapy after CRS and HIPEC, the 5-year survival was 75% ($p = 0.0374$). Significant prognostic variables were age, gender, treatment administered, peritoneal cancer index, and completeness of cytoreduction by the multivariate analysis. These authors concluded that long-term regional chemotherapy was associated with improved survival in patients with MPM.

6   Evolution of Surgical Treatments

Optimal cytoreduction of all visible malignancy is essential for treatment of MPM for maximal long-term benefit. Up to six peritonectomy procedures may be required (Sugarbaker 2017; Deraco et al. 2009). The visceral resections and parietal/visceral peritonectomy procedures that one must utilize to adequately resect all visible evidence of disease are shown in Table 3.1. Their utilization depends on the distribution and extent of invasion of the malignancy disseminated within the peritoneal space. Normal peritoneum is not excised, only that which is implanted by cancer.

Table 3.1 Peritonectomy procedures and resections that are combined to complete a cytoreduction procedure

Peritonectomy	Resections
Anterior parietal peritonectomy	Old abdominal incisions, umbilicus, and epigastric fat pad
Left upper quadrant peritonectomy	Greater omentectomy and spleen
Right upper quadrant peritonectomy	Tumor on Glisson's capsule of the liver
Pelvic peritonectomy	Uterus, ovaries, and rectosigmoid colon
Omental bursectomy	Gallbladder and lesser omentum
Mesenteric peritonectomy	Visceral peritoneum of small and large bowel

7   Rationale for Peritonectomy Procedures and Visceral Resections

Peritonectomy procedures are necessary if one is to successfully treat MPM with curative intent. Peritonectomy procedures are used in the areas of visible cancer progression in an attempt to leave the patient with only microscopic residual disease. Isolated tumor nodules on parietal peritoneum may be removed using electroevaporation. Involvement of the visceral peritoneum frequently requires resection of a portion of the stomach, small intestine, or colorectum. Layering of cancer on a parietal or visceral peritoneal surface or a portion of the bowel requires peritonectomy or bowel resection for complete removal.

8   Locations of Malignant Peritoneal Mesothelioma

Peritoneal implants of MPM involve the visceral peritoneum in greatest volume at three anatomic sites (Carmignani et al. 2003). These are sites where the bowel is anchored to the retroperitoneum and peristalsis causes less motion of the visceral peritoneal surface. The rectosigmoid colon, as it emerges from the pelvis, is a nonmobile portion of the bowel. Also, it is located in a dependent site and therefore is frequently layered by peritoneal metastases. Usually, a complete pelvic peritonectomy requires stripping of the pelvic sidewalls, the peritoneum overlying the bladder, the cul-de-sac, and resection of the rectosigmoid colon. The ileocecal valve is another area where there is limited mobility. Resection of the terminal ileum and a small portion of the right colon are often necessary. A final site often requiring resection is the antrum of the stomach which is fixed to the retroperitoneum at the pylorus. Tumor coming into the foramen of Winslow accumulates in the subpyloric space and may eventually cause intestinal obstruction as a result of gastric outlet obstruction (Sugarbaker 2002).

9 Electroevaporative Surgery

In order to adequately perform peritonectomy, the surgeon must use electrosurgery (Sugarbaker 1994). The electrosurgical handpiece uses a ball tip that allows the tissue surfaces beneath the peritonectomy to be contoured (Valleylab, Boulder, CO). The smooth surface is then able to be resurfaced by peritoneum (Fig. 3.1). Peritonectomies and visceral resections using traditional scissor and knife dissection will unnecessarily disseminate a large number of tumor cells within the abdomen. High-voltage electrosurgery leaves a margin of heat necrosis that is devoid of viable malignant cells. Not only does electroevaporation of tumor and normal tissue at the margins of resection minimize the likelihood of persistent disease, but also it minimizes blood loss. In the absence of electrosurgery, profuse bleeding from stripped peritoneal surfaces may occur.

10 Abdominal Exposure

The abdominal cavity is opened through a midline incision from xiphoid to pubis. The old abdominal incision is widely excised including the umbilicus. The skin edges are secured by heavy sutures to the self-retaining retractor. Traction on the edges of the abdominal incision elevates the structures of the abdominal wall to facilitate their accurate dissection (Fig. 3.2). Strong elevation of abdominal wall helps to avoid damage to bowel loops that are adherent to the anterior abdominal

Fig. 3.1 Ball-tipped electrosurgery is used to dissect and simultaneously provide small vessel hemostasis. Frequent room temperature saline irrigation is needed to prevent heat damage to tubular structures. A margin of heat necrosis from electrosurgical dissection at high voltage helps to prevent local recurrence. Smoke evacuation is required to prevent environmental contamination. (From Sugarbaker (2017) with permission)

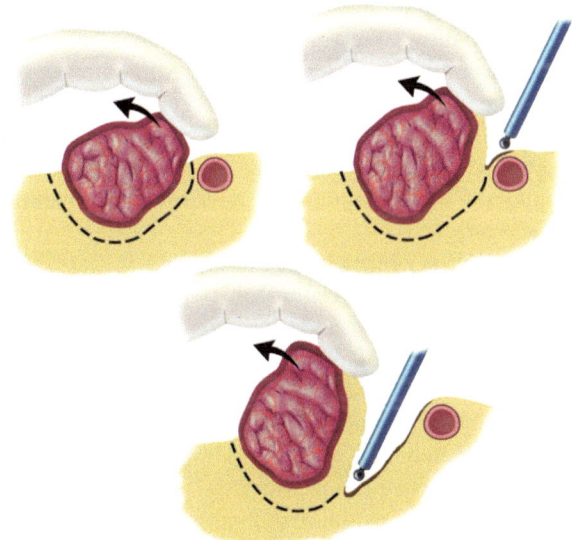

Fig. 3.2 Elevation of the edges of the abdominal incision. Skin traction on a self-retaining retractor facilitates dissection of abdominal wall structures and minimizes the likelihood of damage to bowel loops adherent to the abdominal wall. (From Sugarbaker (2017) with permission)

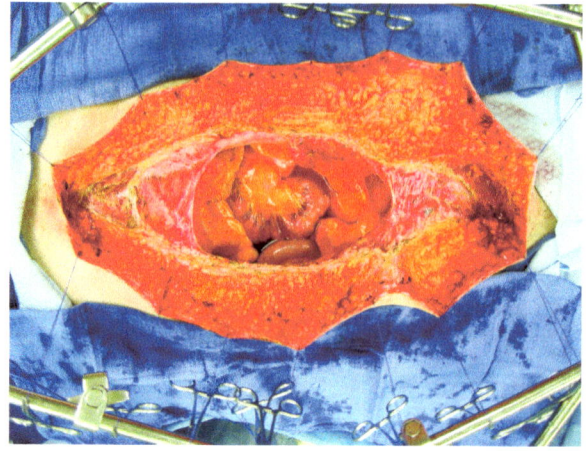

wall (Sugarbaker 2008; De Lima Vazquez and Sugarbaker 2003a). This is especially important in patients who have had prior surgery. Generous abdominal exposure is achieved through the use of a Thompson Self-Retaining Retractor (Thompson Surgical Instruments, Inc., Traverse City, MI).

11   Total Anterior Parietal Peritonectomy

As the peritoneum is dissected away from the posterior rectus sheath, a single entry into the peritoneal cavity in the upper portion of the incision (peritoneal window) allows the surgeon to assess the requirement for a complete parietal peritonectomy (Fig. 3.3). Usually, MPM nodules are palpated on the parietal peritoneum. If so, a complete dissection may be indicated to achieve a complete cytoreduction (De Lima Vazquez and Sugarbaker 2003b). If the parietal peritoneum is not involved by PM, except for the small defect in the peritoneum required for this peritoneal exploration, the remainder of the peritoneum is maintained intact.

The self-retaining retraction system is steadily advanced along the anterior abdominal wall. This optimizes the broad traction at the point of dissection of the peritoneum from its underlying tissues. The dissecting tool is the ball tip, and smoke evacuation is used continuously (Sugarbaker 1994). It is most adherent directly overlying the transversus muscle. In some instances, dissection from inferior to superior aspects of the abdominal wall facilitates clearing in this area. The dissection blends in with the right and left subphrenic peritonectomy superiorly and with the complete pelvic peritonectomy inferiorly. As the dissection proceeds beyond the peritoneum overlying the paracolic sulcus (line of Toldt), the dissection becomes more rapid with the loose connections of the peritoneum at this anatomic site.

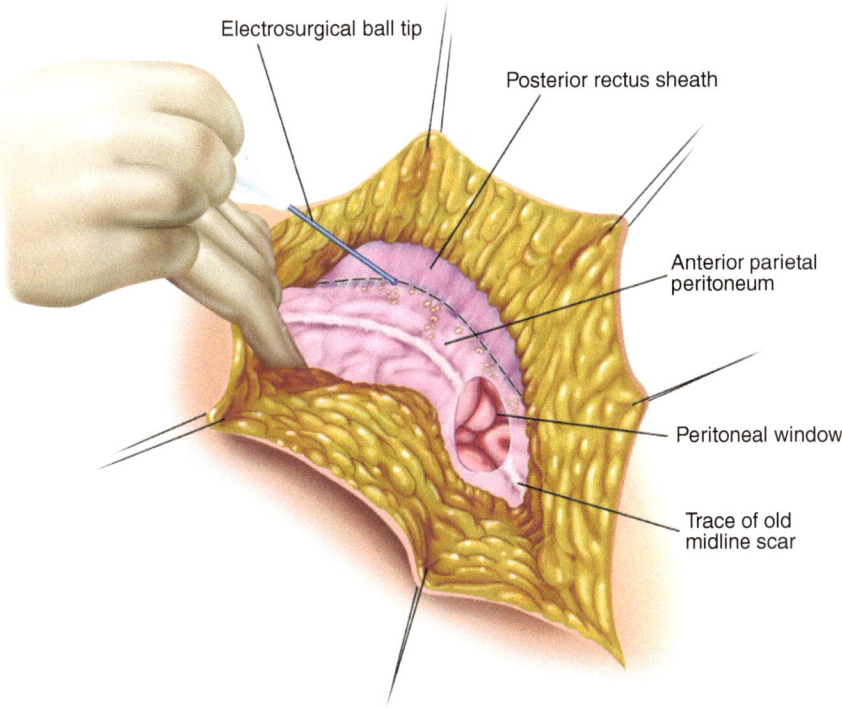

Electrosurgical ball tip

Posterior rectus sheath

Anterior parietal peritoneum

Peritoneal window

Trace of old midline scar

Fig. 3.3 Peritoneal window is necessary to assess the need for total anterior parietal peritonectomy. (From Sugarbaker (2017) with permission)

12   Left Subphrenic Peritonectomy

The peritonectomy procedures are greatly facilitated by the self-retaining retractor that provides continuous exposure of all quadrants of the abdomen including the pelvis. The epigastric fat and peritoneum at the edge of the abdominal incision are stripped off the posterior rectus sheath. Strong traction is exerted on the tumor specimen throughout the left upper quadrant in order to separate tumor from the diaphragmatic muscle, the left adrenal gland, and the superior half of the perirenal fat. The splenic flexure of the colon is severed from the left abdominal gutter and moved medially by dividing the peritoneum along Toldt's line. Dissection beneath the hemidiaphragm muscle is performed with ball-tipped electrosurgery, as well as by blunt dissection (Fig. 3.4). Numerous blood vessels between the diaphragm muscle and its peritoneal surface must be visualized and individually electrocoagulated before their transection or unnecessary bleeding will occur as the severed blood vessels retract into the muscle of the diaphragm. The plane of dissection is

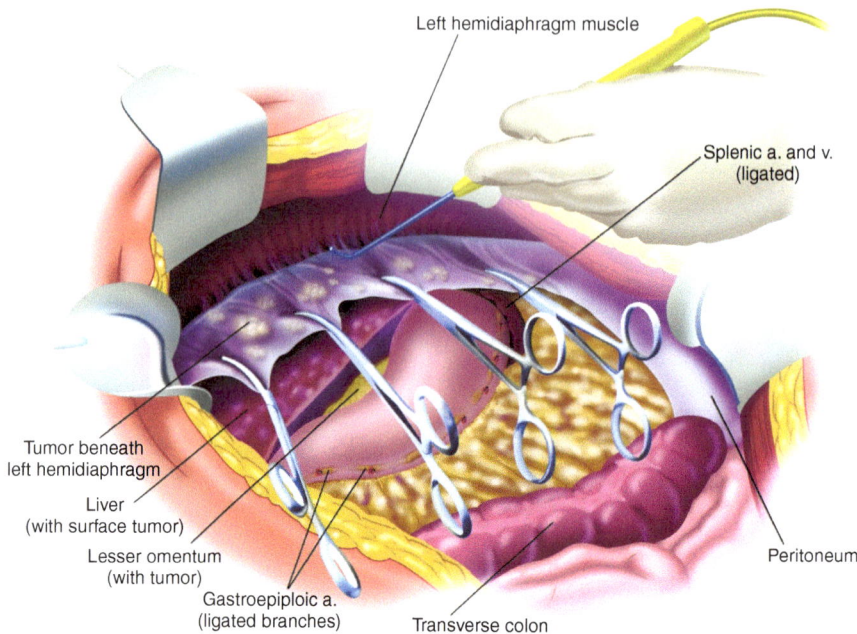

Left hemidiaphragm muscle

Splenic a. and v. (ligated)

Tumor beneath left hemidiaphragm

Liver (with surface tumor)

Lesser omentum (with tumor)

Gastroepiploic a. (ligated branches)

Transverse colon

Peritoneum

Fig. 3.4 Peritoneal stripping of the undersurface of the left diaphragm. (From Sugarbaker (2017) with permission)

defined using ball-tipped electrosurgery on pure cut, but all blood vessels are electrocoagulated before their division.

13 Greater Omentectomy and Possible Splenectomy

To free the mid-abdomen of a large volume of tumor, the greater omentectomy-splenectomy is performed. The greater omentum is elevated and then separated from the transverse colon using electrosurgery. This dissection continues beneath the peritoneum that covers the transverse mesocolon in order to expose and avoid the lower border of the pancreas. The branches of the gastroepiploic arcade to the greater curvature of the stomach are ligated in continuity and then divided.

Because the left upper quadrant peritonectomy has been completed, the structures deep beneath the left hemidiaphragm can be elevated. Therefore, under direct vision, the short gastric vessels are transected. With traction on the spleen, the peritoneum superior to the pancreas may be stripped from the gland bluntly or by using electrosurgery. If the peritoneum covering the pancreas is free of cancer implants, it remains intact. The splenic artery and vein at the tail of the pancreas are ligated in continuity and proximally suture ligated. Great care is taken not to traumatize the body or tail of the pancreas.

14 Right Subphrenic Peritonectomy

Peritoneum is stripped from beneath the right posterior rectus sheath to begin the peritonectomy in the right upper quadrant of the abdomen. Strong traction on the specimen is used to elevate the hemidiaphragm into the operative field. Again, ball-tipped electrosurgery on pure cut is used to dissect at the interface of tumor and normal tissue. Coagulation current is used to divide the blood vessels between diaphragm and peritoneum as they are encountered and before they bleed.

15 Stripping of Tumor from Glisson's Capsule

The stripping of tumor from the right hemidiaphragm continues until the bare area of the liver is encountered. At that point, tumor on the superior surface of the liver is electroevaporated until the liver surface is cleared (Fig. 3.5). With ball-tipped electroevaporative dissection, a thick layer of tumor may be bloodlessly lifted off the liver surface by moving beneath Glisson's capsule (high-voltage pure cut electrosurgical dissection). Isolated patches of tumor on the liver surface are electroevaporated with the distal 2 cm of the ball tip bent and stripped of insulation ("hockey-stick" configuration). Ball-tipped electrosurgery is also used to extirpate tumor from attachments of the falciform ligament and round ligament.

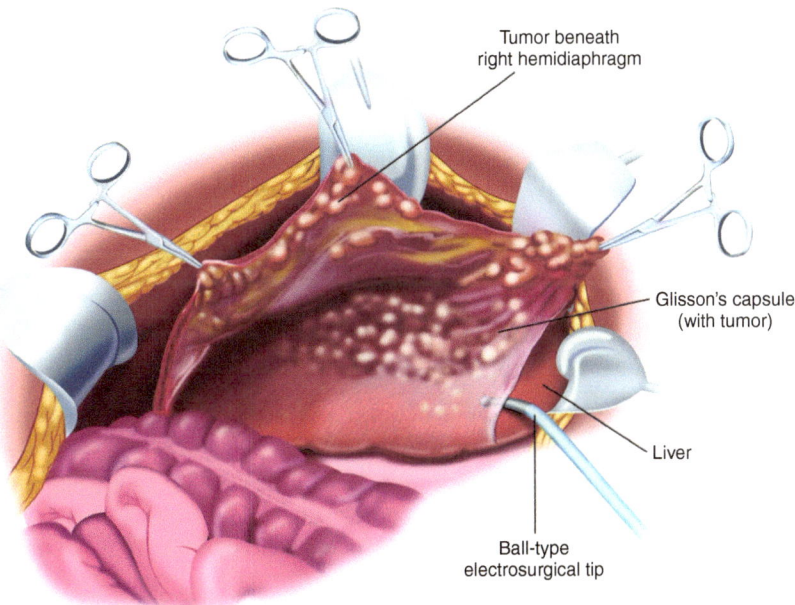

Tumor beneath right hemidiaphragm

Glisson's capsule (with tumor)

Liver

Ball-type electrosurgical tip

Fig. 3.5 Electroevaporation of tumor from the liver surface with resection of Glisson's capsule. (From Sugarbaker (2017) with permission)

Tumor from beneath the right hemidiaphragm, from the right subhepatic space, and from the surface of the liver forms an envelope as it is removed en bloc. The dissection is greatly facilitated if the tumor specimen is maintained intact. The dissection continues laterally on the right to encounter the perirenal fat covering the right kidney. Also, the right adrenal gland is visualized and carefully avoided as tumor is stripped from the right subhepatic space. As the peritoneal reflection at the posterior aspect of the liver is divided, care is taken not to traumatize the vena cava or to disrupt the caudate lobe veins that pass between the vena cava and segment 1 of the liver.

16   Lesser Omentectomy and Cholecystectomy with Stripping of the Hepatoduodenal Ligament

The gallbladder is removed in a routine fashion from its fundus toward the cystic artery and cystic duct. These structures are ligated and divided. The hepatoduodenal ligament is characteristically heavily layered with tumor. After dividing the peritoneal reflection onto the liver, the cancerous tissue that coats the porta hepatis is bluntly stripped using a Russian forceps from the base of the gallbladder bed toward the duodenum. The right gastric artery going to the lesser omental arcade is preserved (Fig. 3.6). To continue resection of the lesser omentum, the surgeon separates the gastrohepatic ligament from the fissure that divides liver segments 2 and 3 from segment 1. Ball-tipped electrosurgery is used to electroevaporate tumor from the surface of the caudate process. Care is taken not to traumatize the anterior surface of the caudate process, for this can result in excessive and needless blood loss. The segmental blood supply to the caudate lobe is located on the anterior surface of this segment of the liver, and hemorrhage may occur with only superficial trauma. Also, care must be taken to avoid an accessory left hepatic artery that may arise from the left gastric artery and cross through the hepatogastric fissure. If the artery is embedded in tumor or its preservation occludes clear exposure of the omental bursa, the artery is ligated as it enters the liver parenchyma. It is resected as part of the hepatogastric ligament.

17   Circumferential Resection of the Hepatogastric Ligament and Lesser Omental Fat by Digital Dissection

The triangular ligament of the left lobe of the liver was resected in performing the left subphrenic peritonectomy. This completed, the left lateral segment of the liver is retracted left to right to expose the hepatogastric ligament in its entirety. A circumferential electrosurgical release of this ligament (lesser omentum) from the fissure between liver segments 2 and 3, and the left caudate lobe, and from the arcade of right gastric artery to left gastric artery along the lesser curvature of the stomach is required. After electrosurgically dividing the peritoneum on the lesser curvature of the stomach, digital dissection with extreme pressure from the surgeon's thumb

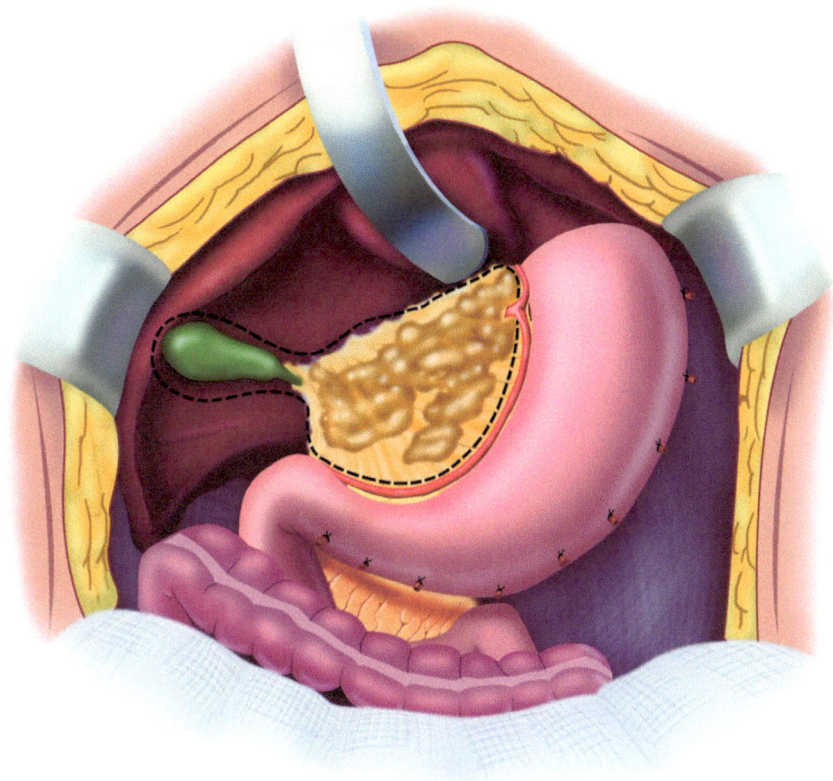

Fig. 3.6 Lesser omentectomy and cholecystectomy with stripping of the anterior and posterior (if necessary) aspect of the hepatoduodenal ligament. (From Sugarbaker (2017) with permission)

and index finger separates lesser omental fat and tumor from the vascular arcade. As much of the anterior vagus nerve is spared as is possible. The tumor and fatty tissue surrounding the right and left gastric arteries are split away from the vascular arcade. In this manner, the specimen is centralized over the major branches of the left gastric artery. With strong traction on the specimen, the lesser omentum is released from the left gastric artery and vein.

18   Stripping of the Floor of the Omental Bursa

A Deaver retractor or the assistant's fingertips beneath the left caudate lobe are positioned to expose the entire floor of the omental bursa (Fig. 3.7). Further electro-evaporation of tumor from the caudate process of the left caudate lobe of the liver may be necessary to achieve this exposure. Ball-tip electrosurgery is used to cautiously divide the peritoneal reflection of the liver onto the left side of the subhepatic

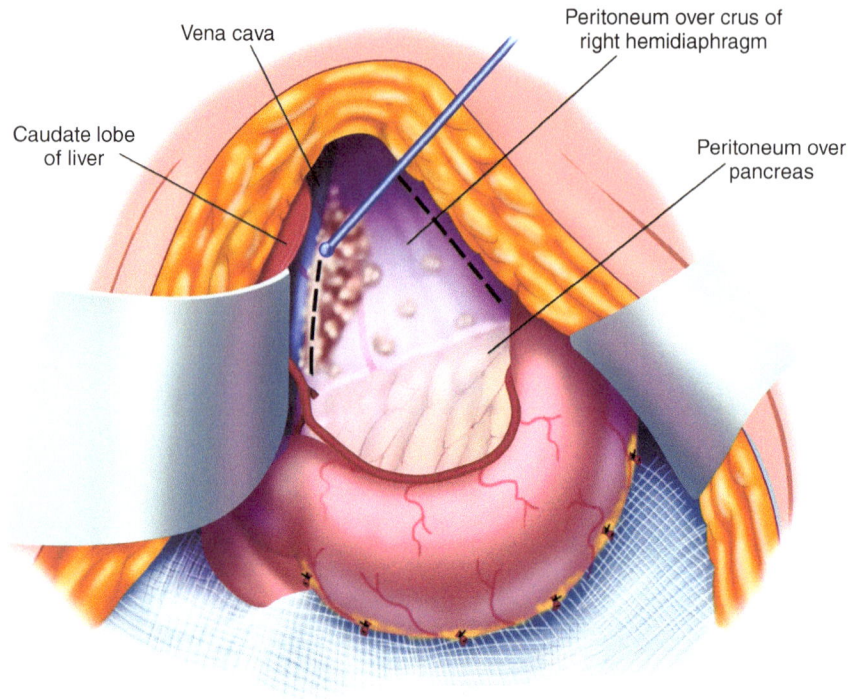

Fig. 3.7 Stripping of the omental bursa after dividing the peritoneal reflection between left caudate lobe and superior vena cava. (From Sugarbaker (2017) with permission)

vena cava. After the peritoneum is divided, Russian forceps assist in a blunt stripping of the peritoneum from the superior recess of the omental bursa, from the crus of the right hemidiaphragm, and from beneath the portal vein. Electroevaporation of tumor from the shelf of liver parenchyma beneath the portal vein that connects right and left aspects of the caudate lobe may be required. Care is taken while stripping the floor of the omental bursa to stay superficial to the right phrenic artery.

In some patients, a large volume of tumor on the posterior aspect of the hepato-duodenal ligament may be difficult to visualize. A ½ inch Penrose drain placed around the portal triad may allow improved visualization beneath these structures. Using a Russian forceps, tearing away the peritoneum beneath the porta hepatis may be necessary under direct visualization.

19   Complete Pelvic Peritonectomy

The tumor-bearing peritoneum is stripped from the posterior surface of the lower abdominal incision, exposing the rectus muscle. After dissecting generously the peritoneum on the right and left sides of the bladder, the urachus is localized and placed on strong traction using a Babcock clamp. The peritoneum with the underlying fatty tissues is stripped away from the surface of the bladder. Broad traction on the entire anterior parietal peritoneal surface and frequent saline irrigation clears the point for tissue transection that is precisely located between the bladder musculature and its adherent fatty tissue with peritoneum. The inferior limit of dissection is the cervix in the female or the seminal vesicles in the male.

The peritoneal incision around the pelvis is connected to the peritoneal incisions of the right and left paracolic sulci (Fig. 3.8). In the female, the round ligaments are divided as they enter the internal inguinal ring. The right and left ureters are identified and preserved. In women, the right and left ovarian veins are ligated at the level of the lower pole of the kidney and divided. A linear stapler is used to

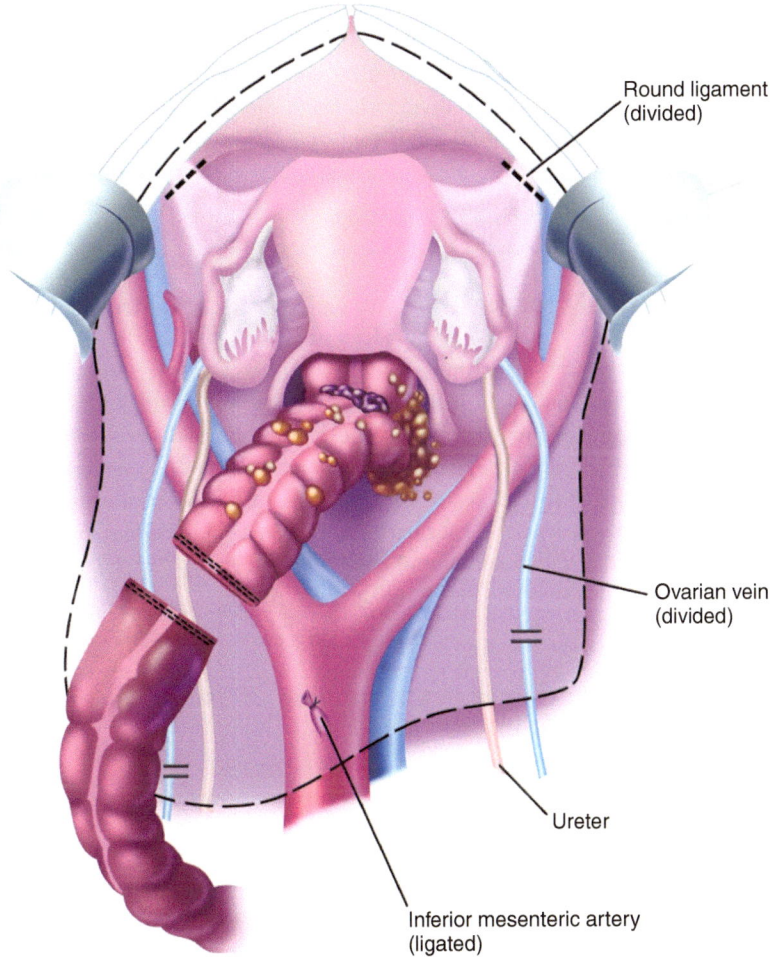

Fig. 3.8 The complete pelvic peritonectomy includes the uterus and ovaries, rectosigmoid colon, and pelvic peritoneum. (From Sugarbaker (2017) with permission)

divide the sigmoid colon just above the limits of the pelvic tumor. The vascular supply of the distal portion of the bowel is traced back to its origin on the aorta. The inferior mesenteric artery is ligated, suture ligated, and divided. This allows one to pack all the viscera, including the proximal sigmoid colon, in the upper abdomen.

20   Resection of Rectosigmoid Colon and Cul-de-sac of Douglas

Electrosurgery is used to dissect at the limits of the mesorectum. The surgeon works in a centripetal fashion. Extraperitoneal ligation of the uterine arteries is performed just above the ureter and close to the base of the bladder. The bladder is dissected away from the cervix, and the vagina is entered. The vaginal cuff anterior and posterior to the cervix is transected using electrosurgery, and the rectovaginal septum is exposed. The perirectal fat is divided beneath the peritoneal reflection so that all tumor that occupies the cul-de-sac is removed intact with the specimen. The rectal musculature is skeletonized using electrosurgery so that a stapler can be used to close off the rectal stump.

21   Vaginal Closure and Low Colorectal Anastomosis

One of the few suture repairs performed prior to the intraoperative chemotherapy is the closure of the vaginal cuff. If one fails to close the vaginal cuff, chemotherapy solution will leak from the vagina. The circular stapled colorectal anastomosis occurs after the intraoperative chemotherapy has been completed. A circular stapling device is passed into the rectum, and the trocar penetrates the staple line. A purse-string applier is used to secure the staple anvil in the distal descending colon. The body of the circular stapler and anvil are mated, and the stapler is activated to complete the low colorectal anastomosis.

22   Optimization of Cytoreduction of Small Bowel and Its Mesentery

The peritonectomy procedures using high-voltage electrosurgery have been applied to the cytoreduction of parietal peritoneal surface malignancy. However, the electrosurgical techniques used in the peritonectomy procedures are not appropriate for the treatment of tumor nodules involving the small bowel. Only a very limited use of electrosurgery on the small bowel itself is possible in order to avoid postoperative fistula. In contrast, small bowel mesentery is an anatomic site for safe use of electroevaporation of cancer nodules.

22.1 Five Types of Small Bowel Involvement by Cancer

CRS with perioperative chemotherapy has been most commonly used for the management of mucinous appendiceal neoplasms, but they have been successfully applied to other tumors, especially colon cancer and diffuse malignant peritoneal mesothelioma. The histological features and the depth of invasion of these different tumors into the bowel wall are not uniform. Based on the extent of the invasion, the size of the tumor nodule and its anatomic location on the bowel wall, small bowel involvement is classified into five types (Bijelic and Sugarbaker 2008):

- Type 1. Noninvasive nodules
- Type 2. Small invasive nodules on the anti-mesenteric portion of the small bowel
- Type 3. Moderate-sized invasive nodules on the anti-mesenteric portion of the small bowel
- Type 4. All sizes of invasive nodules at junction of small bowel and its mesentery
- Type 5. Large invasive nodules

22.2 Techniques Used in Cytoreduction of the Small Bowel

Type 1. Noninvasive nodules. This type of small bowel involvement involves minute nodules of aggressive histology that because of their small size have not invaded past the peritoneum. It would also include large noninvasive nodules of diffuse peritoneal adenomucinosis or nuclear grade I peritoneal mesothelioma (Ronnett et al. 1995; Cerruto et al. 2006). The curved Mayo scissors are used to trim these noninvasive nodules from the surface of the small bowel; this results in a localized removal of peritoneum. Larger nodules are frequently scissor-dissected in a piecemeal fashion to avoid damage to the deeper layers of the bowel wall. Considerable

Fig. 3.9 Type 1 – noninvasive tumor nodules are usually resectable using a curved Mayo scissor. (From Sugarbaker (2017) with permission)

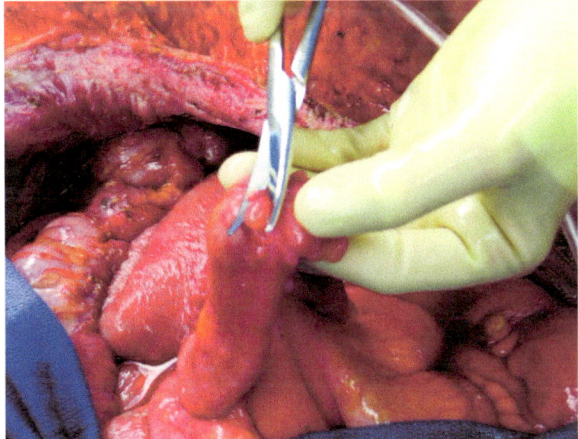

skill acquired over time may be needed to avoid damage to the muscularis propria of the bowel (Fig. 3.9). There is usually no need for seromuscular repair.

Type 2. Small invasive nodules on the anti-mesenteric portion of the small bowel. These invasive nodules do not separate from the muscular layer of the small bowel, and a partial-thickness resection is required. The seromuscular layer is resected leaving mucosa and submucosa intact. This resection is usually performed with a curved Mayo scissor, but occasionally, it may be performed by pure cut electrosurgery with frequent irrigation to cool the resection site. Scissor or knife dissection is preferred. The seromuscular layer is repaired by suture plication after the intraoperative chemotherapy is completed (Fig. 3.10).

Type 3. Moderate-sized invasive nodules on the anti-mesenteric portion of the small bowel. In contrast to small invasive nodules in this location, larger nodules require a full-thickness elliptical resection of the anti-mesenteric portion of the bowel wall. The closure is performed in two layers and at two different times. The first layer is a full-thickness closure using absorbable suture. One suture starts at each corner of the defect, and the sutures are then tied at the midportion of the resection. Following the perioperative chemotherapy, the defect is closed with a second layer of nonabsorbable plication sutures (Fig. 3.11).

Type 4. Small invasive nodules at junction of small bowel and its mesentery. These nodules can sometimes be removed by a localized removal with electrosurgery if sufficiently small and if the vascular supply to the segment of bowel is not compromised. A two-layer repair follows this localized resection. More often, these

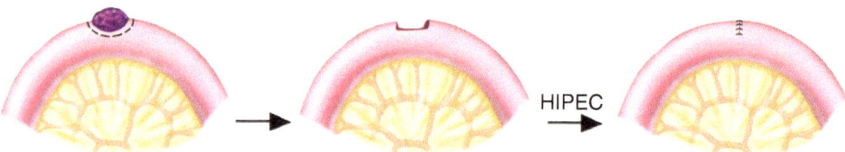

Fig. 3.10 Type 2 – small invasive tumor nodules on the anti-mesenteric portion of the small bowel are resected along with the seromuscular layer. Hyperthermic intraperitoneal chemotherapy is administered prior to suture plication of the defect. (From Sugarbaker (2017) with permission)

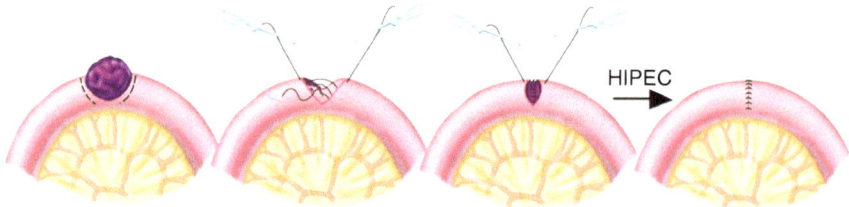

Fig. 3.11 Type 3 – moderate-sized invasive nodules on the anti-mesenteric portion of the small bowel are resected with a full-thickness ellipse. Stay sutures elevate the portion of bowel to be resected. A full-thickness closure with absorbable, running suture allows hyperthermic intraperitoneal chemotherapy to be given. After the intraperitoneal chemotherapy, a second layer of nonabsorbable interrupted sutures is used to plicate the seromuscular layer. (From Sugarbaker (2017) with permission)

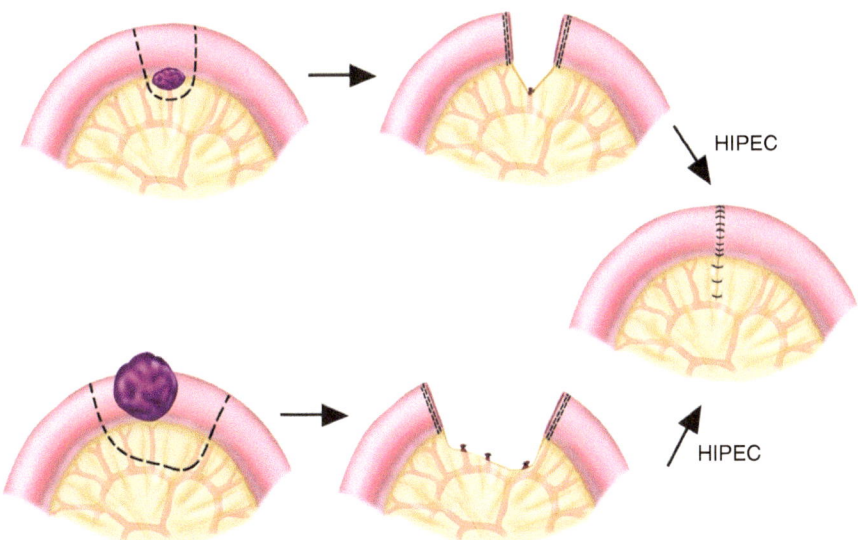

Fig. 3.12 Small invasive nodules at the junction of small bowel and mesentery (Type 4) or large invasive nodules (Type 5) are resected with generous margins using a linear stapler. After hyperthermic intraperitoneal chemotherapy is complete, a two-layer anastomosis is performed. (From Sugarbaker (2017) with permission)

nodules are removed, and the incidence of fistula is reduced by a segmental small bowel resection with end-to-end hand-sewn anastomosis (Fig. 3.12).

Type 5. Large invasive nodules. These lesions require a segmental small bowel resection with generous proximal and distal margins on the bowel wall and on the mesentery. The segment of small bowel and a portion of its mesentery are resected. The bowel is divided and closed using a linear cutter/stapler. The HIPEC is completed prior to a two-layer hand-sewn anastomosis (Fig. 3.12).

23   Follow-Up

After the patient fully recovers from cytoreductive surgery with HIPEC (possibly followed by NIPEC-LT), careful surveillance for disease recurrence is indicated. If disease progression is diagnosed in a timely fashion and it is limited in extent throughout the abdomen and pelvis, a reoperative procedure can greatly benefit these patients. Prolonged survival has been associated with the possibility for the patient to have a second-look (Ihemelandu et al. 2015).

Then the patient enters into follow-up. If the CA-125 was elevated prior to cytoreduction, then it is obtained on a 3-monthly basis for 3 years. CT scans are obtained on a 6-monthly basis for 3 years and then yearly for a total of 10 years.

References

Antman KH, Osteen RT, Klegar KL, Amato DA, Pomfert EA, Larson DA, Carson JM. Early peritoneal mesothelioma: A treatable malignancy. Lancet. 1985;2:977–81.

Antman K, Shemin R, Ryan L, Klegar K, Osteen R, Herman T, Lederman G, Corson J. Malignant mesothelioma: Prognostic variables in a registry of 180 patients, the Dana-Farber Cancer Institute and Brigham and Women's Hospital experience over two decades, 1965-1985. J Clin Oncol. 1988;6:147–53.

Averbach AM, Stephens AD, Sugarbaker PH. Gastric cancer with peritoneal carcinomatosis: Case report and presentation of a pilot treatment plan. Surg Rounds. 1996;19:14–21.

Bijelic L, Sugarbaker PH. Cytoreduction of the small bowel surfaces. J Surg Oncol. 2008;97:176–9.

Brenner J, Sordillo PP, Magill GB, et al. Malignant peritoneal mesothelioma. Am J Gastroenterol. 1981;75:311–3.

Carmignani P, Sugarbaker TA, Bromley CM, Sugarbaker PH. Intraperitoneal cancer dissemination: Mechanisms of the patterns of spread. Cancer Metastasis Rev. 2003;22(4):465–72.

Cerruto CA, Brun EA, Chang D, Sugarbaker PH. Prognostic significance of histomorphologic parameters in diffuse malignant peritoneal mesothelioma. Arch Pathol Lab Med. 2006;130:1654–61.

Chahinian AP, Pajak TF, Holland JF, Norton L, Ambinder RM, Mandel EM. Diffuse malignant mesothelioma. Prospective evaluation of 69 patients. Ann Intern Med. 1982;96(6 Pt 1):746–55.

De Lima Vazquez V, Sugarbaker PH. Xiphoidectomy. Gastric Cancer. 2003a;6:127–9.

De Lima Vazquez V, Sugarbaker PH. Total anterior parietal peritonectomy. J Surg Oncol. 2003b;83:261–3.

Deraco M, Baratti D, Kusamura S, et al. Surgical technique of parietal and visceral peritonectomy for peritoneal surface malignancies. J Surg Oncol. 2009;100:321–8.

Helm JH, Miura JT, Glenn JA, Marcus RK, Larrieux G, Jayakrishnan TT, Donahue AE, Gamblin TC, Turaga KK, Johnston FM. Cytoreductive surgery and hyperthermic intraperitoneal chemotherapy for malignant peritoneal mesothelioma: a systematic review and meta-analysis. Ann Surg Oncol. 2015;22(5):1686–93.

Ihemelandu C, Bijelic L, Sugarbaker PH. Iterative cytoreductive surgery and hyperthermic intraperitoneal chemotherapy for recurrent or progressive diffuse malignant peritoneal metastases: Clinicopathologic characteristics and survival outcome. Ann Surg Oncol. 2015;22(5):1680–5.

Lederman GS, Recht A, Herman T, Osteen R, Corson J, Antman KH. Long-term survival in peritoneal mesothelioma. The role of radiotherapy and combined modality treatment. Cancer. 1987;59:1882–6.

Lederman GS, Recht A, Herman T. Combined modality treatment of peritoneal mesothelioma. NCI Monogr. 1988;6:321–2.

Ma GY, Bartlett DL, Reed E, Figg WD, Lush RM, Lee KB, Libutti SK, Alexander HR. Continuous hyperthermic peritoneal perfusion with cisplatin for the treatment of peritoneal mesothelioma. Cancer J Sci Am. 1997;3(3):174–9.

Markman M. Intraperitoneal therapy in the management of peritoneal mesothelioma. J Infect Chemother. 1993;3:50–2.

Markman M, Kelsen D. Intraperitoneal cisplatin and mitomycin as treatment for malignant peritoneal mesothelioma. Reg Cancer Treat. 1989;2:49–53.

Markman M, Kelsen D. Efficacy of cisplatin-based intraperitoneal chemotherapy as treatment of malignant peritoneal mesothelioma. J Cancer Res Clin Oncol. 1992;118:547–50.

Markman M, Cleary S, Pfeifle C, Howell S. Cisplatin administered by the intracavitary route as treatment for malignant mesothelioma. Cancer. 1986;58:18–21.

Moertel CG. Peritoneal mesothelioma. Gastroenterology. 1972;63:346–50.

Mongero LB, Beck JR, Kroslowitz RM, Argenziano M, Chabot JA. Treatment of primary peritoneal mesothelioma by hyperthermic intraperitoneal chemotherapy. Perfusion. 1999;14:141–6.

Moore MLG, Savaraj N, Feun LG, Donnelly E. Successful therapy of peritoneal mesothelioma with intraperitoneal chemotherapy alone. A case report. Am J Clin Oncol. 1992;15:528–30.

Park BJ, Alexander HR, Libutti SK, Wu P, Royalty D, Kranda KC, Bartlett DL. Treatment of primary peritoneal mesothelioma by continuous hyperthermic peritoneal perfusion (CHPP). Ann Surg Oncol. 1999;6(6):582–90.

Pfeifle CE, Howell SB, Markman M. Intracavitary cisplatin chemotherapy for mesothelioma. Cancer Treat Rep. 1985;69:205–7.

Piccigallo E, Jeffers LJ, Reddy KR, Caldironi MW, Parenti A, Schiff ER. Malignant peritoneal mesothelioma. A clinical and laparoscopic study of ten cases. Dig Dis Sci. 1988;33:633–9.

Plaus WJ. Peritoneal mesothelioma. Arch Surg. 1998;123:763–6.

Ronnett BM, Zahn CM, Kurman RJ, Kass ME, Sugarbaker PH, Shmookler BM. Disseminated peritoneal adenomucinosis and peritoneal mucinous carcinomatosis: A clinicopathologic analysis of 109 cases with emphasis on distinguishing pathologic features, site of origin, prognosis, and relationship to "pseudomyxoma peritonei". Am J Surg Pathol. 1995;19:1390–408.

Sebbag G, Shmookler B, Chang D, Sugarbaker PH. Peritoneal mesothelioma. Abstract presented at 36th Congress of the American Society of Clinical Oncology (ASCO), New Orleans, 20–23 May 2000.

Sugarbaker PH. Dissection by electrocautery with a ball tip. J Surg Oncol. 1994;56:246–8.

Sugarbaker PH. The subpyloric space: An important surgical and radiologic feature in pseudomyxoma peritonei. Eur J Surg Oncol. 2002;28:443–6.

Sugarbaker PH. Circumferential cutaneous traction for exposure of the layers of the abdominal wall. J Surg Oncol. 2008;98:472–65.

Sugarbaker PH. An overview of peritonectomy, visceral resections, and perioperative chemotherapy for peritoneal surface malignancy. In: Sugarbaker PH, editor. Cytoreductive surgery & perioperative chemotherapy for peritoneal surface malignancy. Textbook and video atlas. 2nd ed. Woodbury: Cine-Med Publishers; 2017.

Sugarbaker PH, Chang D. Long-term regional chemotherapy for patients with epithelial malignant peritoneal mesothelioma results in improved survival. Eur J Surg Oncol. 2017;43(7):1228–35.

Sugarbaker PH, Fernandez-Trigo V. Evolution of local-regional treatment strategies in a curative approach to patients with malignant peritoneal mesothelioma. Surg Rounds. 1996;19(9):369–75.

Sugarbaker PH, Jablonski KA. Prognostic features of 51 colorectal and 130 appendiceal cancer patients with peritoneal carcinomatosis treated by cytoreductive surgery and intraperitoneal chemotherapy. Ann Surg. 1995;221(2):124–32.

Sugarbaker PH, Turaga KK, Alexander HR Jr, Deraco M, Hesdorffer M. Management of malignant peritoneal mesothelioma using cytoreductive surgery and perioperative chemotherapy. J Oncol Pract. 2016;12(10):928–35.

Verschraegen CF, Key CR, Hassan R. Clinical presentation and natural history of mesothelioma: abdominal. In: Pass HI, Vogelzang NJ, Carbone M, editors. Malignant mesothelioma. New York: Springer; 2005. p. 391–401.

Vidal-Jove J, Sweatman TW, Israel M, Graves T, Litwin FP, Davidson ED, Sugarbaker PH. A curative approach to malignant peritoneal mesothelioma. A case-report and review of the literature. Reg Cancer Treat. 1991;3:269–74.

Yan TD, Welch L, Black D, Sugarbaker PH. A systematic review on the efficacy of cytoreductive surgery combined with perioperative intraperitoneal chemotherapy for diffuse malignant peritoneal mesothelioma. Ann Oncol. 2007;18:827–34.

Yan TD, Deraco M, Baratti D, Kusamura S, Elias D, Glehen O, Gilly FN, Levine EA, Shen P, Mohamed F, Moran BJ, Morris DL, Chua TC, Piso P, Sugarbaker PH. Cytoreductive surgery and hyperthermic intraperitoneal chemotherapy for malignant peritoneal mesothelioma: multiinstitutional experience. J Clin Oncol. 2010;27:6237–42.

Radiation Therapy

4

Andreas Rimner

1 Integration of Radiation Therapy into Multimodality Management Regimen

MPM remains a therapeutic challenge with poor prognosis. Many patients present with advanced disease, have numerous comorbidities or poor performance status, and are therefore only eligible for best supportive care and palliative management. For those who are diagnosed at an operable stage, a multimodality approach of chemotherapy, surgery, and radiation therapy is commonly applied. The combination of all the three treatment modalities carries a significant risk for toxicity for the patients and calls for sophisticated treatment planning in high volume medical centers with experience in treating the disease given the challenging and complex nature of MPM.

Two types of surgical resection have been most commonly used in the management of resectable MPM. An extrapleural pneumonectomy (EPP) is the most comprehensive radical surgery and involves an en bloc resection of the lung, pleura, pericardium, and diaphragm. Somewhat surprisingly, even after such an extensive surgery as an EPP, up to 80% of patients still experience local intrathoracic recurrence indicating that additional adjuvant therapy may be needed to reduce the significant risk of local recurrence. In addition, EPP is associated with significant morbidity and mortality, thus being applicable to only a subset of patients with excellent functional status and operability.

A less complete resection but an alternative associated with lesser morbidity and mortality is a lung-sparing pleurectomy/decortication (P/D) which involves resection of the parietal and visceral pleura, with or without resection of the pericardium

A. Rimner (✉)
Department of Radiation Oncology, Memorial Sloan Kettering Cancer Center,
New York, NY, USA
e-mail: rimnera@mskcc.org

© Springer Nature Switzerland AG 2019
M. Hesdorffer, G. E. Bates-Pappas (eds.), *Caring for Patients*
with Mesothelioma: Principles and Guidelines,
https://doi.org/10.1007/978-3-319-96244-3_4

and diaphragm while the lung is spared. Given that P/D is a less comprehensive oncologic surgery and by default is assumed to leave microscopic cells behind, the case for adjuvant therapy is even stronger.

Somewhat surprisingly early retrospective comparisons of EPP and P/D revealed higher morbidity, decreased quality of life (QOL) and worse overall survival with EPP when compared to P/D (Flores et al. 2008). The Mesothelioma and Radical Surgery (MARS) trial was designed to prospectively assess the feasibility to randomize patients to EPP versus no EPP after induction chemotherapy (Treasure et al. 2011). Fifty patients were randomized, and with a median survival of 14.4 months in patients randomized to EPP, there was no significant difference in survival between patients undergoing EPP vs. no EPP. However, this trial was neither designed nor powered for a survival endpoint and has been heavily criticized for multiple reasons, including its high mortality rate in patients who underwent EPP (18%). A large meta-analysis on 1512 patients undergoing a P/D and 1391 undergoing EPP confirmed the finding of worse survival after EPP (Taioli et al. 2015). Taken together, these studies have led to the increased use of P/D in the surgical management of MPM. Nevertheless, EPP may still have a role in the surgical treatment of MPM, i.e., in particularly fit patients whose tumor cannot be removed without a pneumonectomy.

Most mesothelioma experts will agree that – no matter which surgical technique is used – macroscopic complete resection (MCR) is the goal of cytoreductive surgery in patients with MPM and has been associated with favorable outcomes in appropriately selected patients (Rice et al. 2011). The choice of surgical approach and technique is dependent on the individual patient's presentation, tumor extent, and medical fitness and should be applied in a highly individualized manner.

Given the high risk of disease progression even in patients with early-stage MPM, surgical resection has typically been used as a part of a multimodality treatment approach, combined with systemic or intrapleural chemotherapy, pre- or postoperative 3D conformal RT, or intensity-modulated radiation therapy (IMRT). In this chapter we will describe the radiation therapy options that may be used in the EPP and P/D setting as well as other indications beyond patients who are surgical candidates.

2   Radiation Therapy

RT has been used to improve locoregional intrathoracic tumor control, as local failure rates remain high at up to 80%, even after macroscopic complete resections. Targeting the entire hemithorax in conjunction with surgical resection for early-stage MPM is a challenging task. The anatomy of the thorax and upper abdomen surrounding the diaphragm is complex and difficult to target, with multiple radiation-sensitive organs in or near the radiation field, plus normal organ motion due to respiratory excursion of the diaphragm and cardiac motion.

In the past conventional radiation therapy techniques were available using a combination of photons and electrons to target the hemithorax from a limited number of beam angles, mostly the front and back. However, these treatments – while technically feasible – did not optimally spare normal organs at risk and were associated with significant toxicities and disappointing locoregional control rates.

Substantial technological improvement in radiation oncology over the past 15 years has allowed RT delivery from multiple beam angles, even a hemicircular or full circular arc around the patient, based on three-dimensional treatment planning, using improved dose calculation algorithms and much improved imaging techniques during the treatment delivery. The most notable of these novel techniques include intensity-modulated radiation therapy (IMRT), volumetric modulated arc therapy (VMAT), and proton radiation therapy. With these it has become more feasible to adequately spare normal organs at risk and reduce the incidence and severity of radiation-associated short- and long-term toxicities.

Beyond targeting the hemithoracic pleura as part of a multimodality approach for early-stage MPM, RT can be used for the palliative treatment of painful metastases or critical areas in need of local tumor control, such as the airways, esophagus, or large blood vessels. The appropriate RT technique in those clinical scenarios very much depends on the target shape and location, the anatomy surrounding the tumor, the desired RT dose, the clinical urgency to start treatment, and the patient's functional status. Frequently, simpler techniques may be appropriate in those settings. Simpler techniques may also be used for prophylactic tract irradiation of surgical incisions or chest tube tracks.

2.1   Radiation Therapy in the Setting of EPP

For a long time, it was believed that RT to the entire hemithorax would not be feasible, as the large field that is required to treat the entire pleura would be too toxic. It was first attempted in patients who had undergone an extrapleural pneumonectomy (EPP), since an EPP completely removes the lung on the involved hemithoracic side completely which is thus no longer subject to potentially life-threatening inflammation from radiation therapy. At first, a conventional photon/electron technique was used to target the hemithorax, block the abdominal organs at risk and the heart for left-sided tumors, and supplement the RT dose to the anterior and posterior chest wall with electron fields (Yajnik et al. 2003). One advantage of this approach was the avoidance of oblique angles that would increase the exposure of the contralateral lung to ionizing radiation and the risk of radiation pneumonitis. In 2001, Rusch and colleagues presented results from a phase II trial of using this conventional hemithoracic RT to a median dose of 54 Gy after complete resection, mostly EPP, to determine feasibility and to estimate rates of local recurrence and survival (Rusch et al. 2001). The results demonstrated a low local relapse rate of only 13% and median survival of 17 months The same conventional hemithoracic RT technique was tested in combination with neoadjuvant pemetrexed and cisplatin followed by EPP and postoperative RT to the hemithorax and shown to be feasible and effective (Krug et al. 2009). Median survival in the overall patient population was 16.8 months, while patients completing the entire treatment regimen of all three modalities had a median survival of 29.1 months. The 2- and 3-year survival rates were 37% and approximately 20%, respectively.

Three-dimensional conformal radiation therapy (3D-CRT) and especially intensity-modulated radiation therapy (IMRT) were developed to allow more conformal dose delivery to the tumor and more effective sparing of OARs, even in anatomically challenging areas. However, there is a higher chance of delivering low to intermediate doses of RT to a larger volume of OARs if not tightly controlled. Early reports of postoperative IMRT after EPP in MPM patients were associated with severe toxicities. In a small study by Allen and colleagues, 6 of 13 patients died from radiation pneumonitis (Allen et al. 2006). In subsequent analyses higher mean lung dose and the volume of the contralateral single remaining lung receiving 5, 10, and 20 Gy were associated with an increased risk of radiation-induced pneumonitis (Rice et al. 2007a; Kristensen et al. 2009). A mean lung dose of <8.5 Gy was recommended by some, and low-dose volume within the lung should be minimized (Krayenbuehl et al. 2007). Later studies on IMRT after EPP demonstrated improved outcomes when more carefully controlling the lung dose to the contralateral single remaining lung (Rice et al. 2007b). Local failure was only noted in 13% of patients who underwent EPP and IMRT. This study demonstrated that IMRT after EPP is feasible, safe, and efficacious. Moreover, increasing experience with these conformal techniques was shown to lead to improved target coverage and decreased toxicity rates (Patel et al. 2012). Taken together, these studies demonstrate that patients with good performance status and pulmonary and renal function, in the absence of distant disease, can be treated with IMRT, when the dose to the contralateral lung is kept to a minimum level to minimize the risk of radiation pneumonitis.

The routine use of high-dose hemithoracic RT in a multimodality treatment approach after EPP and chemotherapy has been questioned by the results from the SAKK 17/04 trial in 2015 (Stahel et al. 2015). The multi-institutional, randomized phase II trial compared the survival of MPM patients who received RT and no RT, after completing chemotherapy and EPP. The RT techniques used were 3D-CRT or IMRT. Somewhat in contrast to previously published promising results, no significant difference in median overall survival between those who received radiotherapy (19.3 months) and those that did not (20.8 months) was observed. Therefore, the authors concluded that RT after EPP poses an additional treatment burden without any clear benefit for the patient. However, there were multiple criticisms of this study, including significant patient drop-off, early closure to accrual, and insufficient power for the intended endpoints and for the use of three different radiotherapy fractionation regimens, to name a few. Only 23 patients received RT as prescribed, and there was no central plan review of target coverage and compliance to dosimetric constraints of organs at risk. As previously demonstrated, these factors can be associated with potentially severe toxicities that could very much affect the toxicities, survival, and outcomes of the study. Thus, it is difficult to conclude much about the role of adjuvant hemithoracic RT after EPP from this study (Rimner et al. 2016a).

Preoperative hemithoracic IMRT prior to EPP has been pioneered by the Princess Margaret Hospital in Toronto and shown some of the best results in resectable MPM patients (de Perrot et al. 2015). Patients are treated with 25 Gy in five fractions with concomitant boost of 5 Gy to areas at risk over the course of a week, followed by EPP within 1 week. In their first experience, they selected patients with the prognostically favorable epithelioid histologic type and resectable clinical T1-3N0M0 stage. All 62 patients enrolled in the study were able to complete the treatment, and it was associated with an operative mortality of 1.6%, an overall treatment-related mortality of 4.8%, and no bronchial stump leaks. The median overall survival on an intention-to-treat basis was 36 months. In this subgroup of patients, they observed a median overall survival of 51 months and disease-free survival of 47 months with this regimen, mostly without chemotherapy. Patients with biphasic subtype had median overall survival of 10 months. Furthermore, the treatment time was reduced from about 6 months in traditional multimodality approaches to less than 2 weeks with the SMART approach. These promising results will have to be validated by an independent institution. One of the challenges with this preoperative hemithoracic IMRT approach may be the difficulty to accurately predict tumor resectability because of the limitations in the current clinical and radiographic staging tools for MPM that are frequently associated with significant discrepancies between clinical and pathologic staging. Furthermore, meticulous coordination between the surgeons and radiation oncologist involved will be needed, as the completion of EPP after IMRT is essential to avoid serious radiation pneumonitis. Excellent expertise in radiation oncology and surgery is needed to coordinate treatment so rigorously that patients undergo the mandatory EPP shortly after completion of RT would avoid the risk of potentially life-threatening radiation pneumonitis. Yet, the excellent results might be explained by factors other than simply patient selection and the sequence of treatment. The use of hypofractionated preoperative RT, as used on this protocol, might potentially have additional activating effects of the immune system, besides cytotoxic effects. A potential immunomodulation of preoperative RT, as well as synergisms with checkpoint inhibitors or other immunotherapies, should thus be subject to future human and animal studies.

2.2 Adjuvant Radiation Therapy After P/D

As the use of EPP has gradually declined in recent years in favor of less radical, lung-sparing approaches such as P/D, many patients now present for consideration for adjuvant RT with two intact lungs. This required the development of a RT technique that allows sparing of both lungs in an attempt to avoid severe radiation toxicity. The conventional RT technique used in the setting of EPP was initially also tested in patients who had undergone a lung-sparing P/D. The post-EPP technique was modified with the addition of a lung block to spare the ipsilateral intact lung (Gupta et al. 2005). The median RT dose achieved was only 42.5 Gy, as a more effective RT dose was prohibited by the inability of the conventional technique to meet dosimetric normal organ constraints. This might also be the reason for the discouraging results with a 1-year local control rate of 42%, a median survival of 13.5 months, and nevertheless quite high rates of toxicity with 28% grade 3–4 toxicity and two patients with possible grade 5 cardiac and pulmonary toxicities. Tumor recurrences occurred particularly in areas of match lines between the blocks on the photon fields and the edge of the electron fields, indicating the unsatisfactory precision in delivering the radiation with this technique.

When IMRT became available, it allowed further development of a technique that would be able to more precisely control dose delivery without match lines and sufficient sparing of organs at risk. The feasibility of performing IMRT after P/D was first demonstrated by Rosenzweig and colleagues in 2012, in a series of 36 patients receiving palliative IMRT in unresectable MPM without severe side effects (Rosenzweig et al. 2012). All patients were planned with a PET/CT scan to aid target delineation. Treatment was delivered up to a total dose of 50.4 Gy with a median dose of 46.8 Gy. The median survival was 26 months in patients who underwent P/D and IMRT, with a 1- and 2-year survival of 75% and 53%, respectively. For patients who did not have surgery, the median survival was 17 months, with a 1- and 2-year survival of 75% and 21%, respectively. Grade 3 or 4 radiation pneumonitis was observed in 20% of patients, though all but one recovered. Other studies described similarly good clinical outcomes without excessively high risks of toxicity using a tomotherapy technique (Minatel et al. 2014).

The high precision of IMRT requires more detailed knowledge of the anatomy of the thorax and the diaphragm, state-of-the-art diagnostic imaging tools, information about the pathologic findings at the time of surgery, 4D CT scan to assess the respiratory tumor motion, and image-guided RT delivery. The use of 18-fluorodeoxyglucose (FDG) PET has been shown to improve target delineation and thereby improve local control (Fodor et al. 2011). Furthermore, detection of lymph node involvement not demonstrated on computed tomography may be visualized on FDG-PET scans leading to more accurate staging (Pehlivan et al. 2009). A failure-pattern analysis of 67 patients treated with P/D and adjuvant hemithoracic IMRT revealed that the majority of local failures occurred in sites of gross disease, stressing the need for macroscopically complete surgical resection (Rimner et al. 2014). In patients who were treated with P/D versus those who underwent only a partial pleurectomy or those who had unresectable MPM, the median time to in-field local failure was prolonged (14 months vs. 6 months), and 1- and 2-year actuarial in-field local failure rates were lower (43% and 60% vs. 66% and 83%, respectively). With increasing experience fewer failures at the radiation field margins and decreased toxicity were observed, suggesting an improvement in target delineation and RT planning.

A prospective phase II study on the feasibility of hemithoracic intensity-modulated pleural radiation therapy (IMPRINT) after chemotherapy and P/D demonstrated that a planned dose of 50.4 Gy in 28 fractions can safely be administered, with 30% of the patients developing grade 2 or higher radiation pneumonitis, all of which improved promptly on prednisone, while no grade 4 or 5 pneumonitis was observed (Rimner et al. 2016b). The most common side effect observed was severe fatigue that could last for several months.

When comparing the outcomes of this modern trimodality regimen of chemotherapy, lung-sparing P/D, and adjuvant IMPRINT with historical patients treated with P/D and adjuvant conventional RT without chemotherapy, modern trimodality therapy was associated with improved survival rates (Shaikh et al. 2017). This suggested that trimodality combination therapy including platinum/pemetrexed therapy, improvements in surgical technique and staging, as well as modern IMPRINT result in better survival rates than bimodality therapy with P/D and conventional RT.

A comparison of the clinical outcomes of patients receiving P/D and adjuvant IMRT to EPP and adjuvant IMRT yielded favorable results for the P/D and adjuvant IMRT group with a median overall survival of 28.4 vs. 14.2 months and progression-free survival of 18.9 months vs. not reached (Chance et al. 2015).

Given the complexity and operator dependence of the IMPRINT technique, an ongoing phase II study is testing the safety and exportability of this technique to multiple other centers with experienced radiation therapy departments and high volume of mesothelioma patients (clinicaltrials.gov: NCT00715611). This study was developed with strict radiation planning criteria, central contour, and plan review for every single patient.

Arc therapy, e.g., volumetric modulated arc therapy (VMAT), and helical tomotherapy are rotational RT techniques that deliver radiation from even more beam angles than IMRT. Both techniques allow for the delivery of RT in a highly conformal way, therefore ideally suited for spherical or circular targets and are of particular interest in MPM. For patients with intact lungs after P/D or pleural biopsy, it was shown that tomotherapy allows for the safe delivery of 50 Gy in 25 fractions to the entire hemithorax, including chest-wall incisions and drain sites and excluding the intact lung with promising survival rates (Minatel et al. 2014). Only 7% of the patients treated with this regimen reportedly developed a grade 3 pneumonitis within 5 months after treatment. Other studies have indicated that the use of VMAT may lead to significantly better sparing of OARs compared to static-field IMRT, in an even shorter time (average delivery time 5 min vs. 15 min) (Dumane et al. 2016). Thereby, toxicity may be further reduced and dose escalation achieved.

The use of proton therapy also holds potential benefits for the treatment of MPM. As compared to photon treatment, there is no exit dose with proton therapy. Thus, proton therapy may be another future option to deliver precise radiation confined to the pleural target volume with effective sparing of normal organs, as was shown in planning studies (Krayenbuehl et al. 2010). A case series about intensity-modulated proton therapy (IMPT) for MPM patients with intact lungs showed promising early results (Pan et al. 2015). The investigators described their clinical experience with robust planning and evaluation, dose verification, simulation, image-guided setup, and adaptive planning at their institution and demonstrated that IMPT is feasible for routine clinical practice in MPM treatment. High patient throughput and efficient machine use could be achieved with increased experience. Despite the small sample size (seven patients), a dosimetric benefit compared to IMRT planning could be shown for certain patients. In order to compare clinically relevant outcomes after IMPT to those after IMRT prospective studies with longer follow-up, larger numbers of patients are needed.

2.3   Other Indications for Radiation Therapy

RT has long been used to prevent procedure tract metastases (PTMs) that may occur after invasive diagnostic or therapeutic interventions, e.g., incisions and scars, or around the site of thoracic drains. Most recent data, however, cast doubt over the routine use of prophylactic RT to surgical sites in order to prevent PMS. Clive and colleagues presented results from a randomized phase III study in 2016, indicating that prophylactic RT after pleural interventions did not reduce the incidence of PTM and confers no benefits in terms of symptom control, analgesia use, survival, or quality of life (Clive et al. 2016). Yet, their results indicated that prophylactic RT immediately after surgery might reduce PTMs in two distinct subgroups: patients with epithelioid-only histology and those who did not receive chemotherapy. Future studies ought to address whether a specific subgroup of patients might benefit from the prophylactic treatment.

Apart from its use as part of a multimodality approach in the early-stage setting, palliative RT plays a vital role in treating pain or providing local control in advanced MPM. Even though many patients are treated with analgesics, tumor-related pain can be difficult to control. Various tumor-related factors can cause pain, e.g., tumor infiltration into the chest wall, intercostal nerves, brachial plexus, or bone (MacLeod et al. 2015). An altered microenvironment, with pro-inflammatory cytokines and other factors released by the tumor, may worsen the pain. A wide range of pain medications, from nonsteroidal anti-inflammatory drugs (NSAIDs) to opioids, paracetamol, and adjuvant analgesics for neuropathic pain, as well as topical agents, such as lidocaine patches, is used. Palliative RT is an effective and simple tool to treat pain, locally control tumor invading critical organs, and allow decreased needs for other pain management strategies such as opioids, thus avoiding many of the drug-related side effects. Standard palliative fractionation is acceptable. Whether higher doses may result in better palliation is currently assessed in an ongoing trial (SYSTEMS-2) which is testing whether dose escalation from 4 to 6 Gy per fraction will result in better palliation.

MPM is a disease with highly variable presentation. Thus, no one treatment approach will be applicable to all MPM patients. Radiation therapy can play a role in early-stage as well as advanced-stage MPM. In the early-stage setting, the combination with other multimodality therapies appears to be key for optimal treatment outcomes. Typically, RT in the early-stage setting requires a unique set of experience and expertise when aiming to treat the entire hemithorax, whether before or after EPP or after P/D. These treatments should only be performed at centers of excellence with significant experience with these challenging treatment modalities, ideally as part of a prospective protocol. RT techniques have vastly improved over the past decade with significantly improved imaging, dosimetry and precision of delivery. These have resulted in substantially decreased risks for toxicities. Nevertheless despite all technological improvements, hemithoracic RT remains a high-risk procedure with substantial toxicity and needs to be carefully done with close patient monitoring by a strong supportive care team that is familiar with the typical toxicities of the multimodality treatment and management of the disease. Palliative RT is frequently technologically less challenging yet a powerful tool to improve patient's quality of life and decrease pain. It should thus be a consideration by any multidisciplinary team when treating patients with MPM. Multiple prospective trials on the role of RT in this challenging disease are ongoing and will provide further optimization of RT techniques and more insight into how to best combine RT with other treatment modalities.

References

Allen AM, Czerminska M, Jänne PA, Sugarbaker DJ, Bueno R, Harris JR, et al. Fatal pneumonitis associated with intensity-modulated radiation therapy for mesothelioma. Int J Radiat Oncol Biol Phys. 2006;65(3):640–5.

Chance WW, Rice DC, Allen PK, Tsao AS, Fontanilla HP, Liao Z, et al. Hemithoracic intensity modulated radiation therapy after pleurectomy/decortication for malignant pleural mesothelioma: toxicity, patterns of failure, and a matched survival analysis. Int J Radiat Oncol Biol Phys. 2015;91(1):149–56. PubMed PMID: 25442335. Epub 2014/12/03. Eng.

Clive AO, Taylor H, Dobson L, Wilson P, de Winton E, Panakis N, et al. Prophylactic radiotherapy for the prevention of procedure-tract metastases after surgical and large-bore pleural procedures in malignant pleural mesothelioma (SMART): a multicentre, open-label, phase 3, randomised controlled trial. Lancet Oncol. 2016;17(8):1094–104.

de Perrot M, Feld R, Leighl NB, Hope A, Waddell TK, Keshavjee S, et al. Accelerated hemithoracic radiation followed by extrapleural pneumonectomy for malignant pleural mesothelioma. J Thorac Cardiovasc Surg. 2015. PubMed PMID: 26614413. Epub 2015/11/29. Eng.

Dumane V, Rimner A, Yorke ED, Rosenzweig KE. Volumetric-modulated arc therapy for malignant pleural mesothelioma after pleurectomy/decortication. Appl Radiat Oncol. 2016;5(4):24–33.

Flores RM, Pass HI, Seshan VE, Dycoco J, Zakowski M, Carbone M, et al. Extrapleural pneumonectomy versus pleurectomy/decortication in the surgical management of malignant pleural mesothelioma: results in 663 patients. J Thorac Cardiovasc Surg. 2008;135(3):620–6.e3.

Fodor A, Fiorino C, Dell'Oca I, Broggi S, Pasetti M, Cattaneo GM, et al. PET-guided dose escalation tomotherapy in malignant pleural mesothelioma. Strahlenther Onkol. 2011;187(11):736–43.

Gupta V, Mychalczak B, Krug L, Flores R, Bains M, Rusch VW, et al. Hemithoracic radiation therapy after pleurectomy/decortication for malignant pleural mesothelioma. Int J Radiat Oncol Biol Phys. 2005;63(4):1045–52.

Krayenbuehl J, Oertel S, Davis JB, Ciernik IF. Combined photon and electron three-dimensional conformal versus intensity-modulated radiotherapy with integrated boost for adjuvant treatment of malignant pleural mesothelioma after pleuropneumonectomy. Int J Radiat Oncol Biol Phys. 2007;69(5):1593–9.

Krayenbuehl J, Hartmann M, Lomax AJ, Kloeck S, Hug EB, Ciernik IF. Proton therapy for malignant pleural mesothelioma after extrapleural pleuropneumonectomy. Int J Radiat Oncol Biol Phys. 2010;78(2):628–34. PubMed PMID: 20385451. Epub 2010/04/14. Eng.

Kristensen CA, Nøttrup TJ, Berthelsen AK, Kjær-Kristoffersen F, Ravn J, Sørensen JB, et al. Pulmonary toxicity following IMRT after extrapleural pneumonectomy for malignant pleural mesothelioma. Radiother Oncol. 2009;92(1):96–9.

Krug LM, Pass HI, Rusch VW, Kindler HL, Sugarbaker DJ, Rosenzweig KE, et al. Multicenter phase II trial of neoadjuvant pemetrexed plus cisplatin followed by extrapleural pneumonectomy and radiation for malignant pleural mesothelioma. J Clin Oncol. 2009;27(18):3007–13.

MacLeod N, Chalmers A, O'Rourke N, Moore K, Sheridan J, McMahon L, et al. Is radiotherapy useful for treating pain in mesothelioma?: a phase II trial. J Thorac Oncol. 2015;10(6):944–50. PubMed PMID: 25654216. Epub 2015/02/06. Eng.

Minatel E, Trovo M, Polesel J, Baresic T, Bearz A, Franchin G, et al. Radical pleurectomy/decortication followed by high dose of radiation therapy for malignant pleural mesothelioma. Final results with long-term follow-up. Lung Cancer. 2014;83(1):78–82. PubMed PMID: 24216141. Epub 2013/11/13. Eng.

Pan HY, Jiang S, Sutton J, Liao Z, Chance WW, Frank SJ, et al. Early experience with intensity modulated proton therapy for lung-intact mesothelioma: a case series. Pract Radiat Oncol. 2015;5(4):e345–53. PubMed PMID: 25572666. Epub 2015/01/13. Eng.

Patel PR, Yoo S, Broadwater G, Marks LB, Miles EF, D'Amico TA, et al. Effect of increasing experience on dosimetric and clinical outcomes in the management of malignant pleural mesothelioma with intensity-modulated radiation therapy. Int J Radiat Oncol Biol Phys. 2012;83(1):362–8.

Pehlivan B, Topkan E, Onal C, Nursal GN, Yuksel O, Dolek Y, et al. Comparison of CT and integrated PET-CT based radiation therapy planning in patients with malignant pleural mesothelioma. Radiat Oncol. 2009;4:35.

Rice DC, Smythe WR, Liao Z, Guerrero T, Chang JY, McAleer MF, et al. Dose-dependent pulmonary toxicity after postoperative intensity-modulated radiotherapy for malignant pleural mesothelioma. Int J Radiat Oncol Biol Phys. 2007a;69(2):350–7.

Rice DC, Stevens CW, Correa AM, Vaporciyan AA, Tsao A, Forster KM, et al. Outcomes after extrapleural pneumonectomy and intensity-modulated radiation therapy for malignant pleural mesothelioma. Ann Thorac Surg. 2007b;84(5):1685–93.

Rice D, Rusch V, Pass H, Asamura H, Nakano T, Edwards J, et al. Recommendations for uniform definitions of surgical techniques for malignant pleural mesothelioma: A consensus report of the International Association for the Study of Lung Cancer International Staging Committee and the International Mesothelioma Interest Group. J Thorac Oncol. 2011;6(8):1304–12.

Rimner A, Spratt DE, Zauderer MG, Rosenzweig KE, Wu AJ, Foster A, et al. Failure patterns after hemithoracic pleural intensity modulated radiation therapy for malignant pleural mesothelioma. Int J Radiat Oncol Biol Phys. 2014;90(2):394–401. PubMed PMID: 25073664. Epub 2014/07/31. Eng.

Rimner A, Simone 2nd CB, Zauderer MG, Cengel KA, Rusch VW. Hemithoracic radiotherapy for mesothelioma: lack of benefit or lack of statistical power? Lancet Oncol. 2016a; in press.

Rimner A, Zauderer MG, Gomez DR, Adusumilli PS, Parhar PK, Wu AJ, et al. Phase II study of hemithoracic intensity-modulated pleural radiation therapy (IMPRINT) as part of lung-sparing multimodality therapy in patients with malignant pleural mesothelioma. J Clin Oncol. 2016b;34(23):2761–8. PubMed PMID: 27325859. Pubmed Central PMCID: PMC5019761. Epub 2016/06/22. Eng.

Rosenzweig KE, Zauderer MG, Laser B, Krug LM, Yorke E, Sima CS, et al. Pleural intensity-modulated radiotherapy for malignant pleural mesothelioma. Int J Radiat Oncol Biol Phys. 2012;83(4):1278–83.

Rusch VW, Rosenzweig K, Venkatraman E, Leon L, Raben A, Harrison L, et al. A phase II trial of surgical resection and adjuvant high dose hemithoracic radiation for malignant pleural mesothelioma. J Thorac Cardiovasc Surg. 2001;122(4):788–95.

Shaikh F, Zauderer MG, von Reibnitz D, Wu AJ, Yorke ED, Foster A, et al. Improved outcomes with modern lung-sparing trimodality therapy in patients with malignant pleural mesothelioma. J Thorac Oncol. 2017. PubMed PMID: 28341225. Epub 2017/03/28. Eng.

Stahel RA, Riesterer O, Xyrafas A, Opitz I, Beyeler M, Ochsenbein A, et al. Neoadjuvant chemotherapy and extrapleural pneumonectomy of malignant pleural mesothelioma with or without hemithoracic radiotherapy (SAKK 17/04): a randomised, international, multicentre phase 2 trial. Lancet Oncol. 2015. PubMed PMID: 26538423. Epub 2015/11/06. Eng.

Taioli E, Wolf AS, Flores RM. Meta-analysis of survival after pleurectomy decortication versus extrapleural pneumonectomy in mesothelioma. Ann Thorac Surg. 2015;99(2):472–80. PubMed PMID: 25534527. Epub 2014/12/24. Eng.

Treasure T, Lang-Lazdunski L, Waller D, Bliss JM, Tan C, Entwisle J, et al. Extra-pleural pneumonectomy versus no extra-pleural pneumonectomy for patients with malignant pleural mesothelioma: clinical outcomes of the Mesothelioma and Radical Surgery (MARS) randomised feasibility study. Lancet Oncol. 2011;12(8):763–72.

Yajnik S, Rosenzweig KE, Mychalczak B, Krug L, Flores R, Hong L, et al. Hemithoracic radiation after extrapleural pneumonectomy for malignant pleural mesothelioma. Int J Radiat Oncol Biol Phys. 2003;56(5):1319–26.

Part II

Therapeutic Treatments: Chemotherapy, Biotherapy, and Immunotherapy

Chemotherapy and Standard Treatment Options

5

Mary Hesdorffer and Gleneara E. Bates-Pappas

1 Background

Remarkable advances in cancer interventions over the last 20 years have given rise to a social credo that medical research, given enough resources and time, will find a cure for cancer. However, the development of new cancer treatments is fraught with challenges on many fronts – ethical, scientific, and economic. Malignant mesothelioma faces unique challenges when it comes to drug development and approval. Despite the small study population and limited resources, there have been positive advancements that have established several treatment standards.

In 2003, Vogelzang and colleagues conducted a randomized phase 3 study of pemetrexed in combination with cisplatin enrolling 456 chemotherapy-naïve patients. Patients received either cisplatin and pemetrexed or cisplatin alone (Vogelzang et al. 2003). Results demonstrated intravenous 500 mg/m² pemetrexed, and 75 mg/m² cisplatin had a response rate of 41.3% compared to cisplatin alone with 16.7% and a median survival of 12.1 months compared to 9.3 with cisplatin alone. In 2004, the FDA approved the combination as a standard first-line treatment (Zauderer et al. 2014). While this trial provided valuable gains for the treatment of MPM, the modest increase on survival did not provide patients with significant improvement in quality of life.

The original version of this chapter was revised. The correction to this chapter can be found at https://doi.org/10.1007/978-3-319-96244-3_21

M. Hesdorffer (✉)
Mesothelioma Applied Research Foundation, Alexandria, VA, USA
e-mail: mary@curemeso.org

G. E. Bates-Pappas (✉)
City University of New York, Graduate Center, New York, NY, USA
e-mail: gbates@gradcenter.cuny.edu

It is important to mention however that:

1. The study has never been repeated, and it is unusual for the FDA to approve a new treatment on the basis of a single study – an exception was made here because it was recognized that a repeat large study in a rare disease would delay approval by a number of years.
2. The study was marred and interrupted by a number of cardiac deaths due to initial lack of prophylaxis by folic acid and vitamin b12.
3. The difference in overall survival between the two arms was less than 3 months (Goudar 2008; Vogelzang et al. 2003; Bearz et al. 2012).

In 2016, the Mesothelioma Avastin Cisplatin Pemetrexed Study (MAPS), a randomized phase 3 trial with 448 newly diagnosed pleural mesothelioma patients who had not previously received treatment was conducted in France by the France Cooperative Thoracic Intergroup (IFCT) from 2008 to 2014 (Zalcman et al. 2016). Patients were randomly assigned to one of two treatment arms: intravenous 500 mg/m^2 pemetrexed plus 75 mg/m^2 cisplatin or intravenous 500 mg/m^2 pemetrexed plus 75 mg/m^2 cisplatin with 15 mg/kg bevacizumab (PCB).

Zalcman and colleges reported a significant increase in survival among patients who received the combination of pemetrexed, cisplatin, and bevacizumab (Avastin). Of the 448 patients, 223 received PCB; the median survival was 18.8 months compared to the 16.1 months for the 225 patients who received pemetrexed and cisplatin alone.

Despite the promising results, the combination of pemetrexed, cisplatin, and bevacizumab was not approved by the FDA for use in the United States. However, several countries in Europe have received approval. While the data shows the combination increased survival by 4 months, it has not been fully elucidate whether the carful section of newly diagnosed, chemotherapy-naïve patients exhibits unique or different biological characteristic that may contribute to the positive response rate. Nonetheless, it is listed as recommended for front-line therapy by many who publish disease-specific guidelines which often times drive insurance decisions to cover non-FDA-approved treatments.

In May 2019 based in part upon the results of the Stellar Trial, the FDA granted device approval to NovoTTF-100L System in combination with pemetrexed and a platinum-based therapy for frontline treatment in unresectable, metastatic or locally advanced malignant pleural mesothelioma. Novocure's system NovoTTF-100L utilizes electric fields tuned to specific frequencies to disrupt cell division which is necessary for cancerous cells to multiply. This approval based upon safety is the first approval by the FDA in mesothelioma since 2004. The Stellar Trial Stellar trial was a non-randomized single-arm study conducted outside of the USA which included 80 subjects with a confirmed diagnosis of pleural mesothelioma not eligible for curative-intent surgery. Patients received standard therapy of pemetrexed and a platinum-based therapy and in addition to TTF fields which were administered until radiological verified disease progression was documented. Study results reported an overall survival of 18.2 months and a median progression-free survival of 7.6 months. These results compared against the historical results of the pemetrexed-cisplatin study demonstrate a probable advantage with the addition of the

TTF-100L system. There are no randomized trials to support this conclusion nor are there comparable devices currently approved to treat this patient population.

Toxicities were mainly skin toxicity with 5% requiring treatment interruption. There were no treatment-related deaths nor were there additive toxicity to those that are associated with the use of pemetrexed and a platinum therapy.

2 Chemotherapy Clinical Trials Nursing and Mesothelioma

Malignant mesothelioma, a rare malignancy often attributed to asbestos, has been, until the mid-1990s, virtually refractory to any form of therapy other than surgery and has been characterized by much pain and discomfort and survivals of a year or less (Cinausero et al. 2018). Even at that time, however, it had been noticed that a rare patient or even small phase 1 or 2 clinical trials would exhibit tantalizing responses with reduction in disease and symptoms after some standard chemotherapy drugs, but because of the rarity of disease (less than 3000 new cases per year in the United States), formal randomized control clinical trials had not been done.

Early attempts at chemotherapy with powerful drug such as doxorubicin and mitomycin had shown some symptomatic improvement and objective disease regression accompanied by significant cardiac and hematologic side effects. Better-tolerated drugs such as gemcitabine, methotrexate and its derivatives, and 5-fluorouracil, alone or combined with cisplatin or carboplatin, constituted an acceptable regimen that induced clinical responses and symptom improvement in up to 30% of patients—an encouraging result, but one that did not translate into prolongation of survival (Tomek et al. 2003). Nevertheless it was used routinely in both the adjuvant setting after tumor resection and treatment of advanced unresectable disease.

3 Chemotherapy Symptoms and Tolerability

Pemetrexed, although well tolerated in the main, can rarely produce unusually severe pulmonary toxicity and occasional bone marrow and renal impairment. Cisplatin has a 4% incidence of grade 3–4 ototoxicity and a 10% or more incidence of grade 2+ renal toxicity. Carboplatin is more benign but nevertheless can induce prolonged thrombocytopenia and moderately severe peripheral neuropathy. Vinorelbine invariably produces some peripheral neuropathy. Gemcitabine is mainly toxic to the bone marrow (US Department of Health and Human Services [HHS], National Institutes of Health [NIH], National Cancer Institute [NCI] 2018).

Older drugs, rarely used, include doxorubicin and mitomycin-C which have occasionally been effective when all others have failed. In doses used in mesothelioma, the main toxicity is to the bone marrow. However doxorubicin may precipitate cardiac toxicity, and mitomycin can cause a hemolytic uremic syndrome (HHS, NIH, NCI 2018).

Because of the unsatisfactory overall gains in mesothelioma treatment from chemotherapy alone, there are strong attempts today to introduce experimental regimens which employ immunotherapy maneuvers or drug enhancers (Table 5.1).

Table 5.1 Chemotherapeutic mechanism of action and common side effects

Agent	Mechanism of action	Example (s)	Common side effects
Platinum-based agent	Cross-linking DNA, inhibit DNA synthesis/ transposition, function, and transcription	Cisplatin, carboplatin, oxaliplatin	Nausea, vomiting, diarrhea, constipation, gas, hair loss, loss in ability to taste food, hiccups, dry mouth, sores in the mouth and throat, dark urine, decreased sweating, dry skin, and other signs of dehydration, pain, burning, or tingling in the hands or feet, pain, itching, redness, swelling, blisters, or sores in the place where the medication was injected, pain, weakness, muscle, back, or joint pain, tiredness, anxiety, depression, difficulty falling asleep or staying asleep
Antimetabolite	Interferes with DNA transcription, synthesis, and function	Methotrexate (Gemzar®), gemcitabine, pemetrexed (Alimta®)	Joint or muscle pain, reddened eyes, swollen gums, hair loss, vomiting, blurred vision or sudden loss of vision, sudden fever, severe headache, and stiff neck, confusion or memory loss, weakness or difficulty moving one or both sides of the body, difficulty walking or unsteady walking, decreased urination, swelling of the face, arms, hands, feet, ankles, or lower legs, hives, itching, skin rash, difficulty breathing or swallowing, constipation, loss of appetite, weight loss, tiredness, dizziness, fast heartbeat, difficulty falling asleep or staying asleep, changes in mood, depression, diarrhea

Table 5.1 (continued)

Agent	Mechanism of action	Example (s)	Common side effects
Topoisomerase inhibitor	Prevents DNA supercoiling, leads to DNA breaks, and interferes with DNA transcription/replication	Doxorubicin (Adriamycin®)	Nausea, vomiting, sores in the mouth and throat, loss of appetite, weight loss, weight gain, stomach pain, diarrhea, increased thirst, unusual tiredness or weakness, dizziness, hair loss, separation of fingernail or toenail from the nail bed, itchy, red, watery, or irritated eyes, eye pain, pain, burning, or tingling in the hands or feet, red discoloration of urine (for 1 to 2 days after dose)
Vinca alkaloid	Inhibits microtubule polymerization, arrest in cell division	Vinorelbine	Nausea, vomiting, diarrhea, loss of appetite, weight loss, change in ability to taste food, sores in the mouth and throat, hearing loss, dizziness, headache, pain, numbness, burning, or tingling in the hands or feet, muscle, joint, or bone pain, hair loss, shortness of breath, cough, constipation, stomach pain, chest pain, irregular heartbeat, pale skin, unusual tiredness or weakness, unusual bleeding or bruising, hives, itching, rash, difficulty breathing or swallowing
Alkylating agent	DNA base pair alkylation, formation of abnormal DNA crossbridges, and mispairing of nucleotides	Mitomycin C	Nausea, vomiting, loss of appetite or weight, sores in the mouth and throat, headache, fainting, blurred vision, hair loss, loss of strength and energy, rash, pain, itching, redness, swelling, blisters, or sores on the skin especially near the injection site, shortness of breath, difficulty breathing, fast, irregular, or pounding heartbeat

US Department of Health and Human Services [HHS], National Institutes of Health [NIH], National Cancer Institute [NCI] (2018)

4   The Future of Chemotherapeutic Treatment

It would be important to point out that patients with biphasic disease, who are missing the P 16 chromosome, have a much worse prognosis than those with epithelioid disease only. Depending upon the makeup of the study population, the data will be skewed one way or the other. The current regimens have not been fully compared with respect to quality of life, although some data does exist.

It's important to note that there is a robust roster of clinical trials and mesothelioma using combinations of immunotherapy agents, immunotherapy/chemotherapy combinations, in vitro molecular or biochemical testing of new drugs and combinations, and better profiling of patient groups.

References

Bearz A, Talamini R, Rossoni G, et al. Re-challenge with pemetrexed in advanced mesothelioma: a multi-institutional experience. BMC Res Notes. 2012;5:482.

Cinausero M, Rihawi K, Sperandi F, Melotti B, Ardizzoni A. Chemotherapy treatment in malignant pleural mesothelioma: a difficult history. J Thorac Dis. 2018;10(Suppl 2):S304–10. https://doi.org/10.21037/jtd.2017.10.19. Review. PubMed PMID: 29507800; PubMed Central PMCID: PMC5830568.

Goudar RK. Review of pemetrexed in combination with cisplatin for the treatment of malignant pleural mesothelioma. Ther Clin Risk Manag. 2008;4(1):205–11.

Tomek S, Emri S, Krejcy K, Manegold C. Chemotherapy for malignant pleural mesothelioma: past results and recent developments. Br J Cancer. 2003;88(2):167–74. http://doi.org.ezproxy.cul.columbia.edu/10.1038/sj.bjc.6600673

U.S. Department of Health and Human Services, National Institutes of Health, National Cancer Institute. A to Z list of cancer drug National Cancer Institute. 2018. Retrieved August 16, 2018, from https://www.cancer.gov/about-cancer/treatment/drugs

Vogelzang NJ, Rusthoven JJ, Symanowski J, et al. Phase III study of pemetrexed in combination with cisplatin versus cisplatin alone in patients with malignant pleural mesothelioma. J Clin Oncol. 2003;21:2636–44.

Zauderer MG, Kass SL, Woo K, et al. Vinorelbine and gemcitabine as second- or third-line therapy for malignant pleural mesothelioma. Lung Cancer. 2014;84:271–4.

Zalcman G, Mazieres J, Margery J, et al. Bevacizumab for newly diagnosed pleural mesothelioma in the Mesothelioma Avastin Cisplatin Pemetrexed Study (MAPS): a randomised, controlled, open-label, phase 3 trial. Lancet. 2016;387:1405–14.

Buerkley Rose

1 Immunotherapy and Mesothelioma

Immunotherapy is a type of systemic treatment that works differently than chemotherapy. Currently, there is no Food and Drug Administration (FDA)-approved immunotherapy for pleural or peritoneal mesothelioma. However, there are several types of immunotherapy currently in clinical trials. The various types of immunotherapy activate the immune system through a specific immune checkpoint blockade. This essentially turns on the immune system, potentially allows it to recognize cancer cells, and attack them.

There are some types of immunotherapy treatments for mesothelioma which are available in clinical trials. The various types of active immunotherapy include, but are not limited to, PD-1 and PDL-1 inhibitors and CTLA4 inhibitors (Calabrò et al. 2015; Oncology Nursing Society 2016). Drugs in both of these classes are given intravenously at different dosages, over different infusion times, and schedules. This is why it is crucial for patients on clinical trials to have a specialized mesothelioma team at a mesothelioma center to administer the immunotherapy correctly, monitor side effects, follow patients safely after the discontinuation of treatment, as well as manage their overall quality of life and mesothelioma symptoms.

2 Clinical Trials Nursing and Mesothelioma

As explained and is evident throughout this book, caring for mesothelioma patients is complex and requires and interdisciplinary team to provide the best possible patient outcomes. Nurses play a critical role in the team and are the frontline to their

B. Rose (✉)
University of Chicago, Chicago, IL, USA
e-mail: brose@medicine.bsd.uchicago.edu

© Springer Nature Switzerland AG 2019
M. Hesdorffer, G. E. Bates-Pappas (eds.), *Caring for Patients
with Mesothelioma: Principles and Guidelines*,
https://doi.org/10.1007/978-3-319-96244-3_6

care. To care for mesothelioma patients, nurses need expertise in oncology and to have experience working with both pleural and peritoneal mesothelioma patients from diagnosis, throughout treatment, during observation, and in end-of-life care. This experience provides a solid foundation, so that when a patient receives an experimental treatment on a clinical trial, they can manage the additional complex adverse events that can occur. Caring for mesothelioma patients receiving immunotherapy on a clinical trial requires detailed communication and education.

When a mesothelioma patient discusses a clinical trial with an oncologist, it can be overwhelming, and nurses play a key role in communicating with patients, educating patients, and guiding them through the process. The clinical trial process involves informed consent, screening, treatment, and a follow-up period. Educating mesothelioma patients on a clinical trial is an ongoing process, but the informed consent process is possibly the most important time to establish communication methods with the patient, establish a trusting nurse-patient relationship, and provide important side effects that must be reported to their care team.

Informed consent is required prior to any patient enrolling on a clinical trial. If a mesothelioma patient is newly diagnosed or received news that it is time for treatment, like immunotherapy on a clinical trial, they can feel overwhelmed and immense anxiety. Clinical trial nurses specialized in mesothelioma can use their skills and experience to assess their patient's learning needs and overcome barriers to learning.

A clinical trial informed consent document can be lengthy and requires a quiet private environment which can be provided in an outpatient oncology clinic, and for mesothelioma patients, in a specialized center for mesothelioma. The informed consent process involves the nurse and oncologist educating the potential participating patient on the risks and benefits of participating in the clinical trial. Education is provided to the patient during the informed consent discussing topic including, but not limited to, what is involved in the trial, why the trial is being done, information about the treatment, side effects of the treatment, schedule and procedures on the trial, cost to the patient to participate, and patient's rights as a participant (Oncology Nursing Society 2016).

It is important that complete transparency is provided to the patient and they verbalize an understanding of all topics discussed, and the patient is given an opportunity to ask questions. The patient may also ask for time to determine whether they would like to participate. At this juncture, it is important to communicate appropriate routes of communication (i.e., paging, telephone, e-mail, etc.) for the patient. This helps establish a trusting nurse-patient relationship so that moving forward they feel comfortable communicating questions or symptoms. It is important to emphasize to patients on the importance of open communication and highlight safety concerns or adverse effects that must be immediately reported. It is important to continue to reiterate the information and adverse effects to report to the patient throughout the screening process, treatment, and in follow-up.

The screening process typically comprises of labs, physical exam, review of medications, diagnostic imaging, biopsies, and other procedures necessary to confirm a patient is eligible for the clinical trial, and it is safe for them to start treatment. Eligibility must be confirmed prior to a patient starting treatment on a clinical trial.

Again, the nurse should review material in the informed consent as well as reeducate mesothelioma patients on side effects to report so that patients are completely prepared to start treatment.

During treatment and follow-up on trial, the clinical trial nurse monitors mesothelioma patients for safety, adverse effects, coordinates their care, and involves the multidisciplinary team in their care (Oncology Nursing Society 2016). It is important for patients to have appointments coordinated with other crucial members of the mesothelioma care team such as but not limited to a palliative care specialist, social worker, psychologist, physical therapist, and surgeon throughout the clinical trial. This optimizes their patient outcomes and overall quality of life. This also pertains to the follow-up period. Even after a patient discontinues treatment, they must still communicate delayed toxicities or side effects of treatment or any new symptoms related to their mesothelioma.

3   Toxicities of Immunotherapy in Mesothelioma Patients

Immunotherapy has completely different side effects from standard chemotherapy, so it is important that a mesothelioma specialized oncologist administers these drugs and that their team feels comfortable managing their toxicities. Immunotherapy toxicities typically occur when an area of the body or organ outside of the mesothelioma becomes inflamed. This can cause generalized fatigue, side effects in the skin, endocrine glands, gastrointestinal tract, lungs, kidneys, and other areas of the body (Calabrò et al. 2015; Kindler et al. 2017; Thompson 2018).

4   Fatigue

The type of fatigue caused by immunotherapy is different than the fatigue caused by chemotherapy. Fatigue with chemotherapy is usually predictable. Immunotherapy can cause different types of fatigue: daily low-level fatigue or intermittent periods of fatigue. Typically, the fatigue does not reach higher than a grade 1 or 2 (Calabrò et al. 2015; Kindler et al. 2017; Thompson 2018). The fatigue usually does not interfere with activities of daily living. The best way to combat this fatigue is for patients to stay active, to exercise within a tolerable threshold, and to take breaks when needed. If extreme fatigue occurs (greater than grade 2), it should be communicated to patients to notify their team immediately seeing as this can be an indicator that a more serious side effect related to the endocrine system is occurring.

5   Skin

Immunotherapy can cause pruritus and rash. These symptoms can be generalized or in localized areas such as the arms, chest, back, or legs. It is important to communicate with patients transparently about their symptoms prior to them initiating any medication. Over-the-counter remedies include topical cream or lotion (without steroids), oral diphenhydramine at night for pruritus, hydroxyzine, or loratadine which can typically manage grade 1 or 2 symptoms. If the rash or itching exceeds a grade 2, then a consultation with a dermatologist experienced in managing immunotherapy-related rashes is essential (Calabrò et al. 2015; Kindler et al. 2017; Thompson 2018). If the rash is severe enough, topical corticosteroids or oral steroids will be prescribed.

6   Endocrine System

Immunotherapy can cause toxicities in the thyroid, adrenal, and pituitary glands. Toxicities of the endocrine system that can occur include adrenal insufficiency, hyperthyroidism, hypophysitis, hypopituitarism, hypothyroidism, thyroid disorder, and thyroiditis (Kindler et al. 2017; Thompson 2018). Symptoms include, but are not limited to, fatigue, headache, visual disturbances, vomiting, joint pain, and confusion. Laboratory values checking thyroid levels as well as other hormones in the body are typically ordered for these patients. It is crucial for a consult with an endocrinologist experienced in diagnosing, differentiating, and treating autoimmune-mediated toxicities. Treatment for patients includes steroids and hormone replacement therapy. It is important that instructions regarding steroid and hormone treatments as well as follow-up are communicated clearly to patients. If addressed early, these toxicities are manageable, but without appropriate diagnosis and follow-up, they can be fatal. Close follow-up is recommended for patients while these toxicities resolve, and careful assessment for recurrence during tapering of steroids or hormones is also recommended.

7   Gastrointestinal Tract

Another area that immunotherapy can cause toxicity is in the gastrointestinal tract. Colitis or inflammation of the bowel can lead to intestinal obstruction or hemorrhage if not treated immediately. Symptoms include, but are not limited to, diarrhea, abdominal pain, and mucus or blood in the stool. Other causes of symptoms should be ruled out initially such as clostridium difficile infection or other infections. Grade 1–2 diarrhea usually involves fluid replacement and the initiation of oral steroids. Consultation with a gastroenterologist as well as endoscopy with biopsy may also be necessary for even grade 1–2 colitis and are absolutely crucial in grade 2 or higher colitis. Intravenous steroids may be necessary as well for grade 2 or higher events as well as hospitalization (Calabrò et al. 2015; Kindler et al. 2017).

8   Liver Toxicity

The liver can also be affected by immunotherapy. Hepatitis, autoimmune hepatitis, and transaminase elevations can occur. Symptoms include, but are not limited to, fever, jaundice, and transaminase elevations in patients. Patients should be carefully assessed for drug-induced liver injury and hepatitis. Oral steroids should be initiated for grade 1 events, and intravenous steroids are usually recommended for grade 2 or higher events. Patients may be hospitalized, and should see hepatology, and if safe, have a liver biopsy to confirm diagnosis. Several steroid tapers may be necessary for resolution for transaminase elevations. Close follow-up and several repeat transaminase levels are necessary in managing these patients. Treatment as well as close follow-up is essential, because if untreated or recurring, this toxicity could be fatal (Kindler et al. 2017; Thompson 2018).

9   Lungs

Pneumonitis, or inflammation in areas of the lung, is a serious and urgent toxicity that can be fatal if untreated. Symptoms include, but are not limited to, new or worsening shortness of breath or cough. Patients should receive immediate attention and get a diagnostic computed tomography (CT) scan or x-ray of the chest for diagnosis. Depending on the severity, patients will need oral or intravenous steroids. Bronchoscopy, hospitalization, or bronchoalveolar lavage may be necessary. Re-treatment after a patient has pneumonitis depends on patient safety, clinical trial restrictions, and also to the discretion of the oncologist (Kindler et al. 2017; Thompson 2018).

10   Kidneys

Nephritis, or inflammation of the kidneys, can be caused by immunotherapy. Symptoms include, but are not limited to, dysuria, hematuria, hypertension, edema, and elevated blood urea nitrogen levels or creatinine levels. Treatment includes fluid replacement with oral and intravenous fluids, steroids, and consultation with a nephrologist. Hospitalization may be necessary as well depending on the severity. Acute renal failure can occur if not treated appropriately (Kindler et al. 2017).

11   Neurologic and Ocular

Immunotherapy can cause ocular toxicity as well as toxicity in the neurologic system. Ocular toxicities can include uveitis – inflammation of the uvea – or iritis, inflammation of the iris of the eye. Symptoms include, but are not limited to, blurred vision and dry eyes. Consultation with an ophthalmologist is crucial. Topical prednisolone acetate suspension and iridocyclitics may be prescribed or even oral steroids depending on the severity. It is important an ophthalmologist experienced in treating autoimmune-mediated eye toxicities works with the treatment team. Patients can continue treatment with grade 1 toxicity, and these are usually reversible if treated immediately and appropriately.

Neurologic toxicity from immunotherapy is rare, but can occur, and needs immediate treatment by a neurologist. Toxicities include autoimmune neuropathy, demyelinating polyneuropathy, Guillain-Barre syndrome, and myasthenic syndrome

(Kindler et al. 2017; Thompson 2018). Oral or intravenous steroids may be necessary. IVIG or other immunosuppressive therapies may be necessary for grade 3 or 4 events. Patients that develop autoimmune neuropathy should follow closely with a palliative care specialist as well for the management of their neuropathy.

12   Cardiac

Immunotherapy can cause cardiac toxicity. These include myocarditis or pericarditis – an inflammation of the heart. Symptoms include, but are not limited to, shortness of breath, chest pain, peripheral edema, and weight gain. A cardiologist should be consulted immediately, and the patient will need to be hospitalized. Intravenous steroids, medications to control heart rate and blood pressure, an echocardiogram, as well as biopsy or pericardial window may be necessary. Patients need close follow-up with their oncologist as well as cardiologist until resolution of their cardiac toxicity (Kindler et al. 2017; Thompson 2018).

13   Other

Immunotherapy has been reported to cause other serious toxicities. These include pancreatitis, allergic reaction, anaphylaxis, cytokine release syndrome, and infusion reactions. Close nursing assessment during and after infusion is important to report to the provider any potential allergic or infusion reaction so it can be treated appropriately per local guidelines (Kindler et al. 2017; Thompson 2018).

14   Caring for Patients During and After an Immune-Mediated Toxicity

Nursing care for patients during and after they experience an autoimmune toxicity requires intense communication and follow-up. Patients often are prescribed a steroid that can taper over a month or more, so providing clear and concise instruction is crucial to their recovery from any toxicity. It is also important that prophylactic antibiotics during steroid therapy as well as other medications that are prescribed are taken correctly by the patient. Telephone follow-up, repeat laboratory values, laboratory value follow-up, follow-up with specialists, and other important assessments must also be appropriately communicated to the patient.

From the time of consent on a clinical trial, a therapeutic and trusting nurse-patient relationship should be established so that a patient feels comfortable asking questions and communicating symptoms or side effects of their treatment (Oncology Nursing Society 2016). Providing patients with a contact card as well as appropriate channels of communication is crucial to patient care. Communicating with the interdisciplinary team treating the patient is also another essential component to their care. Patients need to be educated on exactly what symptoms to report and when to report them. The more educated the patient, the more empowered they are to be active participants in their care and treatment. Communication ultimately makes or breaks whether a patient's toxicity can be appropriately treated and resolved.

15 Caring for Mesothelioma Patients on Immunotherapy: The Big Picture

Mesothelioma patients have complex needs that require care from a specialized multidisciplinary team. The nurse is an essential member of this team that provides and coordinates care, educates, assesses, and monitors patients during and after immunotherapy treatment. A specialized mesothelioma nurse navigates patients throughout the clinical trial process as well as empowers patients to be an active member of their own care team. Mesothelioma patients receiving immunotherapy can have several potential toxicities. Expertise from a specialized mesothelioma multidisciplinary team that can appropriately monitor, treat, and follow those toxicities is absolutely critical. Caring for mesothelioma patients during and after immunotherapy treatment is multifaceted and optimally can be done most successfully by an experienced mesothelioma team.

References

Calabrò L, Morra A, Fosatti F, et al. Efficacy and safety of an intensified schedule of tremelimumab for chemotherapy-resistant malignant mesothelioma. An open-label, single arm, phase 2 study. Lancet Respir Med. 2015;3:301–9.

Kindler H, Karrison T, Carol Tan YH, Rose B, Ahmad M, Straus C, Sargis R, Seiwert T. Phase II trial of pembrolizumab in patients with malignant mesothelioma: interim analysis. J Thorac Oncol. 2017;12:S293. abstract OA13.02.

Oncology Nursing Society. 2016 oncology clinical trials nurse competencies; 2016. Retrieved from https://www.ons.org/sites/default/files/OCTN_Competencies_FINAL.PDF

Thompson J. New NCCN guidelines: recognition and management of immunotherapy-related toxicity. J Natl Compr Canc Netw. 2018;16:594–6. https://doi.org/10.6004/jnccn.2018.0047.

Lisa Bengtson

1 What Is Mesothelin?

In a search for cell surface proteins that are highly expressed on cancers and not in essential tissues, mesothelin, a tumor antigen, was discovered by Ira Pastan and Mark Willingham in the 1990s at the National Cancer Institute (Pastan and Hassan 2014). The normal expression of mesothelin is limited to cells lining the pleural, peritoneum, and pericardium. Mesothelin is a glycoprotein attached to the surface of these cells. The biologic role of mesothelin in healthy cells is unclear (Hassan et al. 2016). Since the normal expression of mesothelin is limited in healthy tissues, it is an attractive target for cancer antibody-based therapy (Pastan and Hassan 2014).

Mesothelin is highly expressed in mesothelioma and pancreatic, ovarian, and lung adenocarcinomas. Expression of mesothelin is correlated with a poorer prognosis in patients with ovarian cancer, lung adenocarcinoma, triple-negative breast cancer, cholangiocarcinoma, and resectable pancreas cancer. Vaccines and antibody-based therapies are being investigated to target mesothelin due to the high expression in these malignancies (Zhao et al. 2016).

2 Treatments Targeting Mesothelin

There have been multiple clinical trials to evaluate anti-mesothelin agents for cancer therapy. Most of the work has been focused on malignant mesothelioma, pancreatic cancer, and ovarian cancer. Malignant mesothelioma is a good target for these therapies because of the high cell surface expression of mesothelin. About 10–15% of malignant mesotheliomas are sarcomatoid, and they do not have the mesothelin

L. Bengtson (✉)
National Cancer Institute, National Institutes of Health, Bethesda, MD, USA
e-mail: lisa.bengtson@nih.gov

© Springer Nature Switzerland AG 2019
M. Hesdorffer, G. E. Bates-Pappas (eds.), *Caring for Patients*
with Mesothelioma: Principles and Guidelines,
https://doi.org/10.1007/978-3-319-96244-3_7

expression targeted by these agents. Immunotoxins, monoclonal antibodies, antibody drug conjugates, vaccines, and chimeric antigen receptor T cells are agents that are being studied in the treatment of mesothelioma (Pastan and Hassan 2014).

3   Immunotoxins

An immunotoxin is an antibody linked to a toxic substance. Some immunotoxins can bind to cancer cells to kill them. SS1P, the first mesothelin-targeted agent to enter clinical trials, is a bacterial toxin. The antibody brings the bacteria to the cancer cell by targeting the mesothelin and kills the cancer. The goal of this trial was to determine the maximum tolerated dose as well as the maximum number of treatments that could be given before the patient developed antibodies to inactivate the toxin. In this first trial, only 10% of the patients could get a second dose due to antibody formation. Due to the expression of mesothelin cells lining the pleura, the dose-limiting toxicities were vascular leak syndrome and pleuritis. A trial was done with SS1P in combination with cisplatin and pemetrexed. The results of this trial showed the drugs can be given together safely with no overlapping toxicities. However, once again, about 90% of the patients developed antibodies to SS1P after one cycle. The most common toxicities from SS1P include hypoalbuminemia, fatigue, hypotension, and edema. Due to the toxicity of pleuritis and potential for pericarditis, immunotoxins are not an appropriate treatment choice for those patients who have had an extra pleural pneumonectomy or have cardiac involvement of their disease. Because the development of antibodies limited the clinical efficacy of SS1P, strategies were developed to avoid this unsuccessfully. Recently, LMB 100, a genetically transformed immunotoxin, has been developed to target mesothelin. LMB 100 is designed to be less immunogenic than SS1P. It also has decreased toxicity. It is currently being studied in the treatment of mesothelioma and pancreatic cancer. The most commonly seen side effects with immunotoxins include vascular leak syndrome, fatigue, fever, hypoalbuminemia, shortness of breath, nausea, and muscular and joint pain. Other potential, but less common side effects include irregular heart rate, infusion-related reaction, increased creatinine, and fluid around the organs. Side effects seen with SS1P which may occur in LMB 100 include inflammation leading to chest pain, shortness of breath, low blood pressure, heart failure, and kidney toxicity. The toxicities with LMB 100 were fewer and less severe than SS1P. The potential development of antidrug antibodies limits the number of effective cycles that can be given to an individual (Zhao et al. 2016).

4   Monoclonal Antibodies

A monoclonal antibody is a protein that is made in the laboratory to bind to a substance in the body. MORAb-009 (amatuximab) is a monoclonal antibody that is being investigated in the treatment of mesothelioma. MORAB-009 binds to the protein mesothelin (https://www.cancer.gov/publications/dictionaries/cancer-terms).

This antibody was well tolerated in the initial phase 1 studies where the maximum tolerated dose was established. The dose-limiting side effects were transaminitis and serum sickness (Hassan et al. 2016). A randomized phase 2 study was done in pancreatic cancer in combination with gemcitabine vs gemcitabine alone. This study was not able to show an advantage with this combined therapy. A non-randomized clinical trial of amatuximab in combination with cisplatin and pemetrexed was done in patients with advanced unresectable pleural mesothelioma. There were no overlapping side effects in this combination. This study showed improvement of overall survival but was not able to show improvement of progression free survival as compared to historical data. This data advocates further study of this combination compared to cisplatin and pemetrexed in patients with advanced pleural mesothelioma (Hassan et al. 2016). The most common side effect from amatuximab is a hypersensitivity reaction. This is demonstrated by fevers, chills, flushing, shortness of breath, hypotension, and pruritis. Other common toxicities for amatuximab are shortness of breath, nausea, vomiting, non-cardiac chest pain, weakness, cough, peripheral neuropathy, and loss of appetite.

5 Antibody Drug Conjugates

An antibody drug conjugate is a substance made up of a monoclonal antibody that is linked to a drug. The antibody binds to proteins or receptors that are found on different cells. The drug then enters those cells and can kill them without harming other cells (https://www.cancer.gov/publications/dictionaries/cancer-terms). Bay94–9343 (anetumab ravtansine) is an antidrug conjugate that is currently undergoing evaluation in patients. Anetumab ravtansine is a human anti-mesothelin antibody conjugated to maytansinoid DM4, which has potential neoplastic activity. The initial study that administered the drug every 3 weeks determined the maximum tolerated dose. The dose-limiting toxicities were keratitis and peripheral neuropathy. These toxicities were reversible and not life-threatening. Approximately half of all the patients studied required a dose reduction. A study was done administering the one-third of the dose weekly. The dose-limiting toxicities were hyperglycemia, hypophosphatemia, and ileus. All trials that followed have administered the dose every 3 weeks (Hassan et al. 2016). A recent study showed that it did not improve survival free progression as compared to vinorelbine (Navelbine). It is currently being studied in combination with cisplatin and pemetrexed as well as a trial evaluating anetumab ravtansine as a treatment for six types of solid tumors and another as a treatment for patients with recurrent platinum-resistant ovarian cancer (Hassan et al. 2016). The most common side effects of anetumab ravtansine include fatigue, nausea, diarrhea, decreased appetite, vomiting, elevated liver function tests, peripheral neuropathy, thrombocytopenia, and infusion-related reaction. Corneal disorders are commonly seen with this drug. This includes changes in the development of corneal microcysts which can be exhibited by dry eye, blurry vision, redness, pain, sensitivity to light, and increased production of tears. These symptoms are treated symptomatically with lubricating drops and steroid drops. In the recent studies, these symptoms required a dose reduction and were resolved. Other potential toxicities that are less common include weight loss, neutropenia, anemia, hyponatremia, increased amylase and lipase, and non-cardiac chest pain (Zhao et al. 2016).

6   Chimeric Antigen Receptor T Cells

Chimeric antigen receptor T cell therapy is treatment where a patient's T cells (a type of immune system cell) are changed in the laboratory to bond to mesothelin. Large numbers of the CAR-T cells are grown in the laboratory and given to the patient by infusion. This is currently under investigation as well as the potential of intrapleural infusions (Hassan et al. 2016). Cytokine release syndrome is a serious side effect that is associated with CAR-T cell therapy. Cytokine release syndrome is a sign that there is a response to therapy because it is the result of T cell activation. This is demonstrated by high fevers, hypotension, and hypoxia. Delirium, confusion, and seizures have also been experienced while the patient is undergoing treatment. These symptoms are reversible and usually seen within the first week. CAR-T cell therapy can also cause B cell aplasia. By targeting the antigens on the surface of B cells it can kill healthy B cells as well as the cancerous cells. This results in risk for infection and may require intravenous immunoglobulin to prevent infection. Another known side effect of CAR-T cell therapy is tumor lysis syndrome. Tumor lysis syndrome is a group of metabolic abnormalities that occur when a large amount of tumor cells are killed off and released into the bloodstream. This can include hyperuricemia, hyperkalemia, hyperphosphatemia, and hypocalcemia (https://www.lls.org/treatment/types-of-treatment/immunotherapy/chimeric-antigen-receptor-car-t-cell-therapy).

7   Vaccines

A vaccine is a substance or group of substances that cause the immune system to respond to a tumor. A vaccine can help the body to recognize and destroy cancer cells (https://www.cancer.gov/publications/dictionaries/cancer-terms).

The first anti-mesothelin vaccine was discovered in the laboratory of Elizabeth Jaffee at Johns Hopkins. In collaboration with Aduro Biotech, they developed a *Listeria monocytogenes* vaccine (LM-mesothelin) that expressed mesothelin. In their studies, they determined that this LM-mesothelin was a priming vaccine in the treatment of pancreatic cancer. This led to studies in other diseases (Hassan et al. 2016).

CRS 207 was developed as a genetically altered live-attenuated double-deleted *Listeria monocytogenes* engineered to stimulate an immune response to mesothelin. CRS 207 was studied in chemotherapy-naïve patients who were not eligible for surgical resection in combination with cisplatin and pemetrexed. Patients received two doses of CRS 207 two weeks apart followed by four to six cycles of cisplatin and pemetrexed. Those patients that had stable disease or achieved a response received two doses of CRS 207 three weeks apart as maintenance. *Listeria* infections, known as listeriosis, can cause diarrhea, abdominal pain, infection in the brain, blood infections, late-term miscarriages, and other infections. CRS 207 is not likely to cause these side effects when administered properly because it has been altered in the laboratory (Hassan et al. 2016). The most commonly seen toxicities include fever, chills, rigors, nausea, fatigue, hypotension, and decreased lymphocytes. These effects usually start during the treatment or two-four hours after the infusion and usually resolve within two days. Other side effects that have been seen include shortness of breath, hypoxia, throat tightness, tachycardia, flu-like symptoms, and pain. Decreases in phosphate levels and increased liver enzymes were also seen. These changes were temporary and resolved without medical intervention. Current studies are evaluating the safety and efficacy of CRS 207 in combination with pembrolizumab in mesothelioma, metastatic and recurrent gastric, gastroesophageal and esophageal cancers.

8   Future

There has been a lot of progress in the development of mesothelin-targeted therapies. This could impact the treatment of patients with solid tumors as well as mesothelioma because mesothelin is highly expressed in many cancers. There are ongoing clinical trials in mesothelioma, metastatic pancreas cancer, and lung adenocarcinoma as well as future trials in gastric cancer, endometrial cancer, cholangiocarcinoma, and triple-negative breast cancer. The toxicities of these drugs may not overlap with chemotherapy and immunotherapy agents. The use of mesothelin-targeted therapies in combination therapies is currently being explored (Hassan et al. 2016).

References

Hassan R, Thomas A, Alewine C, Le DT, Jaffee E, Pastan I. Mesothelin immunotherapy for cancer: ready for prime time? J Clin Oncol. 2016;34(34):4171–9.
https://www.cancer.gov/publications/dictionaries/cancer-terms
https://www.lls.org/treatment/types-of-treatment/immunotherapy/chimeric-antigen-receptor-car-t-cell-therapy
Pastan I, Hassan H. Discovery of mesothelin and exploiting it as a target for immunotherapy. Cancer Res. 2014;74:2907–12.
Zhao X, Subramanyam B, Sarapa N, Golflier S, Dinter H. Novel antibody therapeutics targeting mesothelin in solid tumors. Clin Cancer Drugs. 2016;3(2):76–86.

Care of the Mesothelioma Patient Undergoing Extended Pleurectomy and Decortication

Melissa Culligan and Joseph S. Friedberg

1   Introduction

Malignant pleural mesothelioma (MPM) is currently an incurable cancer, and the role surgery plays in treating it remains an area of intense debate and clinical investigation (McCambridge et al. 2018). The majority of the ongoing clinical investigations focus on combining surgery with an intraoperative adjuvant therapy along with multimodality treatments, either before or after surgery (McCambridge et al. 2018). In appropriately selected patients, these surgery-based multimodality treatment investigations currently represent the best chance of surviving much more than a year with this disease. Surgery alone, even with the most aggressive macroscopic complete resection (MCR) employed, is most assuredly going to fail locally in the absence of additional treatment modalities. The pre- and postoperative treatments that have been combined with surgery for these patients include chemotherapy, immunotherapy, proton therapy, and radiation therapy. The intraoperative adjuvants that are being investigated include hyperthermic chemotherapy lavage, heated povidone-iodine lavage, and photodynamic therapy. To date, no single surgery-based treatment plan has emerged as the standard of care for this disease (Pleurectomy/Decortication 2015; Ambrogi et al. 2018; Friedberg et al. 2017).

Surgical procedures for MPM are aimed at either establishing a diagnosis and symptom palliation or achieving an MCR with curative intent. The two accepted surgical techniques aimed at achieving an MCR with curative intent are extrapleural pneumonectomy (EPP) and extended pleurectomy decortication (EPD). The decision regarding which surgical approach is used depends upon several factors including a patient's clinical presentation, surgeon preference, and institutional preference.

M. Culligan (✉) · J. S. Friedberg (✉)
Division of Thoracic Surgery, University of Maryland School of Medicine, Baltimore, MD, USA
e-mail: MCulligan@som.umaryland.edu; jfriedberg@som.umaryland.edu

© Springer Nature Switzerland AG 2019
M. Hesdorffer, G. E. Bates-Pappas (eds.), *Caring for Patients with Mesothelioma: Principles and Guidelines*, https://doi.org/10.1007/978-3-319-96244-3_8

EPD is generally associated with a lower 30-day mortality than EPP, 1.7% vs 4.5%, respectively, with no statistically significant difference in 2-year survival, 24% vs 25%, respectively. For these reasons, there has been a global trend toward EPD as the preferred procedure whenever possible (Flores 2009). There are inherent challenges associated with the preoperative and postoperative care of patients undergoing lung-sparing surgery, beyond those commonly experienced in the general thoracic surgery patient population. These challenges will be the focus of this chapter (Papaspyros 2014; Murphy and Gill 2017; Williams et al. 2015).

2   Preoperative Preparation

Effectively and holistically preparing patients for general thoracic surgery procedures, now termed pre-habilitation, has become an international trend that is having a positive impact on patient outcomes, decreasing postoperative complications, and improving patient experiences and quality of life after surgery (Sharkey et al. 2017). Pre-habilitation focuses on adequate nutrition, establishing or maintaining a formal exercise/walking program, symptom management, and psychological support (Fiore et al. 2016; Jones et al. 2007). This preparation is aimed at improving a patient's physical, nutritional, and mental well-being prior to surgery in the hopes that they will not only be fit to tolerate the surgical procedure itself but also the postoperative recovery and potential complications, which can be physically and mentally challenging for this patient population. Preparing mesothelioma patients for lung-sparing surgery follows all of the same principles as the general thoracic surgery patients, but mesothelioma patients often have disease-specific problems that can create preoperative challenges and require proactive attention in the days leading up to surgery. These disease-specific problems can include one or more of the following: chest wall pain, pleural effusion, weight loss, decreased appetite, anxiety, depression, decreased strength, and stamina. In addition to supporting patients through the extensive preoperative work-up, thoracic surgery teams also need to focus their attention on reversing the negative impact the mesothelioma is having on a patient's well-being.

3   The Day of Surgery

Some centers admit patients the day before surgery for IV hydration and bowel preparation, but this practice is becoming more and more difficult to implement due to the constraints imposed by insurance companies. The day of surgery is an incredibly stressful day for a patient's family and friends, but most often patients describe the feelings they have as something along the lines of an "outer body experience." Patients have anticipated the day of surgery for what seems to them to be an eternity, and when the day finally arrives, it does not seem real to them. As final preparations are made for surgery, it is important not to lose sight of the mental anguish a patient undoubtedly is experiencing while the surgical team routinely prepares for surgery.

The surgical team should remain calm and positive with all of their patient/family interactions to help promote the same feelings in the patient and their family/friends. It is important to keep in mind that the patient is most likely experiencing the most difficult time in their life and likely about to have their first major surgical procedure.

4   Postoperative Care

4.1   Postoperative Day 0–2

The conduct of the operation and techniques used by the surgeon and anesthesia team are subjects for a different discussion and will not be included in this chapter. At the conclusion of the operation, much of what happens over the next 24–48 hours is based upon the routines and preferences of the surgeon, the length of the surgical procedure, and the hemodynamic stability of the patient during the procedure. The time needed to complete a lung-sparing surgery and successfully achieve a macroscopic complete resection for MPM can range anywhere from 6 to 14 hours. Technically challenging cases tend to take longer, resulting in an increased vulnerability to experiencing intraoperative patient management issues and requiring longer anesthesia time. Intraoperatively, patients can experience significant blood loss requiring blood transfusions, fluid shifts, hemodynamic instability, hypoxia, and cardiac arrhythmias. Other intraoperative issues may arise that are more expected based on the intraoperative adjuvant used at the time of surgery (photodynamic therapy, heated chemotherapy, heat povidone-iodine lavage, fibrinogen spray). The primary focus points of care during the immediate postoperative period will continue, in varying degrees of intensity, throughout the entire hospital stay and include chest tube management, respiratory support/secretion management, pain management, nutrition, fluid management, cardiac monitoring, deep vein thrombosis prevention, mobility, and psychological support (Bolukbas et al. 2012).

Chest Tube Placement and Management Chest tubes are placed at the conclusion of the procedure after careful inspection of the entire hemithorax to confirm hemostasis. Chest tubes serve as surgical drains to evacuate air and fluid from the pleural space as well as to enhance lung expansion after surgery. The number of chest tubes placed is based on a surgeon's preference and experience, but generally two tubes are inserted, one posteriorly and one anteriorly, to meet in the apex. A third flexible silicone drain, like a Blake drain, is placed along the diaphragm extending from the anterior sulcus to the most distal recess of the posterior sulcus. It is preferable to use monofilament sutures to secure the apical chest tubes because these sutures are less reactive and can be left in place in the unfortunate event that one of the tubes needs to remain in place and be converted to a Heimlich valve for management of a prolonged air leak. Each chest tube is place to a separate drainage container to ensure accurate assessment of individual chest tube drainage and air leak status. Patients remain on IV antibiotics until the chest tubes are removed. The rationale for this practice is these patients are at an increased risk of developing empyemas due to the extensive air leaks immediately postoperatively and the risk of prolonged air leaks requiring intervention vs Heimlich valve placement (Friedberg 2013).

In an effort to minimize the air leaks, ventilator management is focused son limiting peak inspiratory pressures, and the suction on the chest tubes is maintained at -10 cm of water pressure until the patient is extubated (Friedberg 2013). This limited amount of chest tube suction supports effective evacuation of fluid and air while limiting the pressure gradient across the lung surface, which minimizes potentiation of the air leaks. Water seal can be tried, but it often results in air accumulation in the chest, and/or subcutaneous emphysema develops. Once a patient is extubated, chest tube suction can be increased if needed to support lung expansion and fluid evacuation (Friedberg 2013).

Extubation Versus Mechanical Ventilation The decision to extubate in the operating room depends on the length of the case, the stability of the patient throughout the operation, and the expansion of the lung at the conclusion of the MCR. If the lung fills the chest cavity and the patient is otherwise stable, the patient is extubated. Vigilant attention to a patient's ability to take deep breaths, cough, and actively participate in airway clearance is critical after patients are extubated. The surgical team should have a low threshold to perform frequent bronchoscopies to help support the patient through this early stage in their recovery (Friedberg 2013).

If the surgeon feels the patient would benefit from positive pressure ventilation to achieve better lung expansion or there are any safety concerns, then the patient is reintubated with a single lumen tube, a bronchoscopy is performed, and the patient is transported to the ICU on a pressure mode ventilator. Effectively ventilating a patient following an EPD is the first major challenge the surgical team faces after the patient leaves the operating room. Parenchymal air leaks following visceral pleurectomy can be significant, and attempting to maintain a patient on a fixed tidal volume can result in hypoventilation. The opposite is true for pressure-cycled ventilation. The lungs essentially function like fish gills after visceral pleurectomy because a significant amount of air can pass through the lungs and out of the chest tubes causing a hyperventilation and hypocarbia situation. Ventilator settings and calculations are confounded by the large air leaks resulting in inaccurate assessment of tidal volumes and minute ventilation. The most effective approach is to keep in mind the impact the air leaks are having and carefully follow arterial blood gases and make ventilator setting adjustments accordingly (Friedberg 2013).

Pain Management Effectively managing postoperative thoracotomy pain is a critical element in caring for this patient population. Without effective and proactive pain control, a cascade of predictable adverse events will ensue that can ultimately lead to a patient not leaving the hospital. A thoracic epidural is placed before the operation begins and is left in place for up to 10 days after surgery. Some patients will experience hypotension related to the sympathetic effect of the epidural during the initial postoperative period. These patients will sometimes be managed with intravenous blood pressure support in an effort to maintain both hemodynamic stability and effective pain control (Yegin et al. 2003).

Fluid Management Fluid management in the early phase of recovery is directly related to the intraoperative blood loss and replacement and the amount of other fluids received during the operation. Vasopressors, blood products, and fluid boluses may be needed to maintain the mean arterial blood pressure ≥65 mmHg and the urine output ≥30 ml/hr. Specific fluid management strategies will also be based upon the intraoperative adjuvant used and the expected effects that particular adjuvant treatment may have on fluid volume status, hemodynamic stability, and organ function/risk. For example, if intraoperative heated chemotherapy is used, there is a risk of acute renal failure, and therefore a fluid management protocol is initiated for renal protection. In the case of intraoperative photodynamic therapy, the chest cavity is essentially healing from burn, and these patients will require larger volumes of intravenous fluids, both colloids and crystalloids (Friedberg 2013).

Cardiac Arrhythmias General thoracic surgery patients are at risk for developing postoperative cardiac arrhythmias, atrial fibrillation in particular. Radical pleurectomy patients are at an even greater risk of this happening when the pericardium has been resected or manipulated in some way as part of achieving a macroscopic complete resection. In addition to careful fluid management, electrolytes are carefully monitored and replaced as needed in an effort to avoid the exacerbation of cardiac irritability (Fernado et al. 2011).

Nutrition Nutritional support is very important to this patient population at this stage in their treatment as their body works to heal multiple parenchymal air leaks and recover from a physically stressful surgery. Specific nutritional recommendations are covered in a separate chapter. For the purpose of this discussion, the specific care is related to nutrition; patients are maintained NPO (nothing by mouth) with a nasogastric tube in place. Total parenteral nutrition is started in the evening on the day of surgery.

Deep Vein Thrombosis (DVT) Prophylaxis The risk of developing a DVT increases after major surgery and in patients with cancer. Pneumatic compression stockings are placed on a patient's lower extremities intraoperatively and remain in place, unless a patient is walking, until the day they are discharged from the hospital. It is important to stress this with the patient and family members so they do not resist using them during their hospital stay and can remind the surgery team to put them back on after walking. When it is deemed safe from a postoperative bleeding perspective, subcutaneous heparin (or another anticoagulant as per institutional preference) is started and continued until discharge.

4.2   Postoperative Day 3: Discharge to Home

Oxygenation/Secretion Management/Airway Clearance As previously stated, vigilant attention to a patient's ability to participate in airway clearance is critical after patients are extubated throughout their entire hospital stay. Once extubated, most patients require supplemental oxygen via nasal cannula. Multiple clinical factors will impair or enhance a patient's ability to oxygenate effectively and mobilize their secretions including pain control, fluid balance, and mobility. As a result of the tumor debulking along the diaphragm and the skeletonization of the phrenic nerve, these patients will have impaired breathing mechanics within their operative hemithorax. The diaphragm is structurally compromised postoperatively, and all patients will have an elevated hemidiaphragm, to some varying degree, visible on their chest x-ray.

Despite even the highest level of motivation on their part, patients often struggle at some point in their recovery. Aggressive secretion management must be employed from the very beginning and continued until a patient is discharged. These maneuvers include chest physiotherapy (manual and the electrically powered VEST), frequent ambulation, incentive spirometry, nasotracheal suctioning, and bronchoscopy. The surgical team should have a very low threshold to perform bedside bronchoscopy, early and often, to avoid patients developing pneumonia or space problems related to poor expansion of their operative lung. Patients should have daily chest x-rays to assess for early radiographic signs of pneumonia. Meticulous intake and output should be recorded in an effort to avoid volume overload that could contribute to pulmonary compromise (Post-operative Care to Promote Recovery for Thoracic Surgical Patients 2016; Gronell et al. 2018).

Chest Tube Management Managing chest tubes after EPD is a challenge due to the inherent air leaks and the re-expansion process of a lung that has been encased with tumor and/or compressed with large volume pleural effusion. Chest tube output should be assessed at least every 4 hours and more frequently if there is a specific concern. The integrity of the chest tube should be assessed every 4 hours to ensure that the chest tube has respiratory variation and that it is a functional tube. Stripping the chest tubes each time chest tube output is measured and recorded is a good practice to adopt. In addition to the volume, the consistency of the chest tube output should be assessed and noted: frank blood, serosanguinous, cloudy, clear yellow, or milky. If a patient has a large volume of chest tube output and it appears cloudy/milky, the surgical team should consider the presence of a chyle leak and send the chest tube fluid for analysis (Post-operative Care to Promote Recovery for Thoracic Surgical Patients 2016; Gronell et al. 2018).

Generally the chest tubes stay on suction for 2–3 days after surgery, and at that point, water seal is attempted. If the lung appears to remain expanded, the leaks tend to decrease fairly quickly, and the tubes can be removed as per the surgeon's routine. The management problem arises when the air leaks persist and the lung does not remain expanded. There are multiple options to consider when faced with a persistent air leak, and they include chemical pleurodesis, blood patch, or insertion of an endobronchial valve designed to stop air leaks. Blood patching uses ~60 ml of autologous blood with a drop of povidone-iodine. This sterile mixture is inserted into the chest tube, and this can be done as many times as needed. If the patient is ready for discharge and the air leak persists despite these interventions, a Heimlich valve can be placed on the end of the chest tube, and the patient can go home. Plans are made to have the patient come back to have the tube removed in the office once the air leak has stopped (Friedberg 2013).

Fluid Management Patients generally experience fluid shifts after surgery, and their volume status needs careful attention. During the early postoperative period, patients tend to need increased volume via intravenous fluids, but at a midpoint in their hospital course, this reverses, and patients require IV or oral diuretics to decrease their lower extremity edema and pulmonary congestion seen on chest x-ray. Each patient is slightly different in his or her ability to manage and/or tolerate these fluid shifts, and it is the surgical team's job to keep a close eye on the patient and be proactive in their fluid management (Post-operative Care to Promote Recovery for Thoracic Surgical Patients 2016; Gronell et al. 2018).

Pain Management The importance of meticulous pain management cannot be stressed often enough. Without it, patients will not be able to adequately and effectively clear their secretions, and they will not be able to walk. The cascade of adverse events that can result from poor pain control after a thoracotomy will predictably result in prolonged hospital stays and the development of multiple avoidable complications, some of which can be fatal. Beyond the use of a thoracic epidural, surgical teams need to consider adjuvant pain control strategies, some of which include patient-controlled analgesia (intravenous narcotics), Lidoderm patches, acetaminophen, oral narcotics, nerve blocks, and cryoanalgesia. Working closely with the acute pain service team to achieve and maintain adequate pain control is a critical element in caring for these patients (Yegin et al. 2003).

After the chest tubes are removed, the focus of pain control becomes determining the combination of medications that the patient will be taking when he or she is discharge to home. Patient education is critical at this point in an effort to make it clear to the patient that pain management at home is just as important as it was in the hospital and that they need to stay in close contact with their surgical team if they are experiencing any problems related to pain once they get home.

Mobility The importance of frequent ambulation is stressed with patients preoperatively as they prepare for surgery, as they recover from surgery in the hospital, and when they go home from the hospital and continue their recuperation. Walking after surgery can be overwhelming to a patient because of all of the lines and connections they have early on in their recovery (chest tubes, epidural, IV fluid, oxygen, cardiac monitors, Foley catheter). For this reason, a "thoracic walker" has been designed and is used by many high volume centers to support and encourage patients to walk after thoracic surgery. These walkers are equipped to hold the chest tube canister, oxygen tank, IV/epidural pumps, cardiac and oxygen saturation monitors, and the Foley catheter bag. It is a rolling walker with handles and arm rests which allows a patient to walk in an erect position and propel the walker forward independently. Patients should walk everyday while they are in the hospital. The frequency and distance will vary for each patient, but plan A is for patients to walk three to four times a day and gradually increase their distance each day (Post-operative Care to Promote Recovery for Thoracic Surgical Patients 2016; Gronell et al. 2018).

Nutrition/Gastric Motility Reestablishing gastric motility after surgery and introducing food and drink to patients who have had a long surgical procedure and are taking narcotics for pain control require careful attention and consideration. As previously stated, these patients are working to heal multiple parenchymal air leaks and regain their strength and stamina; therefore they should be receiving nutritional support immediately postoperatively in the form of total parenteral nutrition (TPN). This practice ensures that while the patient's intestines are waking up, which can vary in the length of time it takes from person to person, there is no delay in providing critical nutrition to support the healing process.

Patients remain NPO until their ability to safely and effectively swallow has been formally evaluated by either a bedside swallow test or a formal swallowing study. Generally, the NGT is removed on postoperative day 1 or 2, after confirming bowel sounds, to allow for a more effective cough. It is critical that a patient does not vomit in the early stages of recovery as their diaphragm is at risk for rupturing related to the extent of diaphragmatic resection done at the time of surgery. Once a patient has been cleared to start taking food and drink by mouth, this process is started with clear liquids, advancing slowly as tolerated. Patients cannot drink or eat while lying in bed. They must be sitting upright and have both feet on the floor. They should not drink large volumes of liquids at one time to avoid gastric bloating. They should never drink through straws or have carbonated beverages to avoid gastric bloating. Caffeine (coffee, tea, chocolate) is restricted until a patient is discharged to home in an effort to avoid developing cardiac arrhythmias (Cardinale et al. 2010). Once a patient is discharged to home, they are instructed to eat frequent, small meals until they have regained their appetite, which can take several weeks to months.

Patients will be started on a bowel regimen as soon as they are able to swallow. The exact regimen will vary at each institution, but the important care point to keep in mind is that narcotics are very constipating, and we need to avoid the complications associated with severe constipation. It is important to make sure a patient is moving his or her bowels at least every 2–3 days while in the hospital and instructed to continue that focus once they are discharged to home.

Psychological Support The anticipatory stress experienced by patients prior to any surgery, let alone a surgery of the magnitude of extended pleurectomy decortication, is difficult to describe unless you have experienced it yourself. People handle this stress in different ways, and it is important for the surgical team to keep this in mind when caring for these patients and their families. It is also critical to keep in mind that mesothelioma patients are most likely going to have additional treatment after they recover from surgery and are facing a deadly disease. Oftentimes patients have been connected, by phone or in person, with other patients who have gone through a similar surgical treatment, which helps them prepare for what to expect before, during, and after surgery. The information and support fellow mesothelioma patients receive from each other is invaluable, and surgical teams should keep this in mind and seek to establish this patient network at their institution.

Sleep is a difficult problem to manage after surgery both while in the hospital and after patients are discharged to home. Providing short periods of uninterrupted quiet time when patients can rest and try to sleep is important. Making sure this happens takes commitment from the entire multidisciplinary team caring for the patient and their family. The prolonged hospital stay contributes to sleep deprivation, and this can lead to anxiety and confusion, especially for older patients. Recognizing the impact sleep deprivation can have on a patient and proactively working to minimize it as much as possible should be done starting on postoperative day 1. If a patient was taking medications to help them to sleep prior to surgery, it is important to either start that medication or a medication that is safe in combination with the pain medication regimen.

5 Conclusion

Caring for patients undergoing lung-sparing surgery for malignant pleural mesothelioma is clinically challenging. Meticulous attention to every detail of their care and anticipating the inherent problems encountered postoperatively will support a patient's successful recovery and ensure that they are discharged home safely from the hospital. If something does not seem right, it most likely isn't and should be investigated and acted upon immediately. When a patient develops a problem in one area, it often has a negative impact on other aspects of their recovery and can quickly escalate to serious if not fatal problems. It takes an experienced, highly skilled, and dedicated multidisciplinary team of experts to care for these patients and their families.

References

Ambrogi M, et al. Diaphragm and lung-preserving surgery with hyperthermic chemotherapy for malignant pleural mesothelioma: a 10-year experience. J Thorac Cardiovasc Surg. 2018;155:1857–66.

Bolukbas S, Eberlein M, Schirren J. Prospective study of functional results after lung-sparing radical pleurectomy in the malignant pleural mesothelioma. J Thorac Oncol. 2012;7(5):900–5.

Cardinale D, Martinoni A, et al. Atrial fibrillation after operation for lung cancer: clinical and prognostic significance. Ann Thorac Surg. 2010;90(2):368–74.

Fernado H, Jaklitsch M, Walsh G, et al. The Society of Thoracic Surgeons practice guideline on the prophylaxis and management of atrial fibrillation associated with general thoracic surgery: executive summary. Ann Thorac Surg. 2011;92:1144–52.

Fiore J, et al. Systematic review of the influence of enhanced recovery pathways in elective lung resection. J Thorac Cardiovasc Surg. 2016;151(3):708–16.

Flores R. Surgical options in malignant pleural mesothelioma: extrapleural pneumonectomy or pleurectomy/decortication. Semin Thorac Cardiovasc Surg. 2009;21(2):149–76.

Friedberg JS. State of the art in the technical performance of lung sparing operations for pleural mesothelioma. Sem Thorac Cardiovasc Surg. 2013;25(2, Summer):125–43.

Friedberg JS, Simone C, Culligan M, Barsky A, Doucette A, McNulty S, Hahn SM, Alley E, Sterman E, Cengel K. Extended pleurectomy/decortication-based treatment for advanced stage, large tumor volume mesothelioma yielding a median survival of 3 years. Ann Thorac Surg. 2017;103(3):912–9.

Gronell J, Holleran C, Mintz E, Wiesel O. Postoperative bedside critical care of thoracic surgery patients. Am J Crit Care. 2018;27(4):328–33.

Jones L, Peddle C, Eves N, et al. Effects of pre-surgical exercise training on cardiorespiratory fitness among patients undergoing thoracic surgery for malignant lung diseases. Cancer. 2007;110(3):590–9.

McCambridge A, et al. Progress in the management of malignant pleural mesothelioma in 2017. J Thorac Oncol. 2018;13(5):606–23.

Murphy D, Gill R. Overview of treatment related complications in malignant pleural mesothelioma. Ann Trans Med. 2017;5(11):235.

Papaspyros S. Surgical management of malignant pleural mesothelioma: impact of surgery on survival and quality of life – relation to chemotherapy, radiotherapy and alternative therapies. ISRN Surg. 2014;1–19.

Pleurectomy/Decortication. Hyperthermic pleural lavage with povidone-iodine, prophylactic radiotherapy and systemic chemotherapy in patients with malignant pleural mesothelioma: a 10-year experience. J Thorac Cardiovasc Surg. 2015;149:558–66.

Post-operative Care to Promote Recovery for Thoracic Surgical Patients. A nursing perspective. J Thorac Dis. 2016;8(Suppl 1):S71–7.

Sharkey A, Bilancia R, Tenconi S, Nakas A, Waller D. Extended pleurectomy decortication for malignant pleural mesothelioma in the elderly: the need for an inclusive yet selective approach. Interact Cardiovasc Thorac Surg. 2017;25:696–702.

Williams T, Duraid H, Watson S, Durkin A, Todd K, Kindler H, Vigneswaran W. Extended pleurectomy and decortication for malignant pleural mesothelioma is an effective and safe cytoreductive surgery in the elderly. Ann Thorac Surg. 2015;100:1868–74.

Yegin A, Erdogan A, Kayacan N, Karsli B. Early postoperative pain management after thoracic surgery: pre- and postoperative versus postoperative epidural analgesia: a randomized study. Eur J Cardiothorac Surg. 2003;24:420–4.

Part III

Supportive Health Care for Treatment

Maintaining a Nutritional Diet During and After Active Treatment

Colleen Norton

1 Causes of Weight Loss in Mesothelioma

Four main factors stick out as the prominent contributors to why patients will lose significant weight around the time of diagnosis and immediately following their diagnosis of mesothelioma. Weight loss is a common side effect that occurs with any cancer diagnosis, not just mesothelioma. Ultimately though, weight loss is inevitable and unavoidable. However, the goal should be not to lose a significant amount of weight or any additional weight throughout the treatment process. Significant loss of weight will interfere with the body's ability to recover and handle treatment and may even inhibit the receiving of treatment.

The first factor that leads to weight loss before and at the time of diagnosis is stress: stress regarding the recurrent health issues that are often misdiagnosed, stress from multiple treatments that have not provided any symptom relief or answers, stress over finally undergoing a biopsy and now having to wait for the final pathology results, stress from *finally* receiving a diagnosis and that diagnosis providing limited information as well as frightening statistics from Internet research, and stress over having to decide on a treatment plan that is the best option for you, your family, and/or your loved ones. All of this stress and worrying can cause you to become disinterested in food or completely lose your appetite. You become so worried about everything surrounding the diagnosis that you forget to eat or you make yourself sick to your stomach. The constant high level of stress on your body almost keeps it in a perpetual state of fight or flight, which in turn leads to an increase in your body's metabolism. Metabolism is your body's ability to break down food and turn it into energy. An increased metabolism means

C. Norton (✉)
The University of Maryland Medical Center, Baltimore, MD, USA

Columbia Surgical Institute, Elkridge, MD, USA
e-mail: cnorton@columbia-surgical.com

© Springer Nature Switzerland AG 2019
M. Hesdorffer, G. E. Bates-Pappas (eds.), *Caring for Patients with Mesothelioma: Principles and Guidelines*,
https://doi.org/10.1007/978-3-319-96244-3_9

your body is burning more calories than you may be taking in with food. This ends up leading to unintentional weight loss.

The second factor that contributes to weight loss before and during the time of diagnosis is what are often referred to as a pleural effusion and ascites. Pleural effusions and ascites are the common symptoms most associated with pleural mesothelioma and peritoneal mesothelioma. A pleural effusion is an abnormal collection of a fluid between the (visceral pleura, lining of the lung, and the parietal pleura, lining of the chest wall) chest wall and the lung. An obstruction, typically the cancer, causes the fluid in the chest to build up which will not only squish the lung but also pushes down on the diaphragm. When the fluid begins to push down on the diaphragm, it will also push down on the stomach. The pressure of the fluid on the stomach leaves the patient feeling fuller faster. This then leads to patients eating less food because they are not as "hungry." On the other hand, ascites is an abnormal accumulation of fluid in the abdominal cavity. Ascites presents with distension of the abdomen as well as weight gain due to the increase in fluid. The outward appearance of a patient suffering from ascites would indicate that they are gaining weight, but it is unfortunately only from the buildup of fluid in the abdominal cavity. Patients experiencing ascites will have a decreased appetite or a feeling of fullness after eating from the weight of the fluid pressing on the stomach. Once either the pleural effusion or the ascites is drained (known as a thoracentesis or paracentesis), it is common to experience weight loss. For reference, a 1-liter bottle of soda weighs a little over 2 pounds. Now imagine 3 liters of fluid has been removed from either the abdomen or the pleural space and that equals over 6 pounds of fluid drained from the body. Combine that removal of fluid with the weight lost from lack of appetite, and the amount of weight lost can now be well over 10 pounds. As you may already know, there will be multiple drainages of pleural effusions and ascites that occur over a span of several months. The total amount of weight lost over that period of time will be significantly more than 10 pounds.

The third factor that leads to weight loss before and during the time of diagnosis is that cancer, especially mesothelioma, in general is highly metabolic. This means that your body will begin to burn more calories than you may be eating on a daily basis. When a patient is not taking in more calories than their body and the cancer are burning throughout the day, this leads to the patient losing a significant amount of weight at very rapid rate. To counteract rapid weight loss from the surge in the body's increased metabolism, one needs to make sure that the amount of daily calories you or your loved one is ingesting is greater than what your body is burning. It is easy to calculate how many calories your body needs on a daily basis. For example, a 60-year-old female that is 5 foot 4, is 150 pounds, and is lightly active throughout the week should eat a minimum of 1700 calories to *maintain* their current weight. Since your body is now fighting cancer and your metabolism is in overdrive, the same female used as an example above should eat 2200–2700 calories a day to not only maintain her current weight but also prevent additional weight loss caused by the cancer (http://www.calculator.net/calorie-calculator.html).

The fourth and final factor that leads to weight loss before and during the time of diagnosis is pain. Pain is often unavoidable and an unfortunate side effect from this cancer that leads to significant weight loss in patients. Attempting to determine an adequate pain control regimen often places patients into a vicious cycle of trying to find what works in order to help keep the pain manageable all the while maintaining adequate intake of food is completely overlooked. Narcotics have a tendency to make individuals drowsy, which often leads to a nap. During the nap, the pain medication wears off, and you wake up in pain. At this point, you are now behind on your pain control and have to chase down the pain in an attempt to control or lessen the pain. The next dose of pain medication is due which of course will help with the pain, and shortly thereafter you are back to needing to take a nap due to the side effects from the narcotics. At any point during this cycle, when do you think an individual is thinking, "I need to eat"? Most often, when the pain is severe enough, the last thing on any one's mind is "I need to eat." It is during this vicious cycle of attempting to make yourself comfortable and the pain tolerable that eating food is often neglected. It is common knowledge that a narcotic should not be taken on an empty stomach, but when the pain is past a certain point, all anyone can concentrate on is getting the pain medication into the system to alleviate the pain. Another reason pain causes weight loss is that when pain reaches a certain level or severity, the thought of eating food churns the stomach. The pain is often so bad it causes a lack of appetite or even nauseated at the thought of eating food.

2   Pre-treatment Diet and Nutrition

Making a full circle back to the initial diagnosis of mesothelioma, I will now detail the importance of diet and nutrition in regard to each treatment. You are consulting for the first time with a mesothelioma specialist to discuss all the treatment options available. During this appointment, a few questions will be asked. Have you lost any weight? How is your appetite? Do you become full quickly when eating? 9 times out of 10, the answer is yes to each question. The topic of adequate diet and nutrition is then discussed at length as well as how to prevent additional weight loss and how to maintain and even gain weight. Before any treatment is to begin, the healthcare provider will stress the importance of a well-balanced diet. Your healthcare provider will address the importance of a diet high in calories that also incorporate a diet high in proteins, fats, and carbohydrates. Proper nutrition from the beginning of treatment will help your body fight infections, decrease the risk of side effects, and improve your body's recovery from each specific treatment.

One of my favorite meals that I suggest to patients that are struggling to keep up with a balanced diet is something that is easy to make and tastes great. This shake can be incorporated in every round of the treatment process.

- 1 cup whole milk (protein and fat) – Fairlife brand milk – 150 calories, *13 grams of protein, 8 grams of fat*, 6 grams of carbohydrates
- 1 scoop whey protein (protein) – Gold Standard whey protein – 121 calories, *24 grams of protein*, 1 gram of fat, 4 grams of carbohydrates

- 1 frozen banana (carbohydrate) – 116 calories, 1.3 grams of protein, *26.9 grams of carbohydrates*, 0 grams of fat
- 1 tablespoon peanut butter (fat and protein) – 99 calories, 3.4 grams of protein, 4 grams of carbohydrates, *7.8 grams of fat*
- *Optional – 1 cup frozen strawberries – 47 calories, 11.7 grams of carbohydrates
- (Patients can substitute the cup of milk and scoop of whey protein for a bottle of Ensure or Boost – nutritional value for a high-protein Boost = 180 calories, 15 grams of protein, 16 grams of carbohydrates, 7 grams of fat.)

Blend all the ingredients together and you have a nutritious and tasty milk shake that is high in calories, protein, carbohydrates, and healthy fats. This shakes' final nutritional value is 486 calories, 41.7 grams of protein, 40.8 grams of carbohydrates, and 17.2 grams of fat. I encourage the addition or substitution of anything that you or your family member may want instead blended into the shake.

Below you will find foods that are high in proteins, good fats, and good carbohydrates to incorporate into your daily diet.

Proteins
Eggs
Greek yogurt
Nuts – almonds, pistachios, cashews, peanuts
Peanut butter
Quinoa
Cottage cheese
Meat – chicken, lean beef, tuna, turkey, and fish (salmon, shrimp, tilapia)
Milk – full fat
Whey protein supplement
Avocado
Hummus
Oats
Quinoa
Lentils – soybeans, chickpeas, kidney beans
Fats
Butter
Whole eggs
Nuts and nut butters
Avocados
Dark chocolate
Cheese
Bacon
Full-fat milk
Full-fat yogurt
Carbohydrates
Fruit – bananas, apples, cantaloupe, grapefruit, blueberries
Sweet potatoes, yams

Vegetables – broccoli, asparagus, spinach
Oatmeal – old fashioned and steel cut
100% whole wheat bread and pasta
Couscous
Pumpkin, butternut squash
Brown rice
Beans and lentils

3   Diet and Nutrition Both Preoperative and Postoperative

Revitalizing your diet after losing weight surrounding the months prior to the diagnosis of mesothelioma will be almost like a full-time job. Nevertheless, to ensure safe surgical candidacy, the surgical team will encourage patients to increase their daily nutritional intake in an attempt to maintain the current weight and even potentially gain weight. A well-balanced diet that is nutrient rich and high in protein before surgery is essential because after surgery, that same nutrient-rich and high-protein diet will be instrumental in facilitating the healing process. Bear in mind the time before surgery is not the time to begin restricting foods from the diet.

Immediately after surgery both pleural and peritoneal patients will be placed on a Nothing by Mouth (NPO) diet for a minimum of 2 days. This is due to the cancer potentially being adhered to specific structures and the process of removing the tumor leaves that organ (e.g., the esophagus, stomach, or small bowel) at a weekend state. Surgeons will not allow the intake of anything by mouth immediately postoperatively in hopes to decrease the risk of further injury to those organs. The reason being that early intake of fluid may cause the patient to become nauseous and vomit which could lead to further insult to the organs that are attempting to heal and cause additional damage. During the first few days of not being able to take anything in by mouth, surgical patients will be started on Total Parenteral Nutrition (TPN) through a central line (a large IV) to provide the patients with their daily nutritional requirements. After a few days of IV TPN, the patient will slowly transition to an oral diet of clear liquids (broth, Jell-O, and water). As soon as they can tolerate the clear liquid diet, they will be transitioned to a full liquid diet and then finally back to a regular diet. At the time the liquid diet is started, most patients have gone days without eating or drinking anything. Patients complain that they are extremely hungry, but when they can finally eat and drink, the meal provided is barely touched. Combine restarting the diet with the barrage of medications ordered by the medical staff and it becomes too difficult to stomach much more than a few bites of food or sips of fluid in the beginning. Subsequently patients also notice a change in their sense of taste after undergoing surgery. The change in taste is typically due to the effects of the anesthesia. The taste buds will return back to normal but that is typically about the time chemotherapy will begin.

After patients are discharged home from the hospital, it is not uncommon that patients now need to recover from their hospitalization admission. There is a lot of catching up on sleep and adjusting to the new normal as well as returning to regular activities of daily living. It is at this time between discharge and the postoperative appointment that patients need to also focus on their nutrition. Countless times patients return to their postoperative appointment and have continued to lose weight. Continuing to lose weight after surgery will interfere with the healing process. The postoperative appointment now includes a lengthy discussion on what to eat and how often to eat. Your surgical team will stress the importance of eating a diet high in calories and proteins to help aid in the tissue healing as well as your general recovery from undergoing surgical intervention. Your overall nutrition during the surgical route will decrease the chance of developing an infection as well as leading to a quicker recovery and healing process.

4   Diet and Nutrition Pre, During, and Post Chemotherapy Treatment

Sustaining an adequate diet for proper nutrition throughout the chemotherapy process may be a little more difficult to maintain due to new side effects that arise. Patients receiving chemotherapy typically complain of nausea, vomiting, mouth sores, and changes to their taste buds. The perception of food while receiving chemotherapy treatment will change drastically during this phase of treatment. These new symptoms will begin to affect the daily nutritional intake because foods will begin to taste off as well as smell unappetizing and often lead to nausea. When food becomes too difficult to swallow, loses its taste, or smells unpleasant, it makes it hard for patients to WANT to eat while receiving chemotherapy. The medical oncologist and medical oncology team will suggest several things to help keep the nutrition on track to include:

- Prescription of an appetite stimulant
- Prescription of an antiemetic (anti-nausea medication)
- Keep a diary of the foods that the patient enjoys eating that hasn't lost its flavor during treatment
- Determine foods that have a pungent smell that causes the patient increased nausea and avoid during treatment
- Determine the foods and snacks that the patient craves and keep in stock
- Have plenty of high-calorie snacks in stock (cheese, peanut butter, nuts)
- Drink plenty of fluids to stay hydrated
- Prepare meals in advance so they can be stored in the freezer for a quick and easy meal
- Eat smaller more frequent meals
- Liquid meal replacement (milkshakes, Boost, soup)
- Consult with a registered dietician or nutritionist

The great thing about the medical oncology team is that they are aware of the increased nausea that causes a decreased appetite and weight loss that occurs during chemotherapy. Patients receiving chemotherapy are placed on an anti-nausea medication in advance as an effort to control the nausea, and the oncology team will involve multiple specialties to help maintain proper nutrition throughout treatment.

5 Diet and Nutrition During Radiation Therapy

Maintaining proper nutrition during radiation therapy may not be as problematic for some patients. Common complaints from patients receiving radiation are nausea and difficulty controlling pain. The radiation oncology team will work with you to help make sure pain and nausea are controlled during the treatment process. Before treatment begins, as well as during treatment, the radiation oncology team will stress consuming enough calories and not necessarily worrying about where the calories are coming from especially if a patient is having a hard time eating. They will also encourage the significance of patients eating an adequate amount of protein to help facilitate tissue healing. Most importantly, patients should remember not to stress through the process of receiving radiation therapy.

6 Maintaining Diet and Nutrition Posttreatments

Once all treatments have concluded, returning to a normal routine can often be daunting. Yet you are not alone in your journey. Your team of specialists and healthcare providers are still available to answer questions and calm your fears. There is no doubt that the whole process of diagnosis, treatment, and recovery has taught you more than you ever thought possible. This includes how to maintain a well-balanced diet provided here in this chapter as well as by multiple healthcare professionals. You have all the tools to continue the proper diet and nutrition throughout the maintenance phase of your disease. Your new diet and nutrition has been followed for months during countless treatments, so it should be easy to continue for the foreseeable future.

Lastly, weight loss is inevitable at some point in the treatment and recovery process. However, proper diet and nutrition throughout every aspect of treatment will aide in overall recovery. It does not matter if you prefer to eat 3–4 meals a day or 5–6 meals a day as long as your body is getting the essential daily calories to prevent additional weight loss. In the end, how many meals you eat to contain the amount of calories needed to prevent weight loss is completely up to you. Only you know how your body functions, and only you will know what will ultimately work for you. Always remember that the better your overall diet and nutrition at the start of treatment, the better your body will handle each treatment.

References

http://www.calculator.net/calorie-calculator.html

10

Richard D. Hemingway

Dedication

In memory of my father, Ron Hemingway, loving husband of Yvonne Hemingway, proud President of USW Local 900, who fought until the end and will always motivate me to support mesothelioma research and those who remain afflicted with this disease. In honor of my mother, Yvonne Hemingway, who by her selfless example, demonstrated grace and honor in supporting and caring for my father in his darkest days.

1 Who Are Physical Therapists?

Physical therapists (PTs) require a high level of education including a graduate degree (either a master's degree or clinical doctorate) and are state-licensed medical professionals. Physical therapists are movement scientists and experts in evaluating and identifying functional limitations and deficits including in gait, proprioception, balance, endurance, posture, cardiovascular and ventilatory systems, respiration, ROM, musculoskeletal deficits, fall risk, sensation, and strength. Physical therapists work across the spectrum promoting health and wellness, prevention, preoperative and post-op treatment, and rehabilitation as well as in palliative care (Kumar and Jim 2010; https://www.apta.org/AboutPTs). PTs help patients reduce pain and restore, improve, or maintain functional mobility often with reduced need for invasive surgery or need for long-term use of prescription medications (including opioids) and their many side effects (https://www.apta.org/AboutPTs). PTs teach patients how to effectively manage or prevent the

R.D. Hemingway (✉)
Brockton Visiting Nurse Association, Brockton, MA, USA

© Springer Nature Switzerland AG 2019
M. Hesdorffer, G. E. Bates-Pappas (eds.), *Caring for Patients with Mesothelioma: Principles and Guidelines*,
https://doi.org/10.1007/978-3-319-96244-3_10

recurrence of their condition to improve their long-term health and symptom burden. Physical therapists can be found throughout the healthcare continuum including hospitals, schools, outpatient facilities, sports teams (including college, amateur, and professional), home care, occupational health clinics, and skilled nursing facilities and in palliative care.

PTs employ evidence-based therapeutic exercise prescription, balance and proprioception training, functional retraining, gait training, skin integrity evaluation, fall risk reduction/prevention, inspiratory muscle training, postural retraining, and chest PT. They also prescribe durable medical equipment (DME) including walkers, canes, AFOs, wheelchairs and pressure-relieving seating recommendations, thermal or electrotherapeutic modalities (within accepted contraindications especially with the oncology and MM population), as well as appropriate manual therapy including, but not limited to, soft tissue mobilization (STM), joint mobilization, deep friction massage (DFM), myofascial release (MFR), and scar mobilization (Fig. 10.1). They may also choose to specialize in pediatrics, orthopedics, sports medicine, geriatrics, cardiopulmonary, neurology, hand therapy, oncology, women's health, or even lymphedema management.

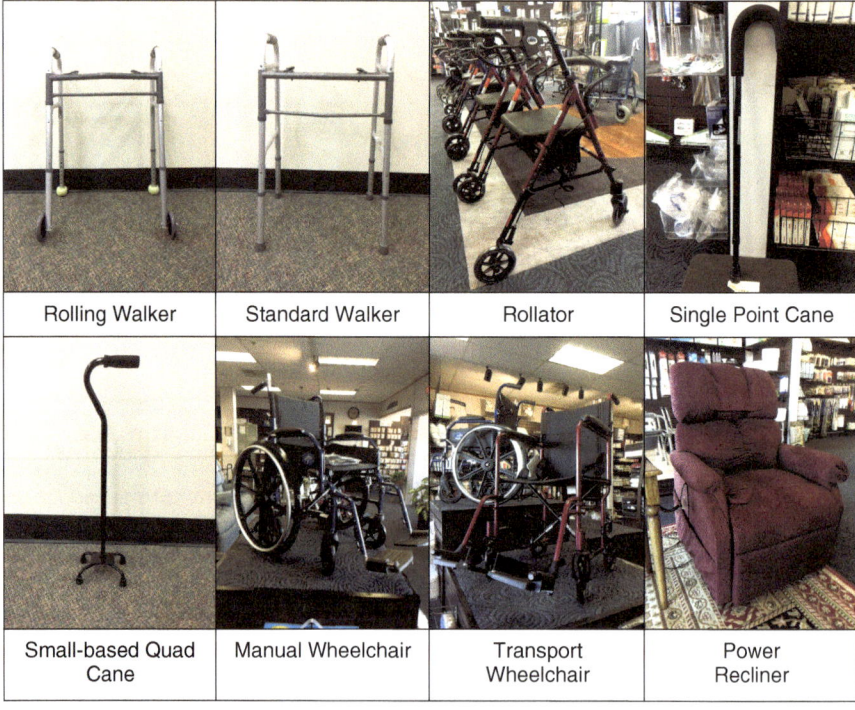

| Rolling Walker | Standard Walker | Rollator | Single Point Cane |
| Small-based Quad Cane | Manual Wheelchair | Transport Wheelchair | Power Recliner |

Fig. 10.1 Examples of durable medical equipment. (Photos courtesy of the author)

2   What Is Mesothelioma?

2.1   Pathophysiology

Malignant mesothelioma (MM) is a rare, often fatal cancer emerging from the mesothelial cells most commonly from the pleura and less frequently from the peritoneal and pericardial cavities as well as from the tunica vaginalis testis (Marinaccio et al. 2010). Malignant pleural mesothelioma (MPM) is most common followed by malignant peritoneal mesothelioma (PMM). MM can be further broken down into histological subtypes including epithelioid, sarcomatoid, biphasic (combination of epithelioid and sarcomatoid), and the rare desmoplastic sarcomatoid variant (Billé et al. 2015; Frontario et al. 2015) (Fig. 10.2). Staging is not a useful prognostic indicator; cell subtype is better (Beebe-Dimmer et al. 2016; Ray and Kindler 2009). The epithelioid subtype is the most common and possessing the best prognosis (Billé et al. 2015; Husain et al. 2017). Sarcomatoid (including desmoplastic) or biphasic type, Eastern Cooperative Oncology Group (ECOG) performance status of 1 or higher, and male sex tend to lead to poor prognosis (Zalcman et al. 2015).

2.2   Etiology

Malignant mesothelioma is most often associated with exposure to asbestos (particularly chrysotile asbestos) through occupational or environmental inhalation (Marinaccio et al. 2010; Beebe-Dimmer et al. 2016; Mazurek et al. 2017; Faig et al. 2015; LaDou et al. 2010). There is a history of exposure >80% in those diagnosed with MM (Faig et al. 2015; Salminen et al. 2013).

The latency period from exposure to asbestos to development of MM is often decades long, from 20 to 50 years (Ray and Kindler 2009; Mazurek et al. 2017; Salminen et al. 2013; LaDou et al. 2010). In the USA, about 3000 new cases of mesothelioma are diagnosed yearly, most often in men, those >65 years old, and Caucasian (Beebe-Dimmer et al. 2016) (Fig. 10.3). Nonetheless, deaths from MM increased for people >85 years old, men and women, African-Americans, Caucasians, Asians and Pacific Islands, and all ethnic groups (Mazurek et al. 2017).

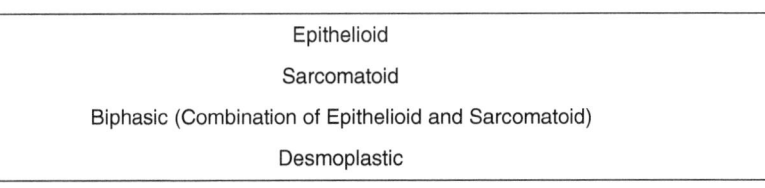

Epithelioid
Sarcomatoid
Biphasic (Combination of Epithelioid and Sarcomatoid)
Desmoplastic

Fig. 10.2 Histological subtypes of mesothelioma (Billé et al. 2015; Frontario et al. 2015)

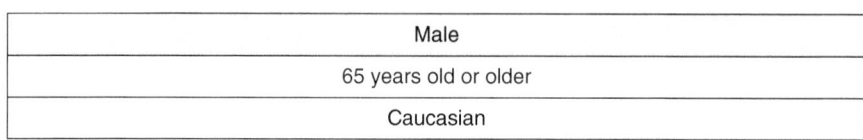

Male
65 years old or older
Caucasian

Fig. 10.3 Demographics – most often diagnosed with mesothelioma. (Beebe-Dimmer et al. 2016)

Although 52 countries have banned all forms of asbestos, it is still produced and exported by several countries including the leader, Russia, as well as China, Brazil, and Canada (LaDou et al. 2010). Due to a 1991 US Fifth Circuit Court of Appeals ruling overturning portions of an EPA standard regarding asbestos, consequently, the following are not banned: asbestos-containing products including, but not limited to, vinyl-asbestos flooring, asbestos-cement shingles, and disc brake pads (Mazurek et al. 2017).

3 Diagnosis

Diagnosis of mesothelioma is difficult and often late in the disease process which may be due to its relative rarity. Its non-specific symptoms usually including dyspnea and/or chest pain for MPM and abdominal distention, abdominal discomfort, and malaise for PMM; and its challenging diagnosis given no specific test for MPM currently exists (Beebe-Dimmer et al. 2016; Ray and Kindler 2009; Husain et al. 2017). In fact, the sensitivity of cytology for the diagnosis of MM is 30–75%, a high false-negative rate (Husain et al. 2017). The "gold standard" for diagnosis of MPM is thoracoscopy which leads to a diagnosis in 98% on patients (Ray and Kindler 2009). For PMM, the most sensitive and specific technique for diagnosis is tissue biopsy with direct immunohistological staining (Frontario et al. 2015).

4 Treatment

Standard treatment includes palliative chemotherapy including pemetrexed with either cisplatin or carboplatin and recent research supporting the use of the immunotherapy drug Avastin (bevacizumab) (Zalcman et al. 2015; Lang-Lazdunski et al. 2015). Disease detected early in patients with good performance status may be candidates for a multimodal approach including surgery with either extrapleural pneumonectomy (EPP) or pleurectomy with decortication (PD), chemotherapy, and/or radiation therapy (XRT) (Ray and Kindler 2009; Lang-Lazdunski et al. 2015).

Diagnosis of malignant peritoneal mesothelioma is also often late in the disease process with similar palliative chemotherapy options as for MPM or, for appropriate patients, cytoreductive surgery (CRS) with hyperthermic intraperitoneal chemotherapy (HIPEC) (Aydin et al. 2015).

Indeed, prognosis remains poor with others reporting median survival of 9–12 months for advanced MPM from time of diagnosis and 12–36 months for localized disease (Billé et al. 2015; Zalcman et al. 2015; Schwartz et al. 2017). For advanced PMM, median survival is 5–12 months (50–60 months when combined with CRS and HIPEC) (Billé et al. 2015; Ellenbogen et al. 2017) (Figs. 10.4 and 10.5).

Mesothelioma Type	Survival
Pleural (diffuse disease)	9-12 months
Pleural (localized disease)	12-36 months
Peritoneal (advanced disease)	5-12 months
Peritoneal (resectable disease)	50-60 months

Fig. 10.4 Predicted median survival by type. (Billé et al. 2015; Zalcman et al. 2015; Schwartz et al. 2017; Ellenbogen et al. 2017)

Fig. 10.5 Malignant mesothelioma (pleural and peritoneal) mean survival (months) without treatment, one treatment modality, and multi-treatment modalities. (Beebe-Dimmer et al. 2016)

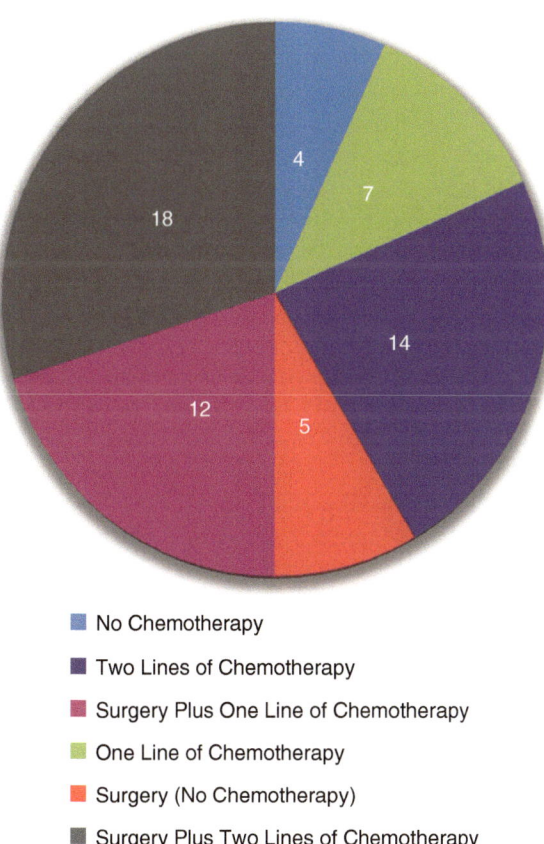

- ■ No Chemotherapy
- ■ Two Lines of Chemotherapy
- ■ Surgery Plus One Line of Chemotherapy
- ■ One Line of Chemotherapy
- ■ Surgery (No Chemotherapy)
- ■ Surgery Plus Two Lines of Chemotherapy

MM was not classified under its own ICD code until the 10th revision was released, making epidemiological study difficult prior to 1999 (Mazurek et al. 2017; Bofetta et al. 2017). Prior to the updated ICD-10, MM was classified under neoplasms of the pleura, under neoplasms of the peritoneum, or under other organs where it rarely occurs (Bofetta et al. 2017).

MM affects some professionals more than others. By industry, this includes shipping (including the Navy) and boat building/repair, while the highest by occupation includes insulation workers (Mazurek et al. 2017; Tata et al. 2008). The age-adjusted death rate is highest in Maine and Washington state (Mazurek et al. 2017).

5   Physical Therapy and Pulmonary Rehabilitation Along the Spectrum

Physical therapy is an adaptive profession with therapists found throughout the medical continuum. The physical therapist is always nearby and available and vital in the recovery and treatment of MM patients.

The PT will need to perform a thorough evaluation of the MM patient upon consultation including, but not limited to, functional mobility including gait, transfers and bed mobility, cancer-related fatigue (CRF), pain, contractures and muscle shortening, deconditioning, postural deficits, fall risk, peripheral neuropathy, and genitourinary dysfunction (Alappattu et al. 2015).

The 6-Minute Walk Test (6-MWT) is a simple and cost-effective functional test that is appropriate for most patients with MM pre-treatment and post-treatment and should be performed according to the American Thoracic Society Guidelines (American Thoracic Society 2002; Rick et al. 2014; Enright and Sherrill 1998; Gijbels et al. 2011). A 30-meter (100-ft) hallway is required per the above guidelines; however, Bohannon et al. used a back-and-forth 15.2 meters (50-ft) which they recognized may be more realistic for most practitioners and found the distance covered in 6 min (6-MWD) comparable to others using a 30-meter hallway (Bohannon et al. 2014). Nonetheless, the 6-MWD is a suitable variable to assess respiratory function (American Thoracic Society 2002; Rick et al. 2014). Moreover, physical therapists should consider assessing the distance walked in 2 min as it is a valid predictor of the 6-MWD whether measured during a 6-MWT or 2-MWT (2-Minute Walk Test) (Gijbels et al. 2011; Bohannon et al. 2014). Nevertheless, the only equipment needed to complete the 6-MWT include a chair if the patient needs to stop, 2 cones to mark the turning points, a tape measure, a clipboard and pen to mark laps, a stopwatch or smartphone with timer, and a 30-meter hallway (American Thoracic Society 2002) (Fig. 10.6). The patient should rate their dyspnea on the Modified Borg Scale before and after the test (Borg 1982). Standing rests are allowed, but if the person must sit, stop the test and mark the distance walked.

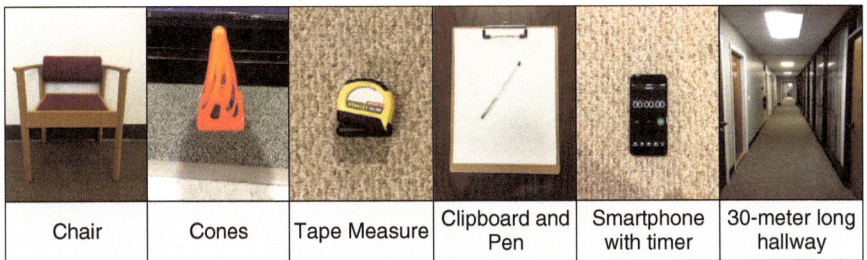

| Chair | Cones | Tape Measure | Clipboard and Pen | Smartphone with timer | 30-meter long hallway |

Fig. 10.6 Items recommended to complete the 6-MWT. (Photos courtesy of the author)

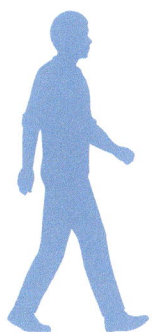

The primary tool of pulmonary rehabilitation is exercise focused on improving endurance (Tiep et al. 2015; Jones et al. 2007). This discussion will focus on the physical therapist's important contributions to the multidisciplinary pulmonary rehabilitation team. This training challenges the full oxygen transport system from the lungs to the tissues (Tiep et al. 2015). Exercise training, often under the supervision of a qualified PT, is the most effective way to reduce or prevent dyspnea on exertion (Shannon 2010).

Pulmonary rehabilitation is appropriate for most MM patients including those undergoing curative or life-prolonging surgeries and those in need of palliative care. For those with MPM, a contributing factor to their functional limitations may be loss of lung volume/capacity due to the tumor in the pleura, surgical removal of lung tissue including EPP, and scarring of the chest wall from the procedure itself as well as the effects of radiation therapy (Tiep et al. 2015). Pulmonary rehabilitation is also appropriate preoperatively as it often improves endurance, strength, gas exchange, and airway clearance (Tiep et al. 2015; Jones et al. 2007; Mujovic et al. 2014).

Moreover, Jones et al. who studied patients undergoing thoracic surgery for malignant lung lesions demonstrated that presurgical exercise training (including a relatively short program of 4–6 weeks) has an extremely low training-associated adverse event rate, small amount of serious adverse events, and high adherence rate (>70%). Indeed, a moderate to high intensity should be considered a safe option for patients scheduled for lung resection including EPP (Jones et al. 2007). Mujovic et al. found improvements in pulmonary function, functional capacity, and dyspnea after an even shorter time period (2–4 weeks) including the best improvement in the sickest patients (i.e., patients with the highest surgical risk) (Mujovic et al. 2014).

Tanaka et al. found that in those undergoing surgery for MPM, exercise capacity and pulmonary function decrease more than limb strength (Tanaka et al. 2017). Although Mujovic et al. studied preoperative pulmonary rehabilitation (PPR) in those with non-small cell lung cancer (NSCLC) and chronic obstructive disease (COPD), PPR will also likely benefit patients with MPM in mitigating these limitations.

6   Preoperative Physical Therapy

Although few studies have been conducted studying the effects of preoperative physical therapy for those undergoing surgery for malignant peritoneal or pleura mesothelioma, several have looked at others undergoing thoracic surgery for lung lesions including non-small cell lung cancer (NSCLC). The results are encouraging including that preoperative exercise training had a beneficial effect on cardiopulmo-nary fitness in those experiencing thoracic surgery for malignant lung lesions (Jones et al. 2007). Also, preoperative physical therapy is likely appropriate for MM patients who are treated first with chemotherapy as Marulli et al. found that induction chemotherapy (IC) improves lung volumes (especially FEV1), oxygen uptake (VO2max), and gas exchanges in those responding to IC (Marulli et al. 2010). They also hypothesized that the pleural mass may lead to atelectasis and reduced chest cage and diaphragmatic expansion leading to weakness in the respiratory muscles (Marulli et al. 2010). Physical therapists should focus most of their treatment on improving inspiratory muscle strengthening including diaphragmatic breathing techniques and endurance training including an aerobic program with a progressive ambulation-based or stationary cycle-based program (Figs. 10.7 and 10.8). Indeed, patients undergoing thoracotomy and lung resection, including EPP, improve their exercise capacity with a preoperative physical therapy or pulmonary rehabilitation program (Nagarajan et al. 2011). In fact, improved exercise capacity is associated with decreased surgical complications (Jones et al. 2007) (Fig. 10.9). These patients may be seen in outpatient physical therapy or a pulmonary rehabilitation clinic or by a home care physical therapist if the patient is homebound. Use of the Modified Borg Scale (MBS) or Rating of Perceived Exertion (RPE) is recommended in this population (Borg 1982).

Inspiratory Muscle Training (Incentive Spirometry, Diaphragmatic Breathing Techniques)	Endurance/Aerobic Training (Progressive Ambulation/Treadmill Program or Cycle-based Program)

Fig. 10.7 Focus of preoperative physical therapy. (Nagarajan et al. 2011)

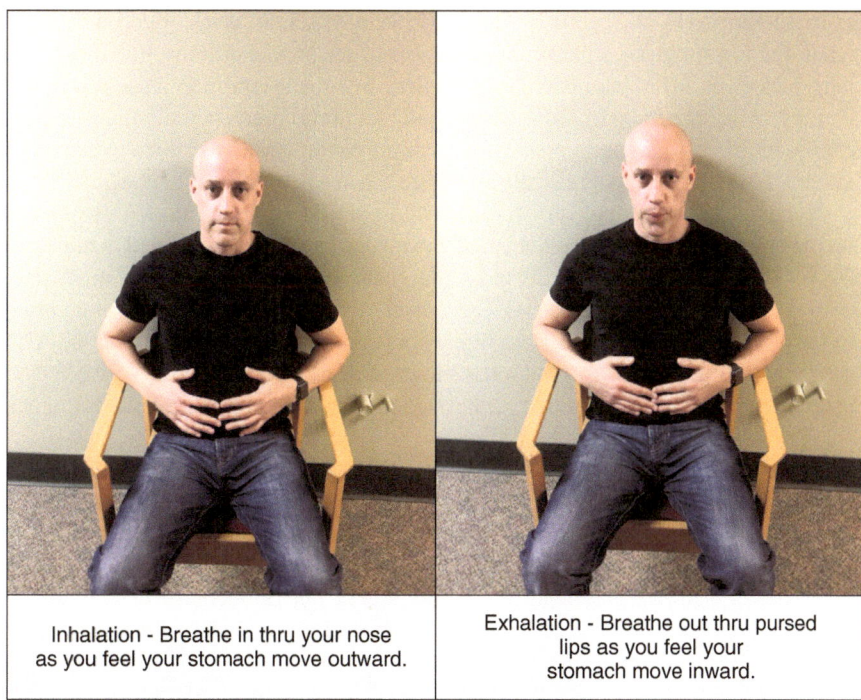

Inhalation - Breathe in thru your nose as you feel your stomach move outward.	Exhalation - Breathe out thru pursed lips as you feel your stomach move inward.

Fig. 10.8 Diaphragmatic breathing. (Photos courtesy of the author)

Improved Pulmonary Function, Improved Functional Capacity
Reduced Dyspnea/SOB
Improved Endurance, Strength, Gas Exchange and Airway Clearance
Moderate to High Intensity is Safe
Low Training-Associated Adverse Event Rate, Small Amount of Adverse Events, High Adherence Rate

Fig. 10.9 Benefits of preoperative pulmonary rehabilitation. (Tiep et al. 2015; Jones et al. 2007; Mujovic et al. 2014)

7   Postoperative Pulmonary Rehabilitation

In their meta-analysis concerning the effects of exercise training on patients with lung cancer who underwent lung resection, Li et al. found insufficient evidence to support the efficacy of this intervention in their target population (Li et al. 2017). However, they warned of careful interpretation of the results due to confounding variables in the studies they assessed including the use of different parameters and exercise forms (Li et al. 2017). On the other hand, Salhi et al. found a 12-week rehabilitation program, combining aerobic and resistance training, for those with lung cancer or MPM combated with radical treatment (surgical resection, radiotherapy, or combination of radiotherapy and platinum-based chemotherapy) significantly improves exercise capacity, muscle strength, and QoL even when those variables significantly decreased following radical treatment (Salhi et al. 2015).

Nonetheless, early recovery (i.e., post-op pulmonary rehabilitation or physical therapy) can reduce the incidence of postoperative complications (Chang et al. 2014). Physical therapists understand that patients, when ambulating, must stand with proper posture and breathe deeper than when at rest, resulting in maximum oxygen uptake and improved maximum expiratory ventilation (Cicutto 2006). Also, a progressive ambulatory program has shown to be an effective component of physical therapy that leads to markedly improved lung function following major thoracic surgery (Kortebein et al. 2008).

Moreover, hospitalized and non-hospitalized patients with MM should be encouraged to increase activity as soon as medically stable (Gill et al. 2004). Kortebein et al. studied a group of healthy older adults (ages 62–75 years old) and investigated the functional impact of 10 days of bed rest in this population (Kortebein et al. 2008). Bed rest may lead to pressure ulcers, DVTs, incontinence, as well as functional decline and disability (Gill et al. 2004). Indeed, bed rest results in a substantial loss of lower extremity strength, power, as well as aerobic capacity (Kortebein et al. 2008). Although their study focused on healthy older adults, it is likely that their findings would be pronounced in the MM population given the similar age demographic when mesothelioma is first diagnosed (Mazurek et al. 2017).

Research demonstrates that lower extremity power is a bigger factor in impaired functional mobility than lower extremity strength (Bean et al. 2003). As people age, muscle power declines more rapidly than strength (Beijersbergen et al. 2017; Reid et al. 2015). In fact, low power was associated with a 2–3 times greater risk for decreased mobility than strength (Bean et al. 2003).

Resistance training is a common tool in physical therapy. It is also an important way, when conducted with increased velocity during the concentric phase (the eccentric phase is performed at normal velocity), to improve lower extremity power via emphasizing both force production and velocity of the movement, and the gains do not diminish after 10 weeks of detraining (Bean et al. 2003; Beijersbergen et al. 2017). Power training can improve function in many ways including gait velocity in that the increased power and modified joint kinematics (e.g., larger joint ROM and rotational velocities) consequently lead to longer and faster strides (Beijersbergen et al. 2017).

A plan of care that addresses power deficits may also lead to a decreased fall risk by improving balance (Pamukoff et al. 2014). Indeed, fallers have less lower extremity power than non-fallers (Perry et al. 2007). Power training may also be a more time-efficient form of resistance exercise as it improves both muscle power and strength, whereas strength training only improves muscle strength, to reduce the effects of sarcopenia often found in MM patients as well as older adults (Marsh et al. 2009) (Fig. 10.10). Marsh et al. demonstrated that modifying a strength training program with the instruction to complete the concentric phase "as fast as

Power Training	Power and Strength Improvements
Strength Training	Strength Improvements Only

Fig. 10.10 Gains seen with different types of interventions. (Marsh et al. 2009)

possible" is a practical, safe, and beneficial intervention to increase lower extremity strength and power in older adults, especially those with mild to moderate self-reported disability (Marsh et al. 2009). In fact, high velocity resistance training, using light resistance at a more rapid pace, may be a more feasible form of power training to address mobility loss (Reid et al. 2015).

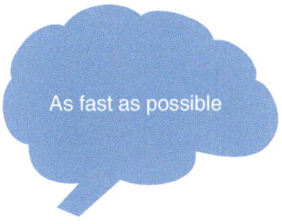

8   Outpatient Physical Therapy and MM

Outpatient clinics tend to be generalized practices which evaluate and treat a myriad of injuries, disabilities, diseases, and impairments. The most frequent neuromuscular impairments described by Alappattu et al. for respiratory cancers include posture, ROM, soft tissue, strength, fatigue, and pain (Alappattu et al. 2015) (Fig. 10.11). In fact, only two other cancer types had higher frequencies of impairments in pain – bone or joint cancers and soft tissue cancers (Fig. 10.12). Overall, for all cancer types, they reported the most frequent impairments included soft tissue, ROM, and strength.

The need for a complete medical history is understood by outpatient PTs, but it is especially important for patients presenting with MM or other cancers. The therapist may not know the nuances of HIPEC, EPP, or P/D, but their extensive training in evaluating the complex patient should leave them well-prepared for the task. Use of the 6-MWT is likely the most appropriate functional test with this patient population. Also, close evaluation of the surgical site, if present, which typically includes the right or left flank for EPP or P/D patients and abdomen for HIPEC patients will likely demonstrate scar and fascial restrictions requiring manual or instrument-assisted mobilization. Those undergoing chemotherapy and/or radiotherapy are appropriate candidates for outpatient physical therapy as well.

Most outpatient therapists do not monitor vital signs as closely as their acute care, inpatient rehabilitation, SNF, or home care colleagues, but it is warranted in this population given the complex nature of MM and the significant proportion with MPM. Hypertension remains in high frequency across all oncological groups, not

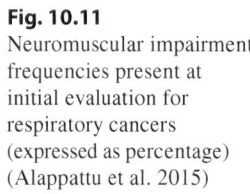
Fig. 10.11
Neuromuscular impairment
frequencies present at
initial evaluation for
respiratory cancers
(expressed as percentage)
(Alappattu et al. 2015)

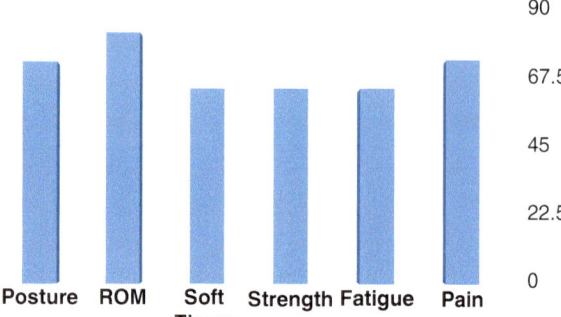

Fig. 10.12 Frequency of
impairment in pain present
at initial evaluation for all
cancers, respiratory, bone or
joint, and soft tissue cancers
(Alappattu et al. 2015)

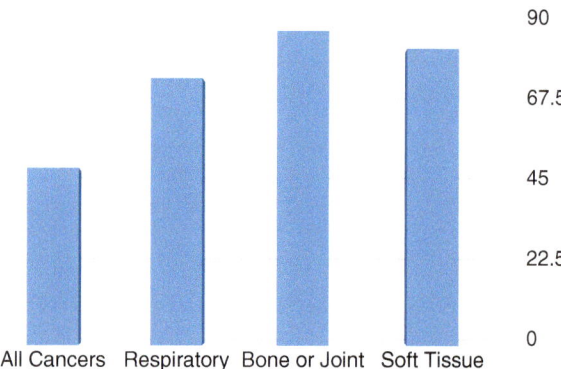

inconsistent with that found across the general population (Alappattu et al. 2015). Before initiating an exercise or treatment program with the MM patient, blood pressure (BP), heart rate (HR), and oxygen saturation (Sats) should be measured. HR monitoring is especially important with those undergoing EPP or P/D given the increased incidence of atrial fibrillation (a-fib) in those undergoing these procedures (Neragi-Miandoab et al. 2008). Of course, a-fib can only be detected via EKG, but if the PT assesses a new onset irregular heart rate, they should contact the surgeon, PCP, or oncologist immediately. As evidenced earlier in this chapter, prime active areas of intervention include endurance training, inspiratory muscle training, and power training.

9   Quality of Life

Measurements of quality of life (QoL) including physical symptoms, social and physical function, as well as lung function parameters that are significantly affected by both surgical approaches to MPM including EPP and P/D. P/D tends to have better QoL outcomes, but the research is likely incomplete (Schwartz et al. 2017). In physical therapy, QoL improvement is just as important as physiological improvement (Salhi et al. 2015). One instrument that physical therapist may employ to assess QoL and symptom burden is the M.D. Anderson Symptom Inventory (MDASI) which has been used across different cancer types (Jones et al. 2007, 2014; Cleeland et al. 2000). It asks the patient to rate the severity, during the past 24 hours, of 13 core disease and treatment-related symptoms (Jones et al. 2014; Mendoza et al. 2011; Wang et al. 2014). For MM patients, given the high incidence of opioids to treat pain, constipation should be added to this core list as well (Cleeland et al. 2000). The ratings are on an 11-point (0–10) numerical rating scale, which is familiar to physical therapists across the setting spectrum (Fig. 10.13). The range is from 0 (not present) to 10 (as bad as you can imagine) (Mendoza et al. 2011; Wang et al. 2014). The rating format is based off the Brief Pain Inventory and Brief Fatigue Inventory, which focus on individual symptoms, are valuable in their own rights, but the MDASI is more comprehensive (Cleeland et al. 2000; Mendoza et al. 2011). The MDASI also assesses how these symptoms interfere with function (Cleeland et al. 2000; Wang et al. 2014) (Fig. 10.14). The symptoms can be averaged (i.e., mean score) or assessed individually (Cleeland et al. 2000; Mendoza et al. 2011; Wang et al. 2014; https://www.mdanderson.org/content/dam/mdanderson/documents/Departments-and-Divisions/Symptom-Research/MDASI_user-guide.pdf). Indeed, scores of 5 or above (on the 0–10 scale), on individual symptom report, indicate a moderate to severe symptom that significantly impairs function (Jones et al. 2014; Mendoza et al. 2011; Wang et al. 2014). One advantage of the MDASI is early detection of symptoms before they become severe to reduce the likelihood of emergency room visits and hospitalization as well as to direct PT treatment toward those symptoms (Cleeland et al. 2000).

Figs. 10.13 and 10.14 MDASI numerical rating scale (Cleeland et al. 2000)

Symptom Rating		Interference Rating	
Numerical Rating	Severity	*Numerical Rating*	Severity
0	"Not present"	0	
1	Mild	1	
2		2	
3		3	
4		4	
5	Moderate	5	
6		6	
7	Severe	7	
8		8	
9		9	
10	"As bad as you can imagine"	10	"Interfere completely"

10   Endurance and Resistance Exercise Relating to Cancer-Related Fatigue

Most patients with cancer encounter a loss of energy and reduced physical performance during the duration of their disease (Salhi et al. 2015; Dimeo et al. 2008;
Horneber et al. 2012). The etiology of decreased physical performance is believed
to be in the cortical and sensorimotor center changes, in the energy metabolism
changes, and in the process of muscle activation (Horneber et al. 2012). Some studies suggest that anywhere from 45% to 70% of patients with cancer experience
fatigue during XRT and chemotherapy or after surgery (Wang et al. 2014; Dimeo
et al. 2008). Fatigue, in fact, is the most frequent and most severely reported symptom by those patients during their course of treatment (Yanez et al. 2013; Wang
et al. 2010; Minton et al. 2012; Mustian et al. 2017; Mendoza et al. 1999). It can be
severe and restricting. Physical therapists know well that inactivity can lead to muscular atrophy and likely contribute to fatigue (Dimeo 2001). Dimeo et al. showed
that an exercise program of even limited duration boosts endurance and increases
functional status but also reduced fatigue in cancer patients (Dimeo et al. 2008).
Moreover, Narayanan and Koshy report that regular physical activity, energy conservation, and even group exercise therapy are effective for cancer-related fatigue
(CRF) (Narayanan and Koshy 2009).

Indeed, patients with MM will likely benefit. Of course, the physical therapy
plan of care (POC) must be individualized. The findings in the literature, even those
studying other cancers, provide appropriate evidence as to where to focus the treatment. In fact, in their meta-analysis comparing pharmaceutical, psychological, and
exercise treatments for CRF, Mustian et al. found that exercise may be most effective for treating CRF during primary treatment, while the combination of exercise
and psychological interventions may be most effective for those who have completed primary treatment; pharmaceutical intervention was not effective during or
after treatment (Mustian et al. 2017).

Moreover, an improved performance status can enhance feelings of control,
self-esteem, and functional independence possibly culminating in better social
interactions; thus, reducing fear and anxiety leading to improved mood and less
psychological stress (Dimeo et al. 2008). The physical therapist should consider
a referral to occupational therapy (OT) for relaxation training and speech-language pathology (SLP) for a cognitive evaluation to assist in treating cancer-
related fatigue including the possible components of lack of concentration and
loss of memory.

11   Side Effects of Radiation Therapy and Chemotherapy

XRT and chemotherapy are known to negatively affect exercise capacity, muscle
strength, and QoL (Salhi et al. 2015). XRT is often associated with neuropathic pain
possibly related to damage to nerve roots, plexus, and/or peripheral nerves
(Stubblefield 2011; Dropcho 2010; Cross and Glantz 2003). Familiar side effects of

chemotherapy include neurotoxicity (i.e., peripheral neuropathy, myelopathy, and cognitive changes), hair loss (not as common with the standard MM chemotherapeutic agents pemetrexed and cisplatin or carboplatin), gastrointestinal dysfunction, nausea, fatigue, and weight loss (Alappattu et al. 2015).

The painful neuropathies commonly associated with cisplatin and carboplatin may last for several months or years which will have to be addressed for MM patients who survive long enough for this to become a significant impairment (Ray and Kindler 2009; Sachs and Weinberg 2009). With further research and clinical trials in the future, more patients will need neuropathy included in their plan of care.

Patients may also experience musculoskeletal consequences of XRT including atrophy, fibrosis, osteopenia or osteoporosis, and muscle spasms and pain (Stubblefield 2011; O'Sullivan and Levin 2003). Therapy focused on these areas including muscular strengthening, stretching, pain relief thru multimodal means, and closed-chain exercises with focus on increasing weight-bearing to stimulate osteoblast activity. The above treatment strategies would likely be effective in alleviating XRT-associated side effects. Heat or cold modalities should not be applied to areas of skin that are insensitive, atrophic, and acutely inflamed or have been irradiated (Santiago-Palma and Payne 2001).

12   Physical Therapy and Palliative Care of Patients with Malignant Mesothelioma

Most people know physical therapists practice in a wide range of locations including inpatient, outpatient, and home-based settings; however, PTs are also an important part of the hospice and palliative care multidisciplinary team. Since the prognosis for most patients with malignant mesothelioma remains poor, palliative care options will be an important component for most of them. Symptom control and maintaining their maximum functional independence are paramount (Mendoza et al. 1999; Santiago-Palma and Payne 2001). PTs address the physical and functional aspects of the patient's condition while seeking to maximize the patient's functional status despite their limitations or symptom burden (Kumar and Jim 2010; Cheville and Basford 2014). The many treatment options, both active and passive strategies of which many are listed earlier in this chapter, are useful in ameliorating effects from terminal MM. Improved quality of life (QoL) is an essential component of the physical therapist's plan of care. In fact, the use of any number of heat or cold modalities or Transcutaneous Electrical Nerve Stimulation (TENS) may assist the therapist in reducing the MM patient's pain as most do not achieve adequate pain control with opioids alone (Kumar and Jim 2010; Salminen et al. 2013; Cheville and Basford 2014).

Goal establishment may be difficult for those in need of palliative care or hospice, but those goals must be realistic and include input from the patient and their caregivers (Santiago-Palma and Payne 2001). The ultimate objective for most physical therapy goals is maximizing functional independence within current limitations. Moreover, the goals may need to be adjusted as their disease progresses.

Physical therapy can be useful in reducing dyspnea, improving breathing control and breathing pattern, as well as improving exercise tolerance in the palliative care of the MM patient thru teaching pursed lip breathing (PLB) and diaphragmatic breathing with the understanding that one hemidiaphragm may be resected for those undergoing P/D or the tumor may limit its ability to assist in the respiratory cycle (Damle et al. 2016; LeGrand 2002) (Fig. 10.15). The PT may use several techniques and interventions at their disposal including supine or sitting positioning, DME prescription including rollators, rolling walkers or canes, gait and stair training, pacing instruction, relaxation and posture, among many others, to assist the patient in reducing dyspnea (Syrett and Taylor 2003; Marciniuk et al. 2011).

Muscular weakness frequently develops as the consequence of MM and its treatment. The patient often becomes sedentary due to the restrictions imposed by the symptoms associated with MM which leads to lower extremity (LE) weakness further leading to a downward spiral and severely limited exercise tolerance (Jones et al. 2016). However, one option, the use of neuromuscular electrical nerve stimulation (NMES), improves dyspnea, muscular strength, and performance of ADLs (activities of daily living) which may benefit those who are not capable of exercise (Marciniuk et al. 2011; Jones et al. 2016; Bausewein et al. 2008) (Fig. 10.16).

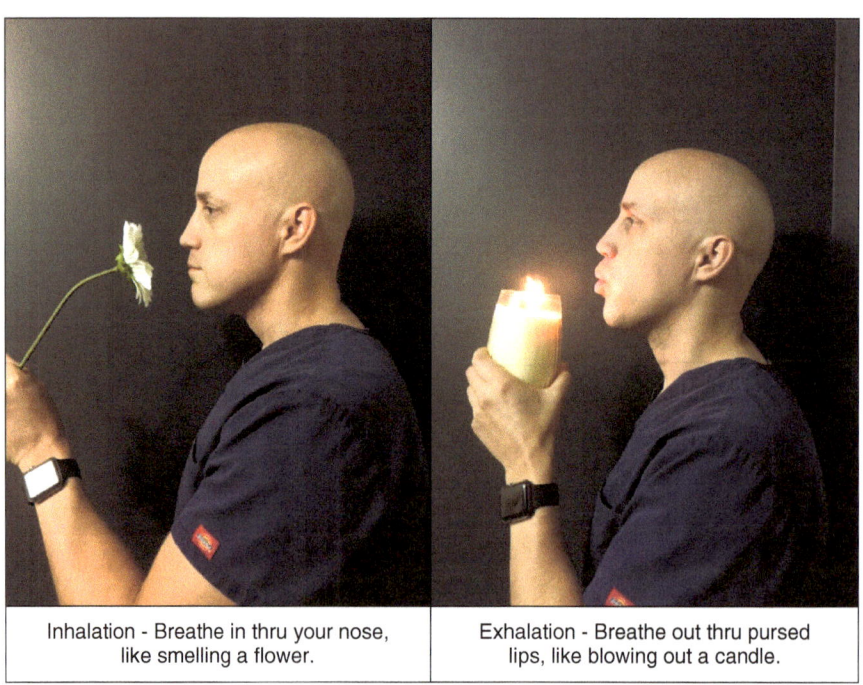

| Inhalation - Breathe in thru your nose, like smelling a flower. | Exhalation - Breathe out thru pursed lips, like blowing out a candle. |

Fig. 10.15 Pursed lip breathing. (Photos courtesy of the author)

Passive Interventions	Active Interventions
TENS/NMES	Endurance/Interval Training
STM/DFM	Gait/Stair Training
PROM	Therapeutic Exercise
Joint Mobilization	PLB/Diaphragmatic Breathing

Fig. 10.16 Passive vs active interventions. (Kumar and Jim 2010; Marciniuk et al. 2011; Jones et al. 2016)

13   Recommendations for Referring Providers

Physical therapists are highly skilled clinicians who are well suited to care for your patient diagnosed with malignant mesothelioma. Whether they are surgical candidates or only candidates for palliative care options, physical therapy should be an option for all of them. As laid out in this chapter, the evidence is clear and supportive of the use of physical therapy along the continuum of care. Indeed, presurgical exercise training (including a relatively short program of 4–6 weeks) has an extremely low training-associated adverse event rate, small amount of serious adverse events, and high adherence rate (>70%), and a moderate to high intensity should be considered a safe option for patients scheduled for lung resection including EPP, even for the sickest patients (Jones et al. 2007; Mujovic et al. 2014).

An immediate postoperative physical therapy consult, while still hospitalized, and avoiding bed rest, can prevent pressure ulcers, DVTs, incontinence, as well as functional decline and disability (Gill et al. 2004). Indeed, this consult can prevent the substantial loss of lower extremity strength, power, as well as aerobic capacity often seen with prolonged immobility (Kortebein et al. 2008).

Whether as an outpatient at the hospital or in a private PT clinic, combining aerobic and resistance training, for those with MPM combated with radical treatment, significantly improves exercise capacity, muscle strength, and QoL even when those variables significantly decreased following radical treatment (Salhi et al. 2015). Indeed, PT has its place in palliative care as well. PTs address the physical and functional aspects of the patient's condition while seeking to maximize the patient's functional status despite their limitations or symptom burden (Kumar and Jim 2010; Cheville and Basford 2014).

The best recommendation for prescribing providers is to refer your patients to physical therapists as soon as possible with the corresponding diagnosis and any restrictions (i.e., lifting restrictions, supplemental O2 needs) that may be needed. Please consider "Evaluate and Treat" as the appropriate wording for this consult. The physical therapist will assess the patient for their limitations and, armed with the above knowledge regarding the appropriate recommendations for care of this population, will develop an appropriate and sound plan of care in collaboration with the medical team including, but not limited to, physicians, nurses, occupational therapists, respiratory therapists, and speech-language pathologists.

References

Alappattu MJ, Coronado RA, Lee D, Bour B, George SZ. Clinical characteristics of patients with cancer referred to outpatient physical therapy. Phys Ther. 2015;95(4):526–38.

American Thoracic Society. ATS statement – guidelines for the six-minute walk test. Am J Respir Crit Care. 2002;166(1):111–7.

Aydin N, Sardi A, Milovanov V, Nieroda C, Sittig M, Nunez M, Jimenez W, Gushchin V. Outcomes of cytoreductive surgery and hyperthermic intraperitoneal chemotherapy for peritoneal mesothelioma: experience of a peritoneal surface malignancy center. Am Surg. 2015;12(81):1253–9.

Bausewein C, Booth S, Gysels M, Higginson IJ. Non-pharmacological interventions for breathlessness in advanced stages of malignant and non-malignant disease. Cochrane Database Syst Rev. 2008;2:CD005623.

Bean JF, Leveille SG, Kiely DK, Bandinelli S, Guralnik JM, Ferrucci L. A comparison of leg power and leg strength within the InCHIANTI study: which influences mobility more? J Gerontol. 2003;58A(8):728–33.

Beebe-Dimmer JL, Fryzek JP, Yee CL, Dalvi TB, Garabrant DH, Schwartz AG, Gadgeel S. Mesothelioma in the United States: a surveillance, epidemiology, and end results (SEER) – Medicare investigation of treatment patterns and overall survival. Clin Epidemiol. 2016;8:743–50.

Beijersbergen CMI, Granacher U, Gäbler M, Devita P, Hortobágyi T. Kinematic mechanisms of how power training improves healthy old adults' gait velocity. Med Sci Sports Exerc. 2017;49(1):150–7.

Billé A, Krug LM, Woo KM, Rusch VW, Zauderer MG. Contemporary analysis of prognostic factors in patients with unresectable malignant pleural mesothelioma. J Thorac Oncol. 2015;11(2):249–55.

Bofetta P, Malvezzi M, Pira E, Negri E, La Vecchia C. International analysis of age-specific mortality rates from mesothelioma on the basis of the international classification of diseases, 10th revision. J Glob Oncol. Published online 11 Aug 2017;1–15.

Bohannon RW, Bubela D, Magasi S, McCreath H, Wang YC, Reuben D, Rymer WZ, Gershon R. Comparison of walking performance over the first 2 minutes and the full 6 minutes of six-minute walk test. BMC Res Notes. 2014;7:269.

Borg GAV. Psychological bases of perceived exertion. Med Sci Sports Exerc. 1982;14(5):377–81.

Chang NW, Lin KC, Lee SC, Chan JYH, Lee YH, Wang KY. Effects of an early postoperative walking exercise programme on health status in lung cancer patients recovering from lung lobectomy. J Clin Nurs. 2014;23:3391–402.

Cheville AL, Basford JR. Role of rehabilitation medicine and physical agents in the treatment of cancer-associated pain. J Clin Oncol. 2014;32(16):1691–702.

Cicutto L. Review: physical training increases cardiopulmonary fitness in asthma and does not decrease lung function. Evid Based Nurs. 2006;9:44.

Cleeland CS, Mendoza TR, Wang XS, Chou C, Harle MT, Morrissey M, Engstrom MC. Assessing symptom distress in cancer patients, the M.D. Anderson symptom inventory. Cancer. 2000;89(7):1634–46.

Cross NE, Glantz MJ. Neurologic complications of radiation therapy. Neurol Clin. 2003;21:249–77.

Damle SJ, Shetye JV, Mehta AA. Immediate effect of pursed-lip breathing while walking during six minute walk test on six minute walk distance in young individuals. Indian J Physiother Occup Therapy. 2016;10(1):56–61.

Dimeo FC. Effects of exercise on cancer-related fatigue. Cancer. 2001;92:1689–93.

Dimeo F, Schwartz S, Wesel N, Voigt A, Thiel E. Effects of an endurance and resistance exercise program on persistent cancer-related fatigue after treatment. Ann Oncol. 2008;19:495–1499.

Dropcho EJ. Neurotoxicity of radiation therapy. Neurol Clin. 2010;28:217–34.

Ellenbogen AL, Barak S, Akin EA. Peritoneal mesothelioma in a young woman: case report of radiopathologic findings and review of the literature. Med Res Innov. 2017;1(2):1–3.

Enright PL, Sherrill DL. Reference equations for the six-minute walk in healthy adults. Am J Respir Crit Care Med. 1998;158:1384–7.

Faig J, Howard S, Levine EA, Casselman G, Hessdorffer M, Ohar JA. Changing pattern in malignant mesothelioma survival. Transl Oncol. 2015;8(1):35–9.

Frontario SCN, Loveitt A, Goldenberg-Sandau A, Liu J, Roy D, Cohen LW. Primary peritoneal mesothelioma resulting in small bowel obstruction: a case report and review of literature. Am J Case Rep. 2015;16:496–500.

Gijbels D, Eijnde DO, Feys P. Comparison of the 2- and 6-minute walk test in multiple sclerosis. Mult Scler J. 2011;17(10):1269–72.

Gill TM, Allore H, Guo Z. The deleterious effects of bed rest among community-living older persons. J Gerontol. 2004;59A(7):755–61.

Horneber M, Fischer I, Dimeo F, Rüffer JU, Weis J. Cancer-related fatigue. Dtsch Arztebl Int. 2012;109(9):161–72.

https://www.apta.org/AboutPTs. Accessed 27 Oct 2017.

https://www.mdanderson.org/content/dam/mdanderson/documents/Departments-and-Divisions/Symptom-Research/MDASI_userguide.pdf. Accessed 29 Oct 2017.

Husain AN, Colby TV, Ordóñez NG, Allen TC, Attanoos RL, Beasley MB, Butnor KJ, Chirieac LR, Churg AM, Dacic S, Galateau-Sallé G, Gibbs A, Gown AM, Krausz T, Litsky LA, Marchevsky A, Nicholson AG, Roggli VL, Sharma AK, Travis WD, Walts AE, Wicks MR. Early online release – guidelines for pathologic diagnosis of malignant mesothelioma. Arch Pathol Lab Med. 2017; https://doi.org/10.5858/arpa.2017-0124-RA.

Jones LW, Peddle CJ, Eves ND, Haykowsky MJ, Courneya KS, Mackey JR, Joy AA, Kumar V, Winton TW, Reiman T. Effects of presurgical exercise training on cardiorespiratory fitness among patients undergoing thoracic surgery for malignant lung lesions. Cancer. 2007;110(3):590–8.

Jones D, Zhao F, Fisch MJ, Wagner LI, Patrick-Miller LJ, Cleeland CS, Mendoza TR. The validity and utility of the M.D. Anderson symptom inventory in patients with prostate cancer: evidence from the Symptom Outcomes and Practice Patterns (SOAPP) date from the Eastern Cooperative Oncology Group. Clin Genitourin Cancer. 2014;12(1):41–9.

Jones S, Man WDC, Gao W, Higginson IJ, Wilcock A, Maddocks M. Neuromuscular electric stimulation for muscle weakness in adults with advanced disease. Cochrane Database Syst Rev. 2016;10:1–64.

Kortebein P, Symons TB, Ferrando A, Paddon-Jones D, Ronsen O, Protas E, Conger S, Lombeida J, Wolfe R, Evans WJ. Functional impact of 10 days of bed rest in healthy older adults. J Gerontol. 2008;63A(10):1076–81.

Kumar SP, Jim A. Physical therapy in palliative care: from symptom control to quality of life. Indian J Palliat Care. 2010;16(3):138–46.

LaDou J, Castelman B, Frank A, Gochfeld M, Greenberg M, Huff J, Joshi TK, Landrigan PJ, Lemen R, Myers J, Soffritti M, Soskolne CL, Takahashi K, Teitelbaum D, Terracini B, Watterson A. Environ Health Perspect. 2010;118(7):897–901.

Lang-Lazdunski L, Billé A, Papa S, Marshall S, Lal R, Galeone C, Landau D, Steele J, Spicer J. Pleurectomy/decortication, hyperthermic pleural lavage with povidone-iodine, prophylactic radiotherapy, and systemic chemotherapy in patients with malignant pleural mesothelioma: a 10-year experience. J Thorac Cardiovasc Surg. 2015;149:558–66.

LeGrand SB. Dyspnea: the continuing challenge of palliative management. Curr Opin Oncol. 2002;14:394–8.

Li J, Guo NN, Jin HR, Wang P, Xu GG. Effects of exercise training on patients with lung cancer who underwent lung resection: a meta-analysis. World J Surg Oncol. 2017;15:158–65.

Marciniuk DD, Goodridge D, Hernandez P, Rocker G, Balter M, Bailey P, Ford G, Bourbeau J, O'Donnell DE, Maltais F, Mularski RA, Cave AJ, Mayers I, Kennedy V, Oliver TK, Brown C. Managing dyspnea in patients with advanced chronic obstructive pulmonary disease: a Canadian Thoracic Society clinical practice guideline. Can Respir J. 2011;18(2):69–78.

Marinaccio A, Binazzi A, Marzio DD, Scarselli A, Verardo M, Mirabelli D, Gennaro V, Mensi C, Merler E, Zotti RD, Mangone L, Chellini E, Pascucci C, Ascoli V, Menegozzo S, Cavone D,

Cauzillo G, Nicita C, Melis M, Iavicoli S. Incidence of extrapleural malignant mesothelioma and asbestos exposure, from the Italian national register. Occup Environ Med. 2010;67:760–5.

Marsh AP, Miller ME, Rejeski WJ, Hutton SL, Kritchevsky SB. Lower extremity muscle function after strength or power training in older adults. J Aging Phys Act. 2009;17(4):416–43.

Marulli G, Rea F, Nicotra S, Favaretto AG, Perissinotto E, Chizzolini M, Vianello A, Braccioni F. Effect of induction chemotherapy on lung function and exercise capacity in patients affected by malignant pleural mesothelioma. Eur J Cardiothorac Surg. 2010;37(6):1464–9.

Mazurek JM, Syamlal G, Wood JM, Hendricks SA, Weston A. Malignant mesothelioma – Unites States, 1999–2015. Morb Mortal Wkly Rep. 2017;66(8):214–8.

Mendoza TR, Wang XS, Cleeland CS, Morrissey M, Johnson BA, Wendt JK, Huber SL. The rapid assessment of fatigue severity in cancer patients. Cancer. 1999;85:1186–96.

Mendoza TR, Wang XS, Lu C, Palos GR, Liao Z, Mobley GM, Kapoor S, Cleeland CS. Measuring the symptom burden of lung cancer: the validity and utility of the lung cancer module of the M.D. Anderson Symptom Inventory. Oncologist. 2011;16:217–27.

Minton SF, Radbruch I, Stone P. Identification of factors associated with fatigue in advanced cancer: a subset analysis of the European palliative care collaborative computerized symptom assessment data set. J Pain Symptom Manag. 2012;43:226–35.

Mujovic NA, Mujovic NE, Subotic D, Marinkovic M, Milovanovic A, Stojsic J, Zugic V, Grajic M, Nikolic D. Preoperative pulmonary in patients with non-small cell lung cancer and chronic obstructive pulmonary disease. Arch Med Sci. 2014;1:68–75.

Mustian KM, Alfano CM, Heckler C, Kleckner AS, Kleckner JR, Leach CR, Mohr D, Palesh OG, Peppone LJ, Piper BF, Scarpato J, Smith T, Sprod LK, Miller SM. JAMA Oncol. 2017;3(7):961–8.

Nagarajan K, Bennett A, Agostini P, Naidu B. Is preoperative physiotherapy/pulmonary rehabilitation beneficial in lung resection patients? Interact Cardiovasc Thorac Surg. 2011;13:300–2.

Narayanan V, Koshy C. Fatigue in cancer: a review of literature. Indian J Palliat Care. 2009;15:19–25.

Neragi-Miandoab S, Weiner S, Sugarbaker DJ. Incidence of atrial fibrillation after extrapleural pneumonectomy vs pleurectomy in patients with malignant pleural mesothelioma. Interact Cardiovasc Thorac Surg. 2008;7:1039–43.

O'Sullivan B, Levin W. Late radiation-related fibrosis: pathogenesis, manifestations, and current management. Semin Radiat Oncol. 2003;13:274–89.

Pamukoff DN, Haakonssen EC, Zaccaria JA, Madigan ML, Miller ME, Marsh AP. The effects of strength and power training on single-step balance recovery in older adults: a preliminary study. Clin Interv Aging. 2014;9:697–704.

Perry MC, Carville SF, Smith IC, Rutherford OM, Newham DJ. Strength, power output and symmetry of leg muscles: effect of age and history of falling. Eur J Appl Physiol. 2007;100(5):553–61.

Ray M, Kindler HL. Malignant pleural mesothelioma. An update on biomarkers and treatment. Chest. 2009;136:888–96.

Reid KF, Martin KI, Doros G, Clark DJ, Hau C, Patten C, Phillips EM, Frontera WR, Fielding RA. Comparative effects of light or heavy resistance power training for improving lower extremity power and physical performance in mobility-limited older adults. J Gerontol. 2015;70(3):374–80.

Rick, Metz T, Eberlein M, Schirren J, Bölükbas S. The six-minute-walk test in assessing respiratory function after tumor surgery on the lung: a cohort study. J Thorac Dis. 2014;6(5):421–8.

Sachs S, Weinberg RL. Pulmonary rehabilitation for dyspnea in the palliative-care setting. Curr Opin Support Palliat Care. 2009;3:112–9.

Salhi B, Haenebalcke C, Perez-Bogerd S, Nguyen MD, Ninane V, Malfait TLA, Vermaelen KY, Surmont VF, Van Maele G, Colman R, Derom E, van Meerbeeck JP. Rehabilitation in patients with radically treated respiratory cancer: a randomised controlled trial comparing two training modalities. Lung Cancer. 2015;89:167–74.

Salminen EK, Silvoniemi M, Syrjänen K, Kaasa S, Kloke M, Klepstad P. Opioids in pain management of mesothelioma and lung cancer patients. Acta Oncol. 2013;52:30–7.

Santiago-Palma J, Payne R. Palliative care and rehabilitation. Cancer. 2001;92(4):1049–52.

Schwartz RM, Watson A, Wolf A, Flores R, Taioli E. The impact of surgical approach on quality of life for pleural malignant mesothelioma. Ann Transl Med. 2017;5(11):230–7.

Shannon VR. Role of pulmonary rehabilitation in the management of patients with lung cancer. Curr Opin Pulm Med. 2010;16(4):334–9.

Stubblefield MD. Radiation fibrosis syndrome: neuromuscular and musculoskeletal complications in cancer survivors. PM&R. 2011;3:1041–54.

Syrett E, Taylor J. Non-pharmacological management of breathlessness: a collaborative nurse-physiotherapist approach. Int J Palliat Nurs. 2003;9:150–8.

Tanaka T, Morishita S, Hashimoto M, Itani Y, Mabuchi S, Kodama N, Hasegawa S, Domen K. Physical function and health-related quality of life in patients undergoing surgical treatment for malignant pleural mesothelioma. Support Care Cancer. 2017;25(8):2569–75.

Tata MJ, Mink PJ, Lau E, Sceurman BK, Foster ED. US mesothelioma patterns 1973–2002: indicators and insights into background rates. Eur J Cancer Prev. 2008;17:525–34.

Tiep B, Sun V, Koczywas M, Kim J, Raz D, Hurria A, Hayter J. Pulmonary rehabilitation and palliative care of the lung cancer patient. J Hosp Palliat Nurs. 2015;17(5):462–8.

Wang XS, Cleeland CS, Mendoza TR, Yun YH, Yang Y, Okuyama T, Johnson VE. Impact of cultural and linguistic factors on symptom reporting by patients with cancer. J Natl Cancer Inst. 2010;102:732–8.

Wang XS, Zhao F, Fisch MJ, O'Mara AM, Cella D, Mendoza TR, Cleeland CS. Prevalence and characteristics of moderate to severe fatigue. Cancer. 2014;120:425–32.

Yanez B, Pearman T, Lis CG, Beaumont JL, Cella D. The FACT-G7: a rapid version of the functional assessment of cancer therapy general (FACT-G) for monitoring symptoms and concerns in oncology practice and research. Ann Oncol. 2013;24:1073–8.

Zalcman G, Mazieres J, Margery J, Greillier L, Audigier-Valette C, Moro-Sibilot D, Molinier O, Corre R, Monnet I, Gounant V, Rivière F, Janicot J, Gervais R, Locher C, Milleron B, Tran Q, Lebitasy MP, Morin F, Creveuil C, Parienti JJ, Scherpereel A, on behalf of French Cooperative Thoracic Intergroup. Bevacizumab for newly diagnosed pleural mesothelioma in the Mesothelioma Avastin Cisplatin Pemetrexed Study (MAPS): a randomised, controlled, openlabel, phase 3 trial. The Lancet. Published online, December 21, 2015.

Rodney Hemingway

Dedication

My dad didn't want to die. He was 61. He and my mom had just built their dream retirement house, a beautiful log home on a lake. Then, in March of 2016, he started to have a persistent cough. He was initially diagnosed with pneumonia. Several courses of antibiotics didn't cure it. After a number of fruitless visits to various physicians, he was finally diagnosed with mesothelioma. That was around June of 2016. He had desmoplastic sarcomatoid mesothelioma. The worst type. Surgeons in Boston tried surgery, but that failed. Dad was on multiple cycles of chemotherapy that worked for only about 6 weeks. Then the tumor stopped responding. He passed away in hospice care in April 2017. He was exposed to asbestos through his work. As a union president, he had seen individuals in his membership suffer from and pass away from this awful disease. I write this for him. I write it for them. My dad was the model of a man I hope 1 day to mold myself into. I love you Dad.

1   Introduction

What is mesothelioma? It is a cancer of the pleural lining of the thorax. The pleura is a thin membrane-like sac that lines the thoracic cavity (Røe and Stella 2015). It affects the lining around the lungs (pleural mesothelioma) or the lining of the abdomen (peritoneal mesothelioma) and is caused by asbestos exposure (Wagner et al. 1960). It is a highly lethal cancer, with a median survival rate of 12 months (Røe and Stella 2015). Asbestos is a plentiful naturally occurring mineral that has been used in everything from shipbuilding to construction products, fire-resistant materials (e.g., jewelry maker gloves), cement, brake pads, and spray-on products such as

R. Hemingway (✉)
Mesothelioma Applied Research Foundation, Washington, DC, USA

© Springer Nature Switzerland AG 2019   121
M. Hesdorffer, G. E. Bates-Pappas (eds.), *Caring for Patients with Mesothelioma: Principles and Guidelines*,
https://doi.org/10.1007/978-3-319-96244-3_11

popcorn ceilings (Becklake et al. 2007). This chapter will discuss how occupational therapy can help patients with mesothelioma recover from treatment or adapt to living with the disease.

The allied health professions of physical and occupational therapy play an important role in the recovery of patients with thoracic cancers like mesothelioma. If a patient has undergone a thoracic-based surgery to treat peritoneal or pleural mesothelioma, it is likely that both rehab disciplines will be indicated during recovery. This chapter will focus on the role that occupational therapy plays in the treatment of mesothelioma.

Rehabilitation services first became critical components of the American healthcare system during the polio pandemic of the late 1800s and mid-1900s (Moffat 2012) in addition to the aftermath of the two world wars. Many individuals endured functional deficits which required them to relearn the basic skills of walking, bathing, dressing, eating, and speaking. This was the interface by which physical therapy and occupational therapy evolved into more widespread use in healthcare. Dunlop (1933) described the meaning of occupational therapy as the use of "interesting work" (p. 6) to assist patients recover from whatever ailed them. The American Occupational Therapy Association (2002) identifies the profession as one that helps patients function in their environments more successfully through the therapeutic use of meaningful activities or occupations. Occupation, simply defined, is any "everyday life activity" (p. 610). In the United States, a master's degree is required for entry-level occupational therapists, and by 2027, all new graduates will require a doctoral-level preparation (aota.org statement on ACOTE decision). In addition to these educational requirements, therapists must also pass a national board certification exam and apply for licensure in their state of practice. In order to maintain good standing with the National Board for Certification in Occupational Therapy (NBCOT) and use the designation of Occupational Therapist Registered (OTR), a therapist must complete 36 units of continuing education credits every 3 years. Additionally, the profession of occupational therapy utilizes an assistant model, who are known as Certified Occupational Therapy Assistants (COTAs). COTAs are associates degree-prepared clinicians and work under the supervision of an OTR. Like OTRs, the professional education for COTAs will be upgraded in 2027 when a bachelor's degree will be required for entry-level clinicians.

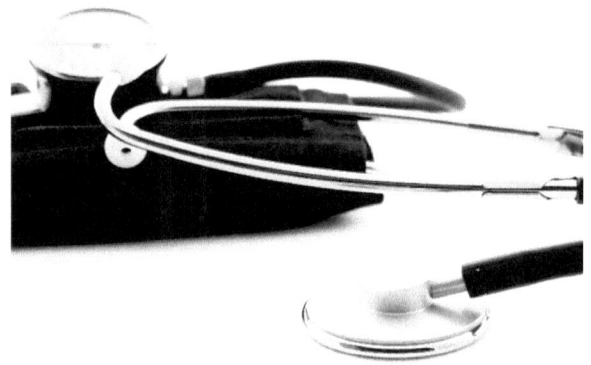

2   Occupational Therapy in the Acute Hospital Setting

Occupational therapy will assess a patient's ability to perform basic activities of daily living (ADLs) such as bathing, dressing, toileting, and transfers. Therapists will utilize these activities as a means of restoring functional endurance and independence. Education on compensatory and adaptive strategies for performing basic self-care tasks will be provided in an attempt to restore some semblance of control over an otherwise unwieldy situation and can help patients gird themselves for the lengthy recovery time ahead of them.

Occupational therapists commonly utilize an assessment tool. One tool that is used by occupational therapists in both the acute and subacute settings to track progress is called the Functional Independence Measure (FIM). It was created by Keith et al. (1987) as a means to track progress across 18 functional areas. Each area is scored on an ordinal scale from 0 to 7. Table 11.1 gives an overview of this grading system.

During this phase of treatment, the occupational therapist will often introduce adaptive equipment to help the patient complete their daily tasks as independently as possible. Some of the equipment a therapist might suggest are reachers, sock aids, long-handled shoe horns, and leg assist devices (Fig. 11.1).

Table 11.1   Terms to describe levels of assistance needed

Level of assistance	% of activity where assistance is required
Dependence (D) [1]	>75%
Maximum assistance (max A) [2]	50–75%
Moderate assistance (mod A) [3]	25–50%
Minimum assistance (min A) [4]	<25%
Supervision (S) [5]	No physical assistance needed, but direct supervision by another person required
Modified independence [6]	Use of adaptive equipment required, but no verbal or physical assistance needed
Independence (I) [7]	Totally independent without need for adaptive equipment

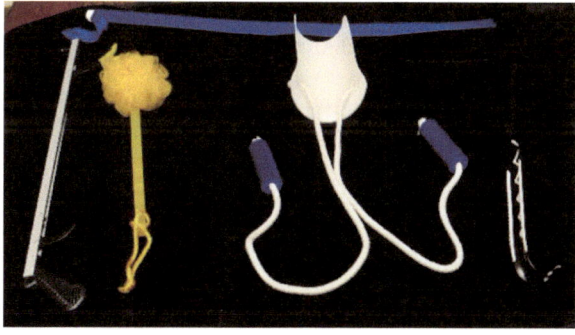

Fig. 11.1   (L–R) Reacher, long-handled loofa, sock aid, long-handled shoe horn. Across top: leg assist

Patients will often transition from acute inpatient rehabilitation to a subacute setting once their medical needs are stabilized. It is in the subacute setting that more frequent and intensive therapy sessions take center stage in the journey toward increased independence and return to daily life.

3   Occupational Therapy in Subacute Rehabilitation

Subacute rehabilitation facilities in the United States can exist as stand-alone locations, can be a component of a large medical campus, or can be a part of a nursing home (also known as a skilled nursing facility or SNF). Rehabilitation is the primary focus in these settings to help patients regain the skills necessary to resume ADLs (activities of daily living) and IADLs (instrumental activities of daily living) as near to their prior level of function as possible.

Occupational therapy (OT) will assess for baseline level of function and focus on advancing independence in the areas of ADLs (dressing, bathing, toileting, self-feeding, and mobility) and IADLs (such as meal preparation, laundry tasks, housekeeping, managing finances and medication management). One tool that is used by occupational therapists in both the acute and subacute settings to track progress is called the Functional Independence Measure (FIM). It was created by Keith et al. (1987) as a means to track progress across 18 functional areas. Each area is scored on an ordinal scale from 0 to 7. These areas of function are typically taken for granted during times of good health; however, these can quickly become overwhelming in the setting of major disease and dysfunction.

OTs are experts at problem-solving ways to modify and grade activities to promote independence and safety. They may work with patients and caregivers to teach compensatory strategies to perform functional tasks, educate on adaptive equipment and durable medical equipment that may be of benefit, provide training on safe techniques for functional transfers and mobility, and educate on energy conservation strategies and breathing techniques during activities. Possible questions that a patient with mesothelioma may wonder are as follows: "How can I dress myself when it's difficult to bend and twist? How can I safely and efficiently prepare a stovetop meal while wearing supplemental oxygen? How can I safely do a load of laundry in the context of my lifting precautions post thoracic surgery? How can my partner and I resume sexual activity in a way that is safe and comfortable for both us?" These are some of the everyday questions that occupational therapy begins to address in the subacute setting.

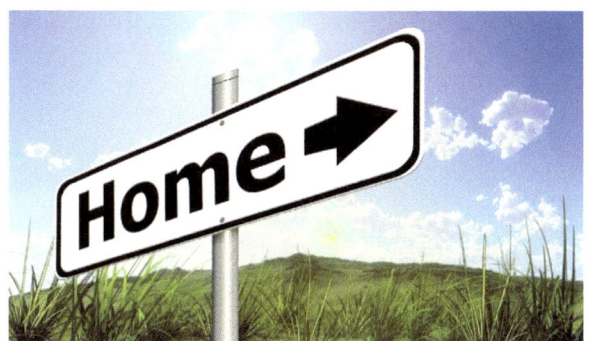

4 Occupational Therapy and Home Care

It is frequently indicated to continue occupational therapy for mesothelioma patients once they transition to their home environment. Home care services under Medicare guidelines are covered if a patient is considered "homebound." The definition of "homebound" can be distilled as "the act of leaving the home is a considerable and taxing effort" (Centers for Medicare and Medicaid). Occupational therapy in the home setting will typically begin with a home safety evaluation, and recommendations will be provided to reduce the likelihood of falls and injury. Environmental recommendations may include removal of scatter rugs, improvement of lighting, and clearing pathways for safe mobility. Occupational therapy will partner with physical therapy in the home safety evaluation with particular focus on bedroom, bathroom, and kitchen accessibility.

4.1 Bedroom Accessibility

The home visiting OT may suggest relocating the patient's bed to the first floor of a residence if it is a multilevel home. Stairs often become a particularly taxing endeavor, and one-level living may be beneficial for mesothelioma patients due the poor endurance and dyspnea associated with the condition. Sleeping positions are also likely to vary for the patient with mesothelioma. In some cases, a standard bed will be sufficient: however, given the weakness that often accompanies a patient with mesothelioma, extra help may be required to get in and out of a standard bed. An OT might recommend a bed assist rail in this instance. This device provides a stable anchor point for the patient to maneuver in and out of bed without the aid of another person.

The use of a *bed wedge* may be suggested if the patient prefers to sleep in their own bed but needs to have their upper body elevated. Sleeping wedges come in many different sizes and angles. The therapist will partner with the patient to determine which type of wedge is most effective (Fig. 11.2).

Another device that can prove quite helpful for patients with mesothelioma is a *bed assist rail*. This piece of equipment provides an anchor for the individual to hold onto when getting into or out of bed. It has utility at all stages of disease progression and treatment. In Figure 11.3, the *bed assist rail* is in white, and a 3:1 commode is positioned next to the bed (Fig. 11.3).

Fig. 11.2 Bed wedge

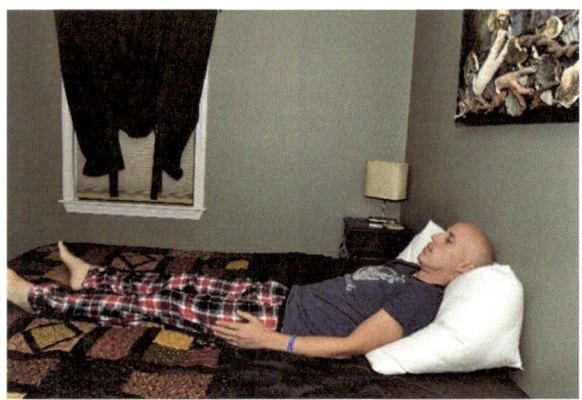

Fig. 11.3 Bed assist rail and bedside commode

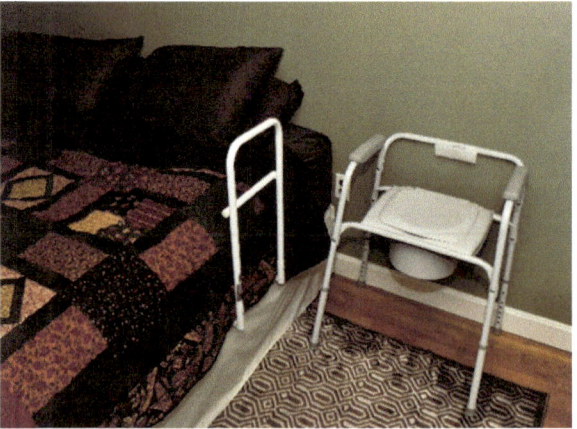

Fig. 11.4 A hospital bed

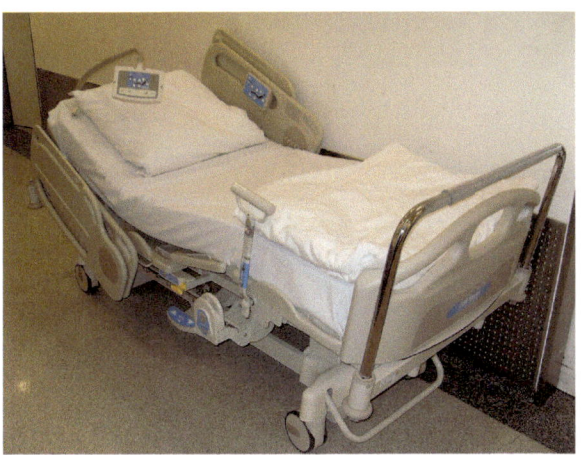

In some cases, a hospital bed may be preferable to increase comfort and ease during bed mobility and transfers. There are two main types of hospital beds: a *semi-electric hospital bed* and a *fully electric hospital bed*. The semi-electric hospital bed has a remote that allows for control of both the head and foot aspects of the bed in order to elevate or flatten the bed to the desired resting position. In most cases, this type of bed is adequate to meet a patient's needs. Fully electric hospital beds add the feature of raising and lowering the height of the entire bed itself. This feature allows for caregivers to adjust the height of the bed in order to maintain proper body mechanics when assisting a patient during sponge baths or repositioning. The semi-electric hospital bed often has a hand crank to make bed height adjustments as well (Fig. 11.4).

An alternative sleeping position for mesothelioma patients may not be supine or semi-supine in the hospital bed, but rather positioned in a recliner chair. As an alternative to the traditional recliner chair, a *lift recliner chair* can be suggested. This chair contains a small mechanized lift apparatus and is remote control operated. It allows a patient to maintain an increased level of independence during transfers and autonomy to adjust the chair to the desired level of incline. Additionally, it can decrease the risk for caregiver injury by minimizing the patient's need for physical assistance during transfers. Also, by adjusting the incline with the remote, pressure relief can be achieved by either the patient or the caregiver (Fig. 11.5).

Fig. 11.5 Lift recliner
chair

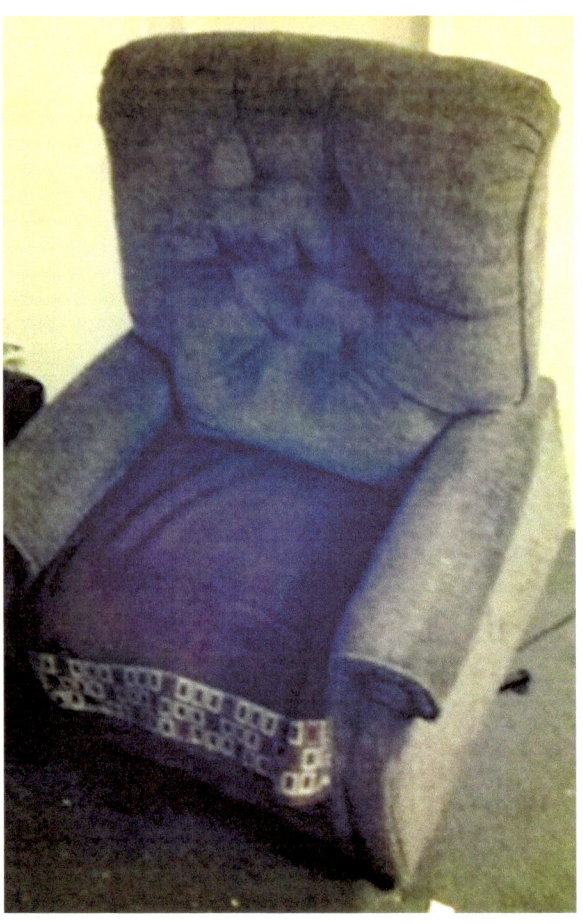

4.2   Bathroom Accessibility

Occupational therapists are specialists in bathroom assessment and modification. Recommendations for durable medical equipment and environmental adaptations may be provided for patients who have undergone thoracic surgery to treat their mesothelioma and present with weakness, deconditioning, balance impairments, or pain. Specific occupational therapy recommendations may vary due to the unique needs of individual patients based on disease progression and environmental factors. Often times a standard height toilet of 13–15 inches presents a challenge for transfers. There are several options to increase the height of a toilet including installation of a *toilet seat riser* or *raised toilet seat*, both of which can be obtained with or without arm rests. The toilet seat riser is often the preferred

Fig. 11.6 Toilet seat riser (also known as an elevated toilet seat)

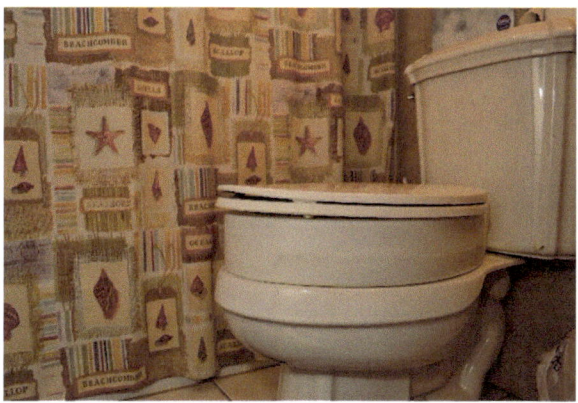

piece of equipment due to a more secure attachment and inconspicuous design. This equipment elevates the toilet between 3 and 4.5 inches and increases ease with sit to stand transfers (Fig. 11.6).

Another option is to obtain a *3-in-1 commode* which can be used bedside or placed over the toilet. The option to use a bedside commode is typically recommended for patients who are unable to safely access the bathroom or have difficulty ambulating to the bathroom during the night. Mesothelioma patients who have severe dyspnea related to disease progression or severe pain with mobility may benefit from a bedside commode (Fig. 11.7).

Therapists may recommend installation of *grab bars* near the toilet and inside the tub or shower unit. Grab bars are utilized to maintain balance, decrease fatigue, and withstand partial body weight during transfers. Steel grab bars should be professionally installed but are the preferred grab bar option for safety (Fig. 11.8).

A *tub assist rail* is a good solution where permanent grab bars are not an option or where they might be temporarily needed. They secure to the edge of the tub with a vice clamp design to offer a secure handhold (Fig. 11.9).

Durable medical equipment such as a shower chair or *tub transfer bench* may be recommended to perform bathing tasks while seated in order to maintain balance and conserve energy. A tub transfer bench is particularly useful if a patient demonstrates difficulty stepping over the threshold of a tub.

As seen in this accompanying picture, a tub transfer bench straddles the tub threshold enabling patients to safely sit on the edge of the bench, lift their lower extremities over the tub threshold while seated, and then slide to the center of the bench (Fig. 11.10).

Other recommendations may include the use of a *handheld shower head* and *nonslip bath mat.* For patients where disease progression is significant, these devices can help the patient to maintain good personal hygiene while minimizing the risk for falls and offsetting effects of progressive dyspnea (Fig. 11.11).

Fig. 11.7 3-in-1 commode (a.k.a. bedside commode) used over the toilet as a toilet safety frame

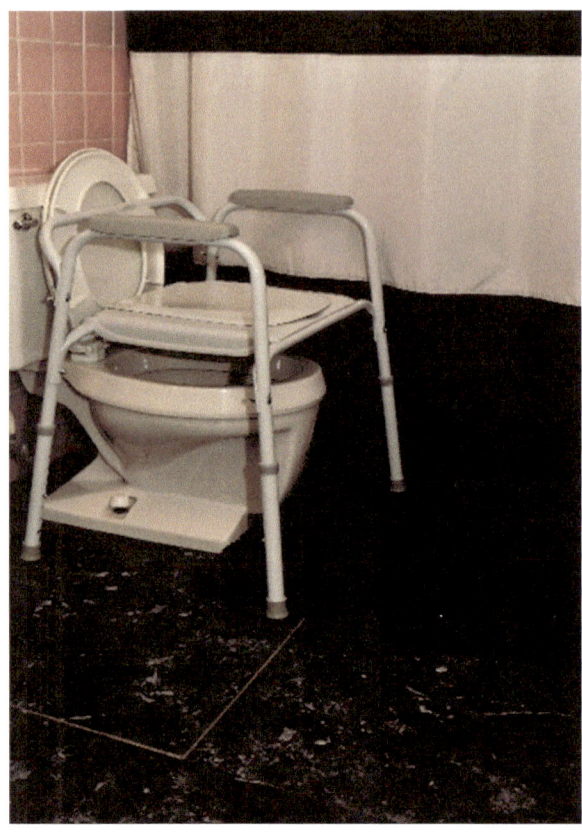

Fig. 11.8 Grab bar installed in bathtub

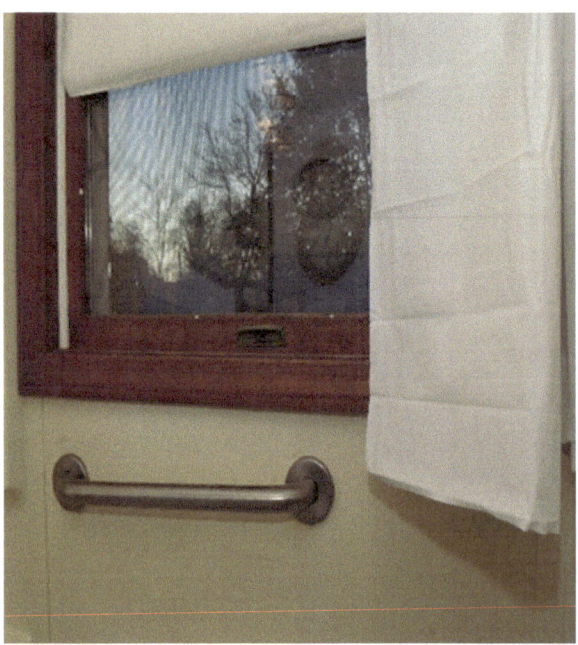

Fig. 11.9 Tub assist rail

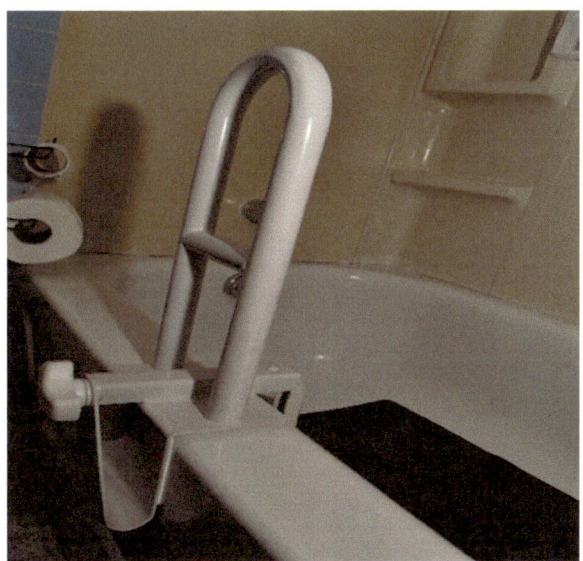

Fig. 11.10 Tub transfer bench

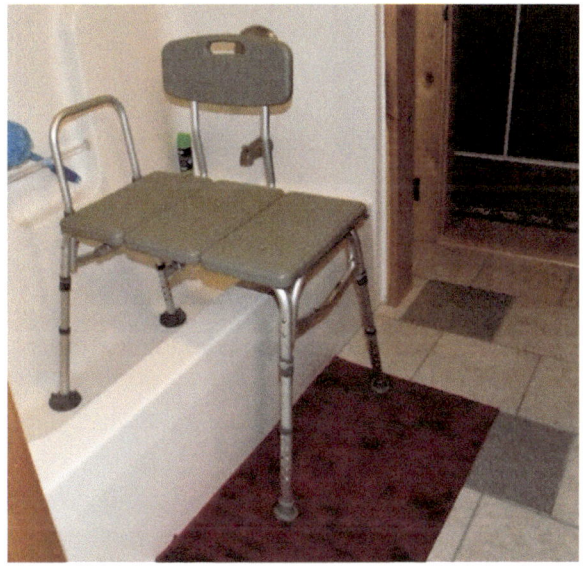

Fig. 11.11 Handheld
shower head

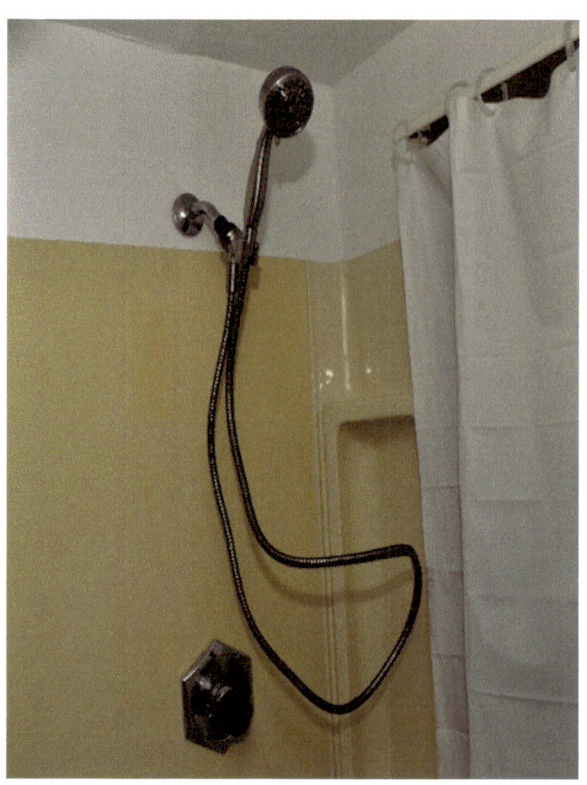

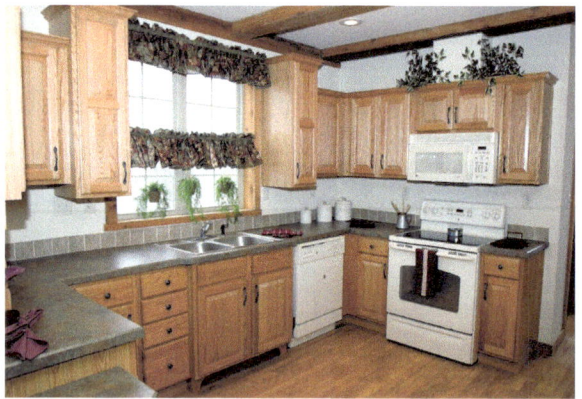

4.3   Kitchen Accessibility

The occupational therapist will assess the storage locations of food stuffs, regularly used plates, bowls, cups, etc. and suggest accessible locations. OT uses the terminology "safe functional reach" to mean the distance an individual can safely extend their arm while maintaining adequate balance to minimize the risk for falls. It is adapted from the definition of functional reach from Whitney et al. (Sept 1998) which "…is the difference in inches between a person's arm length and maximal forward reach with the shoulder flexed to 90° while maintaining a fixed base of support in standing" (p. 667). Factors such as dyspnea level, pain, and limited upper extremity range of motion may all negatively impact a mesothelioma patient's safe functional reach. The functional reach test (Duncan et al., 1990), which measures the functional reach of a patient, can also be used as an outcome measure (Whitney et al. 1998). Education may be required for safe mobility and item transport in the kitchen if learning to utilize an adaptive device such as a rolling walker to compensate for weakness or balance impairments. OTs will teach work simplification and energy conservation strategies for meal preparation and kitchen management.

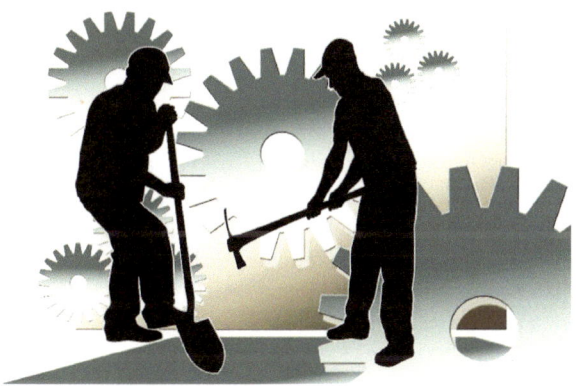

5   Return to Life After Cancer

For oncology patients who achieve remission or stable disease status, occupational therapy will aim to enhance a patient's quality of life (Strong 1987). OT will remain focused on functional outcomes as a measure of success. Reinforcement of work simplification and energy conservation strategies will be a primary focus. OT may suggest that patients create a list of favorite leisure pursuits and then guide them in understanding how their current functional limitations (e.g., ongoing dyspnea, chronic pain, dry mouth, etc.) may impact the resumption of these activities (e.g., golf, running, playing music, etc.). This process, as always, is led by the patient. Schule (2013) identifies engaging in physical activity as a beneficial component of an overall rehabilitation program to build endurance and strength.

Table 11.2 Borg rating of perceived exertion scale (Borg 1982)

Grade	Description
6	
7	Very, very light
8	
9	Very light
10	
11	Fairly light
12	
13	Somewhat hard
14	
15	Hard
16	
17	Very hard
18	
19	Very, very hard
20	

As Strong (1987) states, "When a person loses the ability or desire to perform his or her work, play or self-care activities, dysfunction results. It is such role dysfunction which requires occupational therapy intervention" (p. 4). Therapists will use the role, or occupation, that the patient wishes to resume and will partner with them to develop a plan for doing so. At this stage of treatment, the use of the Borg Scale of Perceived Exertion (see Table 11.2) can be applied and used as a guide for the patient to monitor progress.

The clinician can use the Borg scale (also known as the RPE scale) as a pre-activity check to understand the patient's perception of the challenge at hand. The Borg Scale is also used as a posttest and at other desired time points to monitor progress and functional gains (Crisafulli and Clini 2010).

Since OT is anchored in function, a treatment session will often include components of an actual activity that a patient wishes to resume. For example, if the patient is an avid gardener, the OT may suggest the first step be to create a task checklist of items needed for gardening. Next, a discussion may be had of skills required for participation in the activity of gardening. From the checklist, an OT may suggest modifications, adaptations, and grading of the activity to avoid over-exertion of the patient. For example, this may translate into caregiver assistance with any initial tilling of the soil while the patient acts as supervisor. Having a chair available for needed rest breaks affords the patient the opportunity to gradually restore functional endurance. Once the soil is tilled, the patient might actively participate by dropping seeds onto the soil. This is an example of a meaningful occupation-based activity.

An outpatient occupational therapist may focus on work rehabilitation for patients who have a goal to return to the workplace. First, an assessment of the patient's workplace requirements and job tasks is completed. The patient's goals for returning to work are discussed, a treatment plan is created, and work-centered rehabilitation takes place. Patients can be referred to work rehabilitation clinics where they can gradually reacquire the skills and functional endurance required and expected for resuming work tasks at their job site (AOTA 2017). The OT will utilize an activity analysis model when developing goals and treatment interventions. Activity analysis is "the identification of the demands of the activity and the skills required to perform it" (Joss 2007, p. 301). An occupational therapist may perform back to work assessments as part of a Functional Capacity Evaluation (FCE) which is utilized to determine a patient's fitness for work duties (Suckley 2017). Gibson and Strong (2003) identify the historical use of Functional Capacity Evaluations by Australian occupational therapists for just these types of assessment needs.

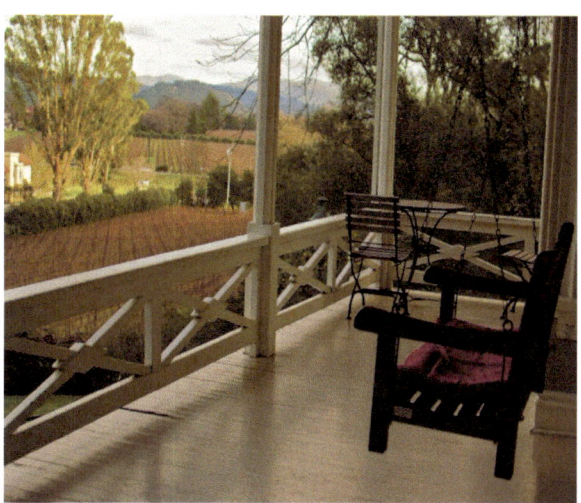

6 Occupational Therapy and Palliative Care

When intervention is no longer primarily curative in intent, palliative care is offered. The goal of palliative care is to improve quality of life through symptom management to minimize pain and discomfort (Morrison and Meier 2004). OT has a role to play for patients and caregivers in this area of treatment as well. While objective measures and clinical evaluation continue to be essential in palliative care, it is also important for treatment to be patient-centered and directed (Cooper 2006). Occupational therapists are always concerned with the "functional implications of symptoms" (Cooper 2006, p. 27), and the clinician will aim to minimize or ease the functional degradation of the patient for as long as possible. This may include revisiting adaptive equipment such as *reachers, sock aids, long-handled sponges, long-handled shoe horns*, etc. that was mentioned earlier in this chapter. The OT will collaborate with the rest of the care team to ensure pressure-relieving surfaces are included with any hospital bed and teach the patient and caregivers about pressure injury prevention strategies. Please see Table 11.3 for pressure injury prevention teaching strategies.

Table 11.3 Pressure injury prevention

Pressure injury prevention strategies
Reposition the patient every 1–2 hours
If the patient is unable to reposition self, utilize pillows, alternating pressure mattress, etc. to help provide pressure relief
Inspect high-risk areas regularly (coccyx, hips, heels)
Encourage the patient to consume as much protein sources and fluids as they can tolerate
Maintain dry/intact skin (includes sweat, urine, loose bowels, etc.)
Use protective underwear if incontinence is a concern and change when soiled

Given the pleural mesothelioma patient's worsening dyspnea in the palliative phase of the disease progression, a reclined position in a chair may provide greater symptom relief than a hospital bed can offer. The previously mentioned *lift recliner chair* is a good option in this instance.

7   Psychosocial Needs

Occupational therapists can offer some unique interventions for the symptom management of depression and anxiety. Patient-directed discussions related to personal hobbies, favorite sports teams, fond memories, etc. may be initiated with encouragement to participate in activities surrounding these areas. Activities might include creating scrapbooks of joyous life events or writing letters to loved ones. For some, it may be empowering them to participate in the writing of their obituary. This can be incredibly difficult for patients, families, and even clinicians but is an often ignored area of care. Engaging in these types of difficult discussions with a therapist can help ease the burden of fear for patients and enable them to manage their mortality with the words that will become their immortal selves. If it is the patient's wish to pursue writing the obituary, an occupational therapist can provide guidance and examples of other obituaries, templates, and suggestions for inclusion (e.g., an award at work, a particularly proud moment, child's schooling, etc.). This author guided his own father in the creation of his obituary, and it was one of the most uncomfortable and difficult things he has ever done. He helped correct the chronology, reminded his dad of an important life event he omitted, and edited spelling errors. Since the passing of his father, he has come to cherish this experience as one of the final projects that he teamed up with his father to complete. Awkward, emotionally raw discussions in palliative care are crucial to ensure the patient's experience is authentic and true to them. Indeed, "the most common complaint made by patients with cancer are about poor communication and inadequate information" (Sowden et al. 2001, p. 193).

The occupational therapist will also look to encourage discussions about spirituality if that is of importance to the patient. It is not the role of the OT to promote a religious experience, but rather to guide the patient to create their own if desired. In functional terms this may be the creation of a small prayer space in the patient's primary room. It may be obtaining access to spiritual music available on demand via speech-activated devices such as the Amazon Echo, Google Home, or Apple HomePod. Perhaps arranging visits from friends or spiritual leaders from their church, synagogue, or temple is what the patient prefers. The occupational therapist will seek to remind the patient to keep these visits brief as end-stage mesothelioma patients become dyspneic very quickly with speech. A functional strategy for managing dyspnea in the context of visiting guests could be the creation of a visual schedule displayed on a wall as a reminder to keep visits under a set time limit, or employing an alarm clock to provide an auditory reminder.

8   Summary

In conclusion, mesothelioma is a very challenging condition for both patient and caregiver. Occupational therapy offers strategies and equipment recommendations to help cope with it. During the recovery phase, occupational therapists can help the patient with mesothelioma restore their ability to be independent in daily life tasks. They can also help prepare the patient to return to work. Given occupational therapy's unique combination of physical and psychosocial rehabilitation components, the discipline is appropriate to be referred into a case of mesothelioma at all phases of care. As treatments emerge that allow more and more patients live longer with the disease, occupational therapy will be there to help them live meaningful and functional lives as possible.

References

American Occupational Therapy Association. Occupational therapy practice framework: domain and process. Am J Occup Ther. 2002;56(6):609–39.

American Occupational Therapy Association. Occupational therapy services in facilitating work participation and performance. Am J Occup Ther. 2017;71(Suppl. 2):7112410010p1–711241 0010p10.

Becklake MR, Bagatin E, Neder JA. Asbestos related diseases of the lung and pleura: uses, trends, and management over the last century. Int J Tuberc Lung Dis. 2007;11(4):356–69.

Borg GAV. Psychophysical bases of perceived exertion. Med Sci Sports Exerc. 1982;14(5):377–81.

Centers for Medicare and Medicaid. https://www.cms.gov/Regulations-and-Guidance/Guidance/Transmittals/downloads/R192BP.pdf

Cooper J. Occupational therapy in oncology and palliative care. West Sussex: Whurr Publishers Limited; 2006.

Crisafulli E, Clini EM. Measures of dyspnea in pulmonary rehabilitation. Multidiscip Respir Med. 2010;5(3):202–10.

Duncan PW, Weiner DK, Chandler J, Studenski S. Functional reach: a new clinical measure of balance. J Gerontol. Nov 1990;45(6):M192–7.

Dunlop WJ. A brief history of occupational therapy. Can J Occup Ther. 1933;1(1):6–10.

Gibson L, Strong J. A conceptual framework of functional capacity evaluation for occupational therapy in work rehabilitation. Aust Occup Ther J. 2003;50:64–71.

Joss M. The importance of job analysis in occupational therapy. Br J Occup Ther. 2007;70(7):301–3.

Keith RA, Granger CV, Hamilton BB, Sherwin FS. The functional independence measure: a new tool for rehabilitation. Adv Clin Rehabil. 1987;1:6–18.

Moffat M. A history of physical therapy education around the world. J Phys Ther Educ. 2012;26(1):13–23.

Morrison RS, Meier DE. Palliative care. N Engl J Med. 2004;350:2582–90.

Røe OD, Stella GM. Malignant pleural mesothelioma: history, controversy and future of a man made epidemic. Eur Respir Rev. 2015;24:115–31.

Schule K. Thirty years of physical activity in oncology in Germany – from the birth of the first rehabilitative cancer sports group until today. Eur Rev Aging Phys Act. 2013;10:61–4.

Sowden AJ, Forbes C, Entwistle V, Watt I. Informing, communicating, and sharing decisions with people who have cancer. Qual Health Care. 2001;10:193–6.

Strong J. Occupational therapy and cancer rehabilitation. Br J Occup Ther. 1987;50(1):4–6.

Suckley N. Assessing fitness for work: a guide. Occup Health. 2017;69(3):22–4.

Wagner JC, Sleggs CA, Marchand P. Diffuse pleural mesothelioma and asbestos exposure in the north western cape district. Br J Ind Med. 1960;17:260–71.

Whitney SL, Poole JL, Cass SP. A review of balance instruments for older adults. Am J Occup Ther. 1998;52(8):666–71.

Respiratory Therapy and Pulmonary Rehabilitation for Mesothelioma Patients

Olivia Chung and Jadmin L. Mostel

Dedication
I dedicate this chapter to my husband John, who has stood by my side through my own battle with Mesothelioma, as well as my supportive immediate family, and to my guardian angels above for protecting me through it all, my mother and grandmother.

Respiratory care in a patient diagnosed with pleural mesothelioma begins with assessing and addressing symptoms, which are most often defined as dyspnea. Those exhibiting dyspnea may experience sensations such as the inability to receive air (air hunger), labored effort to breathe, smothering or suffocating, and/or the feeling of chest tightness (Koelwyn et al. 2012; Williams et al. 2012). As a result, many patients that struggle with the debilitating effects of dyspnea avoid engaging in physical activity, have difficulty breathing at rest, and have an overall lessening of their quality of life (Koelwyn et al. 2012). Pulmonary rehabilitation is a palliative care mechanism that can aid in the relief of symptoms and can help patients regain mobility and confidence while navigating the challenges of pleural mesothelioma (Tiep et al. 2015).

The primary concept of a pulmonary patient is not to see how far the patient can push themselves but rather to build up stamina and endurance of accessory muscle use (Tiep et al. 2015). Setting reasonable and realistic goals for the patient undergoing pulmonary rehabilitation is key to encourage patient rehab and monitor symptom improvement. Patients may feel overwhelmed and hesitant about partaking in physical activity when simply breathing at rest proves difficult; however, exercise rehabilitation seeks to improve symptoms through gas exchange with more efficient

O. Chung
The Valley Hospital, Ridgewood, NJ, USA

J. L. Mostel (✉)
Johns Hopkins Bloomberg School of Public Health, Baltimore, MD, USA

© Springer Nature Switzerland AG 2019
M. Hesdorffer, G. E. Bates-Pappas (eds.), *Caring for Patients with Mesothelioma: Principles and Guidelines*,
https://doi.org/10.1007/978-3-319-96244-3_12

oxygen uptake and carbon dioxide elimination on a long-term scale with the goal of reducing and managing dyspnea symptoms (Tiep et al. 2015).

Pulmonary rehab patients are encouraged to monitor pulse oxygen levels and heart rate at rest, before, during, and after exercising, as well as anytime they may be experiencing shortness of breath. Ideally, patients are asked to check and monitor these vital signs to see if they require inhaled medication such as bronchodilators (rescue inhalers, metered-dose inhalers, or nebulizer treatments) to dilate the bronchial tubes and administer supplemental oxygen therapy or if patients have anxiety or stress-related hyperventilating. Portable pulse oximeters, which are small, battery-operated devices, provide a noninvasive mean to produce an oxygen level and heart rate reading. Once patients can determine a "baseline" of their resting heart rate and pulse ox readings, respiratory therapists and pulmonary rehabilitationists can set goals for the patient's target heart rate and sp02 levels during exertion (Tiep et al. 2015).

To measure how hard a patient is working to breath is determined by a scale of exertion, or the "RPE scale" (see Occupational Therapy and Mesothelioma chapter for further discussion).

1   Exercising and Pulmonary Rehab

There are an array of modalities or exercise equipment that can build a patient's endurance. Not all patients will use the same tools, but all will have similar goals: stretching and easing the muscles into activity, performing aerobic exercise and reaching maximum established heart rate, lightweight training and cooling down stretches, and giving the heart and lungs a chance to come back to their "resting" measurements. In most pulmonary rehabs, treadmills can be used for patients who can confidently walk safely and are not fall risks. For patients who are unsteady, are very weak, or have other ailments preventing them from being a "free walking" candidate, other equipment can be provided for the patient to sit but be able to maintain aerobic exercise promotion. Patients are encouraged to also exercise upper body strength with the aid of arm ergometers and repetitive exertion of lightweight training for the triceps, biceps, and deltoid muscles (Koelwyn et al. 2012).

Proper relaxation, stress, and emotional support also play a significant role in pulmonary rehabilitation, as such emotions have a direct effect on the nature of one's respiratory status. The sensations of dyspnea are not limited to only unpleasantness of physical symptoms but are also emotional and behavioral in patients due to its crippling nature (Koelwyn et al. 2012). Patients often feel a loss of confidence, increased anxiety, and an overall decrease in mental well-being from the effects of dyspnea. It is recommended for patients to use pursed-lip and diaphragmatic breathing as an exercise to reduce the air trapping caused by anxiety and hyperventilation (Tiep et al. 2015). Pursed-lip breathing is a form of "breath training" that emphasizes the patient to take slow, deep breaths through the nose and to exhale out through tight lips. This maneuver engenders a slower heart rate, improves oxygenation levels, and lowers the respiratory rate. This exercise allows for retaining carbon dioxide to be released as the exhalation time is prolonged and allows for the patient's airways to gain positive expiratory pressure causing the patient inflation. This method has a calming effect and can stabilize respiratory tachypnea in a matter of minutes.

2 Avoiding Exacerbation

Patients can abide by physician's orders and remain compliantly active but there may be a time when exacerbation occurs. An exacerbation, or flare-up of symptoms, is one that can present itself at any given time. Some signs and/or symptoms of an exacerbation include but are not limited to increased shortness of breath at rest, coughing, sputum production, increased heart rate without exertion, chest pain, swelling, and fluid retention. Signs and symptoms of an exacerbation should be addressed and treated immediately to prevent further sickness, discomfort, and even hospital admittance. With rehab specialists, patients should discuss the avoidance of large crowds especially during cold and flu seasons, nicotine and second-hand smoke intake, cologne, perfume, strong-smelling cleaning or aerosol products, dust-accumulating items, and allergens that can induce hyper-reactive airways or further irritation of one's lung incapacities. In addition, patients wearing protective masks during cleaning as well as avoiding inhalation and close contact with strong smelling chemicals can avoid complications of lung aggravation (Williams et al. 2012).

In all, pleural mesothelioma patients experiencing breathing challenges may be helped by respiratory therapists and pulmonary rehabilitationists. It is important to address symptoms with medical practitioners to lessen the debilitating effects of dyspnea and to increase the quality of life of patients diagnosed with pleural mesothelioma. The palliative care offered by these specialists can significantly improve a patient's quality of life as they navigate treatment and can be equipped with care techniques for long-lasting self-care.

References

Koelwyn GJ, et al. Exercise therapy in the management of dyspnea in patients with cancer. Curr Opin Support Palliat Care. 2012;6(2):129–37. PMC. Web. 12 June 2018.
Tiep B, et al. Pulmonary rehabilitation and palliative care for the lung cancer patient. J Hosp Palliat Nurs. 2015;17(5):462–8. PMC. Web. 12 June 2018.
Williams AC, et al. Dyspnea management in early stage lung cancer: a palliative perspective. J Hosp Palliat Nurs. 2012;14(5). https://doi.org/10.1097/NJH.0b013e31825e4250. PMC. Web. 12 June 2018.

Palliative Care Services for Mesothelioma Patients

13

Schuyler Cunningham and Hunter Groninger

1   Introduction

People living with mesothelioma and other forms of cancer need and deserve holistic supportive care that focuses on alleviating distressing symptoms, providing person-centered support with medical decision-making and, when indicated, optimal end-of-life care. As a malignancy, mesothelioma is no exception in terms of needs and opportunities.

Palliative care is defined as interdisciplinary care that focuses on alleviating distress in people with a serious, progressive illness and their caregivers. Distress can be of any modality – physical, psychological, social, or existential/spiritual – reflecting the ways in which such an illness experience, such as mesothelioma, affects the whole person and their community (World Health Organization 2017).

Since the relatively recent inception of the field of palliative care (sometimes called palliative medicine, to emphasize medical interventions), scholarship has demonstrated clear impact on a variety of patient-centered outcomes, including improved management of pain, cough, dyspnea, cancer-related fatigue, depression, and anxiety, among others. The World Health Organization definition of palliative care correctly emphasizes that these supportive interventions should be available to patients and caregivers throughout the disease trajectory and implemented according to the needs of the individual (World Health Organization 2017).

As discussed elsewhere in this book, patients with mesothelioma, particularly in more advanced stages, are at high risk of distressing symptoms, low quality of life

S. Cunningham (✉)
Cancer Trauma Project, Washington, DC, USA
e-mail: schuyler@cancertrauma.com

H. Groninger
Georgetown University Medical Center, Washington, DC, USA
e-mail: hunter.groninger@medstar.net

© Springer Nature Switzerland AG 2019   143
M. Hesdorffer, G. E. Bates-Pappas (eds.), *Caring for Patients with Mesothelioma: Principles and Guidelines*,
https://doi.org/10.1007/978-3-319-96244-3_13

and functional status, psychosocial stressors, and death. In this chapter, we provide an overview of palliative care specific to the mesothelioma experience.

2   A Brief History for Context

The word *palliative* is derived from the Latin verb *palliare* – to cloak. Coined in 1973 by Canadian oncology surgeon Dr. Balfour Mount, the term emphasizes intention to shield or protect individuals from suffering associated with a life-threatening illness. The first hospital-based palliative medicine services were developed in Canada in the mid-1970s and in the United States in the late 1980s. Since then, hospital-based palliative services have continued to grow by almost 200% in the past 15 years now numbering over 1500 programs in the United States (Dumanovsky et al. 2016).

Between 80% and 90% of hospitals with at least 300 beds now have some form of palliative care clinical service; among smaller hospitals with greater than 50 beds, at least 55% have palliative services (Dumanovsky et al. 2016). In 2000 24.5% of hospitals with more than 50 beds had a palliative care program as compared to 75% in 2015 (Dumanovsky et al. 2016).

The growth of palliative care has primarily occurred in the context of cancer care. Initially focusing efforts on patients with very advanced illness, often at the end of life, palliative assessments and interventions have moved farther upstream in the disease trajectory, sometimes even being initiated at the time of diagnosis of disease or at least of progressive staging, which is the growing consensus of the literature (Gaertner et al. 2011; Temel et al. 2010).

3   When to Integrate Palliative Care for Mesothelioma

Gaertner et al. (2011) attempted to integrate palliative care into medical care by taking the WHO recommendations for palliative care a step further. They did this by seeking to identify the time point of integration for palliative care for different diseases, recognizing disease processes differ, and by further defining the clinical terms associated with palliative care to provide more guidelines for providers. Their work developed standard operating procedures for 19 different malignancies, which include a recommended time point for palliative intervention per malignancy (Gaertner et al. 2011).

Most relevant to the mesothelioma population is the literature that provides guidelines for people with lung cancer. The literature recommends that palliative care be integrated after staging of a malignancy and at the start of treatment, especially systemic treatment, and immediately after diagnosis of a metastasis or relapse (Dumanovsky et al. 2016; Gaertner et al. 2011). A consensus seems to be emerging among providers that referring patients to palliative care only after there are no more medical options is too late (Gaertner et al. 2011; Temel et al. 2010). Additionally, it is recommended that palliative care be provided at the same location as patients' treatment (e.g., in oncology clinics) to increase integration of care (Gaertner et al. 2011).

4 Improved Outcomes with Early Integration of Palliative Care

People living with cancer have particularly benefitted from this upstream shift with better symptom management aimed to improve functional status and quality of life. Temel et al. (2010) published a landmark study of people with metastatic non-small cell lung cancer and found that such early palliative care plus usual disease-modifying therapies had improved symptom control and depression compared to controls who did not receive early palliative care along with anticancer therapy. Moreover, they reported that the group that had early integration of palliative care received less chemotherapy and longer hospice care at the end of life (Temel et al. 2010). These findings have been confirmed in the literature (Gaertner et al. 2011).

The most striking finding from this study was that patients in the palliative care arm actually had improved mortality compared to controls, by 2.7 months (Temel et al. 2010). This may have been due to more effective treatment of depression, better management of symptoms, or less need for hospitalization. This unexpected finding at least begins to debunk the myth that palliative care leads to shorter life span. One clear result of this study has been widespread interest in palliative care expansion: recent guidelines from the American Society of Clinical Oncology recommend palliative care consultation for patients with notable symptom burden and with metastatic disease (Smith et al. 2012).

5 The Connection Between Hospice and Palliative Care

For both historical and clinical reasons, palliative care is often closely associated with hospice care – this association deserves important qualifications. In both North America and Europe, the modern hospice movement was designed to provide holistic end-of-life care to patients dying from terminal illnesses. The modern concept of "hospice" – originally in medieval times, a place of rest for travelers en route to a religious pilgrimage – was coined and first implemented by Dr. Cicely Saunders in Great Britain in the 1960s, where she founded St. Christopher's Hospice in London.

In the United States, hospice care started as a grassroots nursing movement modeled on Dr. Saunders's attention to "total pain" – that is, the physical, psychological, social, and existential forms of suffering that come with a terminal illness. There, the Medicare Hospice Benefit was created in the early 1980s, formally introducing hospice care as an insurance benefit to Medicare recipients. In subsequent decades, hospice services have grown remarkably in the United States, in general providing care to over 40% of eligible Medicare decedents, with an associated cost to Medicare of over $13 billion per year (Centers for Medicare and Medicaid 2014).

Both hospice care and palliative care emphasize interdisciplinary care of patient and caregivers and expert management of pain and other symptoms associated with advanced disease and facilitated communication and support to patients and caregivers, particularly around complex medical decision-making.

A critical distinction between hospice care and palliative care relates to patient eligibility criteria. Hospice care is designed for people who are dying from their respective illness: hence it is a prognosis-dependent service. The overwhelming majority of hospice providers in the United States require that a patient has a prognosis of 6 months or fewer before they are eligible to enroll in hospice care. This timeframe is driven by Medicare Part A requirements and is the general guideline followed by hospices (Gaertner et al. 2011).

By contrast, palliative care is designed for people with a serious progressive illness who have specific needs for symptom management, supportive counseling, and/or assistance with medical decision-making: hence it is a need-dependent service. Understanding this distinction is important when introducing either service to patients and caregivers – patients who need palliative care consultation may decline or resist this beneficial intervention under the incorrect assumption that they have a limited prognosis.

6   Palliative Care Providers

Medicine, nursing, social work, and other clinical disciplines have initiated subspecialty training pathways for developing content expertise and board certification. Gaertner et al. (2011) suggest a dedicated palliative care team with at least a physician, nurse, and social worker or psychologist (Gaertner et al. 2011).

Palliative care trained providers have a unique set of skills and experiences that are recognized by various national organizations that set standards for practice. A provider that holds a palliative care credential demonstrates their dedication and expertise to the field.

- Physicians can obtain the Certificate of Added Qualification in hospice and palliative medicine through the American Board of Medical Specialties and American Osteopathic Association and American Academy of Hospice and Palliative Medicine.
- The National Association of Social Workers (NASW) offers a Certification in Hospice and Palliative Care Social Work (CHP-SW) for social workers in hospice and palliative care settings.
- Nurses can certify their skills by obtaining the Certified Hospice and Palliative Care Nurse (CHPN) certification and/or an Advanced Certified Hospice and Palliative Nurse (ACHPN) certification.
- Board Certified Chaplains can obtain a certification in hospice and palliative care. This is represented by the initials BCC-HPCC.

7 Goals of Care

Goals of care are always established in the context of treating a medical condition. Goals of care can vary widely depending on what treatments and clinical trials are available and the performance status of the patient. At this point in time, mesothelioma is considered incurable, but the length of time that people are living with mesothelioma is increasing due to better treatments and clinical trials. This reality makes including palliative care in the treatment of mesothelioma essential. The goals of care are the underlying agreements between patient, caregivers, and providers about how to treat the disease toward an agreed upon end, including death.

Goals of care in the context of mesothelioma need to include not only the medical interventions available to patients but the interventions geared toward sustaining and improving quality of life. Some targets for goals of care can include the following. Much of this comes from the *Oxford Textbook of Palliative Social Work*, but the authors have updated and refined that information (Altilio and Otis-Green 2011).

- *Extend Life* – This can include all interventions known to extend one's life with mesothelioma, including clinical trials when applicable. At the end of life, this often means titrating down or stopping aggressive therapy that may cause more harm than benefit.
- *Symptoms Alleviation and Relief* – The goal of symptom relief is to improve quality of life as defined by the patient and caregivers. Common symptoms include anorexia, cough, dyspnea, fatigue, pain, anxiety, depression, traumatic stress, and spiritual distress.
- *Regain Normal Function* – This goal is defined as setting a baseline for normal functioning, which might be functioning before a surgery or after chemotherapy or immunotherapy. Often times this goal, when broken out, includes items such as return to ability for the patient to perform all activities of daily living, return to work, and/or engage in physical activities. However, it can also include talking to loved ones before death, seeing family and friends, or planning end-of-life rituals.
- *Improve Function* – If the disease and/or treatment has impacted a person's functioning (e.g., mental health, motor skill, respiratory status, performance status, etc.), palliative care can be used to restore or improve the lost function(s). Some interventions include medications that target nerve damage that might be caused by treatment, the use of a wide variety of pain and antiemetic medications, medications that can improve appetite and mood, and counseling interventions such as cognitive behavioral therapy for addressing anxiety or trauma-informed therapy to address traumatic responses to past treatments like surgery. These interventions may relieve symptoms that are debilitating and improve a patient's ability to function in a way that improves their quality of life regardless of performance status.

• *Allow a Natural Death* – No one knows the right time to withdraw care so a patient can die a natural death. It is too much to ask a single person, caregiver, or provider to make the decision to withdraw treatments that might extend life. Usually these decisions are made with the patient, caregivers, and medical team together. Nonetheless, planning for a natural death is a reasonable goal of care. Palliative care providers can assist in facilitating conversations about the efficacy of further treatment or the plan for quality of life when treatment is no longer working to assist the treating medical teams, patients, and caregivers to process their preoccupations with stopping treatment, especially when treatment may do more harm than benefit.

8   Palliative Care Needs in the Mesothelioma Experience

In general, mesothelioma is an aggressive malignancy affecting serosal surfaces, most commonly the pleura. For a variety of reasons – location of primary disease, aggressive nature, and side effects of treatments – the patient experience with mesothelioma lends itself to benefit from the best supportive care. To date, relatively few studies have focused specifically on the intersection of mesothelioma and palliative care. Nevertheless, in addition to extrapolating some commonalities with similar malignancies such as non-small cell lung cancer, current evidence indicates important indications for palliative care interventions.

8.1   Symptom Management

Applying the Lung Cancer Symptom Scale (LCSS) to patients with mesothelioma, Hollen et al. (2004) provide one of the earliest data sets to describe physical symptomatology in this population en route to validating a new tool, the LCSS-Meso (Hollen et al. 2004). In this study, 495 patients from 19 countries were included if they had a diagnosis of malignant pleural mesothelioma with surgically unresectable disease, no prior chemotherapy, and a performance status ≥70% using the physician-rated Karnofsky Performance Status (KPS) scale. At baseline (prior to chemotherapy administration), the median patient age was 61 (range 19–85), 92% were Caucasian, and most were either from western Europe (49%) or the United States (24%). Most patients enrolled in the study with a KPS between 80% and 90%, and most (79%) had stage III or IV disease.

The course of the study observed these patients through one of two ongoing clinical trials evaluating either a randomized trial comparing pemetrexed plus cisplatin versus cisplatin alone or a single-arm phase II trial evaluating pemetrexed alone. In all studies, LCSS-Meso data collection repeated at day 40 and day 82.

Results underlined mesothelioma as a highly symptomatic disease. At baseline, 92% of enrolled patients experienced at least three symptoms (Hollen et al. 2004). Patients commonly reported pain (85.3% reporting), dyspnea (89.1%), fatigue (93.7%), anorexia (86.5%), and cough (74.9%) (Hollen et al. 2004). Eighty-five percent of patients reported experiencing all four of the major physical symptoms assessed: pain, dyspnea, anorexia, and fatigue (Hollen et al. 2004). This level of symptom burden remained fairly consistent throughout the study, with ongoing negative impact on global quality of life and interference with activities.

These findings reflect those of a prospective observational study of 56 patients admitted to a home-based palliative care program (Mercadante et al. 2016). There, patients also reported pain, dyspnea, anorexia, weakness, and poor well-being in high frequency and intensity. Median survival time was about 2.5 months, suggesting late referral to these supportive care services (Mercadante et al. 2016).

With this early window into the mesothelioma experience, a brief overview of highly prevalent symptoms is discussed here. This overview will focus on disease-related etiologies of symptom distress, a focus on therapy-related etiologies being outside the scope of this chapter. Note that the common symptom pain is discussed at length elsewhere in this book.

8.1.1   Cough

Uncontrolled cough is not only distressing itself but can be associated with dyspnea, nausea/vomiting, anorexia, insomnia, pain, and impaired communication. In patients with cancer in the chest cavity, disease progression affecting nerves, pleura, bronchi, and bronchioles can cause cough. A thorough workup, including a medication review, is essential.

Optimal treatment includes management of the underlying disease. However, in most cases, a symptom-targeted approach is indicated as well. Sometimes – recurrent malignant pleural effusion, for example – surgical interventions are indicated to palliate recurrent or refractory cough. In most cases, medical strategies are the mainstay of treatment.

Clinicians are encouraged to target the underlying etiology whenever possible. Nevertheless, very often management requires trial and error. Centrally acting antitussive gabapentin is thought to calm sensitized nerves in a manner similar to painful peripheral neuropathy (Ryan et al. 2012). Anecdotal reports of amitriptyline, paroxetine, and benzodiazepines have been reported. Peripherally acting antitussive benzonatate is considered to anesthetize stretch receptors in the pulmonary tree; randomized controlled trials are lacking. A variety of other agents have been reported, with variable evidence, anticholinergics such as hyoscyamine and scopolamine and expectorants such as guaifenesin, and nebulized local anesthetics have been described (Estfan and LeGrand 2004; Lingerfelt et al. 2007).

Opioid therapies – including but not limited to codeine, morphine, and dextromethorphan – are thought to act centrally through *mu* and *kappa* opioid receptor agonism that mitigates cough (Homsi et al. 2001; Center for Advancing Palliative Care 2017). All opioids have antitussive properties; choices of specific opioids for cough are by convention alone, rather than evidence. For patients already using opioids, experts generally recommend employing the same one for cough rather than introducing another opioid for a different symptom.

8.1.2 Dyspnea

In progressive mesothelioma, dyspnea can be related to restrictive pulmonary processes from pleural disease, pulmonary failure related to intraparenchymal disease, pleural cavity fluid collections, and even severe abdominal ascites from peritoneal disease (Dudgeon 2013). In addition to primary disease management, which may improve the underlying etiology at least temporarily, the clinician's approach to dyspnea follows models used in other malignant diseases.

Treating hypoxia with supplemental oxygen may be beneficial. It is important to remember that dyspnea is a subjective symptom. Patients with normal oxygen saturations may complain of dyspnea that certainly deserves assessment and management; in such cases increasing superficial airflow with an open window or a fan may lower dyspnea (Puspawati et al. 2017).

As with lung cancer and other malignancies affecting the chest cavity, opioid therapies may prove beneficial to improve dyspnea and even increase function (Gamborg et al. 2013). For patients already prescribed opioids for pain, clinicians are encouraged to use the same opioid; although there is most evidence supporting morphine for dyspnea, any opioid can be used. Similar in approach to cancer pain management, patients who require routine or frequent opioid dosing for dyspnea may benefit from a scheduled long-acting agent. Benzodiazepines may be useful for anxiety related to under-managed dyspnea; however, most dyspnea-related anxiety will be adequately managed by controlling the dyspnea itself.

On occasion, effective dyspnea management requires surgical intervention, particularly with recurrent malignant pleural effusions. In one prospective observational study of 158 patients with pleural effusions, the vast majority experienced symptomatic improvement with therapeutic drainage; the level of symptomatic improvement positively correlated with volume of fluid removed and negatively correlated with number of septations seen on ultrasound (Psallidas et al. 2017).

8.1.3 Fatigue

Cancer-related fatigue (CRF) remains one of the most disabling and under-assessed symptoms associated with mesothelioma (Hollen et al. 2004; Psallidas et al. 2017). Common underlying etiologies are numerous and may include direct disease effects, deconditioning, dyspnea and/or hypoxemia, nutritional imbalance, sleep disturbances, uncontrolled pain, and coexisting psychiatric illness such as depression (Kao et al. 2013). Additionally, mesothelioma disease-modifying therapies including systemic chemotherapy and radiation are known to cause or worsen CRF.

Management of CRF is challenging, given that underlying etiologies are usually multifactorial and effective interventions can be elusive. There are no clinical trials evaluating CRF management strategies specific to mesothelioma. Treatment should target potential causes – for example, management of related pain, dyspnea, or depression. General to CRF, potential interventions include gentle aerobic exercise (e.g., 20–30 cumulative minutes of exercise per day, at least 3 days per week); resistance training may also benefit some patients (Pearson et al. 2016; Brown et al. 2006; Wiskemann et al. 2016). Although little data supports drug therapies for CRF, some success has been reported with psychostimulants (e.g., methylphenidate, modafinil), corticosteroids, and megestrol acetate, as well as the dietary supplement ginseng (Quist et al. 2015; Yennurajalingam et al. 2013; Bruera et al. 1990, 1998).

Education and counseling are particularly important as well. Clinicians should normalize this symptom experience and promote patient and caregiver adjustment to change in social roles and expectations of activity, routine, and schedule. Counseling is beneficial to change in social roles.

9   Psychosocial-Spiritual Care with Mesothelioma

Palliative care providers recognize the interconnections between the body, psyche, and spirit of patients and caregivers. Palliative services should include assessing and addressing each of these domains, in addition to the physical, for both patients and caregivers. Because mesothelioma has a complicated treatment course, which may include travel for care, a significant financial investment, and stress, taking care of the whole person is paramount to ensuring a high quality of life at any stage of the disease.

9.1   Caregiver Support

Providing care to a loved one with mesothelioma can be extremely stressful and can even begin to have negative health consequences for the caregivers (Barton et al. 2013; National Cancer Institute 2014). Palliative care providers integrate the care of the patient with that of the caregivers. Caregivers should be assessed with patients and ensure their quality of life is also optimized.

Many palliative care programs also offer some form of respite care for caregivers so they perform self-care and be restored, allowing them to provide the best care to their loved one without sacrificing their own health. While it is often hard for a caregiver to be separated from the patient, it is essential that caregivers are encouraged and provided opportunities for self-care.

9.2   Communication

Good patient/provider communication empowers patients, caregivers, and providers. Often times, patients and caregivers underrepresent how much they understand about the course of treatment or their treatment options so as to bolster the impression their provider has of them. This is called the bias of social desirability or appearing to be or say what you think will please another person. This can lead to many misunderstandings, less adherence to medical care, and lower quality of life. It is recommended that patients and caregivers be encouraged to write questions down and be prepared for meetings with providers. It is also recommended that providers seek to confirm that the patient and caregivers understand why it was discussed; often this is achieved by asking the patient and/or caregiver to repeat back their understanding of a meeting, decisions, and/or interventions.

9.3   Mental Health

Frequently people with mesothelioma and their caregivers develop mental health symptoms and, in some cases, conditions as a result of the persistent amount of stress and even traumatic stress exposure (Gurevich et al. 2002). The most common mental health symptoms experienced are anxiety, depression, sleeplessness, and symptoms of traumatic stress (Center for Advancing Palliative Care 2017). During active treatment of the disease, it can be difficult to distinguish side effects of treatment and mental health symptoms given there is some frequent overlap. For example, steroids can cause hypomania, sleeplessness, and anxiety, and chemotherapy can cause weight loss, fatigue, and loss of engagement in normal activities that bring meaning, which may be mistaken for depression. Involving the palliative care, and psychiatry when necessary, to assess for emotional distress and more significant symptoms of mental health is a key element to palliative interventions in people with mesothelioma and their caregivers.

Providing phone or online support groups has been shown to be effective for people with mesothelioma. Bates et al. (2016) demonstrated that active participation on a phone-based guided support group was very helpful to respondents and extremely helpful to neutral participants who joined irregularly (Abrahm 2009).

9.4   Spiritual Care

The search for spiritual meaning in the context of a life-limiting and life-threatening disease cannot be understated. The literature suggests that people of faith often cope better with their illness and disease process (Bevans and Sternberg 2010). Leaning on spiritual and religious practices can provide a significant relief from existential questions such as "why me" or "what is God's plan for me/my loved ones." Furthermore, assessing the patient and caregivers for their beliefs and rituals related to death and dying, if they feel the need to discuss forgiveness, repairing or strengthening a relationship, and continuing to participate in religious rituals is essential (Jim et al. 2015). The literature also cautions that, in some cases, spirituality and religion can be upsetting to people with mesothelioma and their caregivers if they leave these questions unexplored and unanswered. Utilizing a chaplain or the patient's religious community is strongly recommended.

10   Palliative Care Insurance Benefits

As is typical in the insurance industry, Medicare is the benchmark for coverage benefits by insurance companies. Medicare Part A covers palliative care when it is linked with hospice care. State Medicaid coverage also includes palliative care when linked to hospice. The details of the coverage can be found at the www.medicare.gov site.

Many other private insurances cover palliative care when it is linked to hospice as well. When a patient enrolls in palliative care linked to hospice, it is usually at the end of life. Under these circumstances, the coverage is quite comprehensive with the idea that the goals of care are comfort care measures only and not treatment. In some cases palliative radiation, chemotherapy, immunotherapies, nutritional support, and antibiotics and/or other interventions are permitted but must be approved by the Medical Director, or delegate, of the organization providing end-of-life care.

To access a benefit for palliative care that is not linked to hospice care, it is recommended to consult the patient's insurance company. Each medical insurance plan is different with different benefits, co-pays, coinsurances, premiums, and deductibles. Most plans do offer some form of palliative care benefit. The only way to be certain of any palliative care benefit is to ask the insurance provider directly for a summary of benefits and work with the treating medical facility. When contacting insurance companies about a palliative care benefit that is not linked to hospice, consider providing patients with ICD and CPT codes. This will likely expedite the inquiry and provide more accurate information to the patient about their benefits.

Inpatient and outpatient palliative care services are often covered as other consult service depending on the treating facility and on the details of the patient's insurance plan. If enrolled on a clinical trial, palliative care may be included with protocol participation.

If a patient is uninsured or a "self-pay" patient, many outpatient nonprofit hospices that also have distinct palliative care teams will provide these services free of charge. In some cases charity care can be provided for end-of-life patients by for-profit hospices, but it usually comes with the requirement that the patient is also enrolled in their hospice program. It is always worth calling a palliative care and hospice provider to see if they will provide care free of charge. Of note, many providers also provide care for patients who are undocumented as immigration status is not a requirement for hospice and/or palliative care.

The palliative care services that are linked to hospice care are often provided in the patient's home or living environment. There are also instances in which palliative care that is linked to hospice is provided as an inpatient, but this is usually reserved for symptom management of significantly debilitating symptoms. Furthermore, inpatient hospice is often done with the goal of having the patient return to their living environment if possible.

These services include:

- Doctor visits – in home and inpatient as needed
- Nursing care – in home and inpatient as needed
- 24/7 call in number for medical advice and in person care as needed
- Medical equipment, also referred to as durable medical equipment (DME), such as home oxygen, hospital bed, bedside commode, shower chair, walker, wheelchair, etc.
- Medications
- Therapy including physical, occupational, and speech-language

- Social work visits
- Nutritional counseling
- Respite care for caregivers
- Aftercare for the surviving caregivers

11   Where Can You Get Palliative Care for Mesothelioma?

Not all inpatient settings have a palliative care team. Likewise, accessing outpatient palliative care depends on access to a program and insurance or another way to cover the cost.

Here are two state-by-state directories that provide a list of palliative care providers:

- https://getpalliativecare.org/providers
- https://www.nhpco.org/find-hospice/pcp

Some of the listings focus on hospice services, but it is always worth calling the provider on the registry closest to a patient home or a provider that the patient and caregivers choose and inquiring about outpatient palliative care services.

References

Abrahm J. Palliative care for patients with mesothelioma. Thorac Cardiovasc Surg. 2009;21(2):164–71.

Altilio T, Otis-Green S, editors. Oxford textbook of palliative social work. Oxford: University Press; 2011.

Barton D, Liu H, Dakhil S, Linquist B, Sloan J, et al. Wisconsin Ginseng (Panax quinquefolius) to improve cancer-related fatigue: a randomized, double-blind trial, N07C2. J Natl Cancer Inst. 2013;105(16):1230–8.

Bates G, Hashmi A, Bressler T, Zajac J, Hesdorffer M, Taub R. Approach to offering remote support to mesothelioma patients: the mesothelioma survivor project. Transl Lung Cancer Res. 2016;5(3):216–8.

Bevans M, Sternberg E. Caregiving burden, stress, and health effects among family caregivers of adults cancer patients. JAMA. 2010;307(4):398–403.

Brown P, Clark M, Atherton P, Huschka M, Sloan J, et al. Will improvement in quality of life (QOL) impact fatigue in patients receiving radiation therapy for advanced cancer? Am J Clin Oncol. 2006;29(1):52–8.

Bruera E, Macmillan K, Kuehn N, Hanson J, MacDonald R. A controlled trial of megestrol acetate on appetite, caloric intake, nutritional status, and other symptoms in patients with advanced cancer. Cancer. 1990;66(6):1279–82.

Bruera E, Ernst S, Hagen N, Spachynski K, Belzile M, et al. Effectiveness of megestrol acetate in patients with advanced cancer: a randomized, double-blind, crossover study. Cancer Prev Control. 1998;2(2):74–8.

Center for Advancing Palliative Care. Palliative care – can religion play a role. 2017. http://www.capcmssm.org/palliative-car-and-religion.html. Accessed 30 Oct 2017.

Centers for Medicare and Medicaid. Services medical hospice payment reform. 2014. https://www.cms.gov/Medicare/Medicare-Fee-for-Service-Payment/Hospice/Downloads/MedicareHospicePaymentReformLiteratureReview2013Update.pdf. Last accessed 31 Oct 2017.

Dudgeon D. Dyspnea in the cancer patient. In: Berger AM, et al., editors. Principles and practice of palliative care and supportive oncology. Philadelphia: Lippincott Williams & Wilkins; 2013.

Dumanovsky T, Augustin R, Rogers M, Lettang K, Meier D, Morrison RS. The growth of palliative care in U.S. hospitals: a status report. J Palliat Med. 2016;19(1):8–15.

Estfan B, LeGrand S. Management of cough in advanced cancer. J Support Oncol. 2004;2:523–7.

Gaertner J, Wolf J, Hallek M, Glossmann JP, Voltz R. Standardizing integration of palliative care into comprehensive cancer therapy – a disease specific approach. Support Care Cancer. 2011;19:1037–43.

Gamborg H, Riis J, Christrup L, Krantz T. Effect of intraoral and subcutaneous morphine on dyspnea at rest in terminal patients with primary lung cancer or lung metastases. J Opioid Manag. 2013;9(4):269–74.

Gurevich M, Devins G, Rodin G. Stress response syndromes and cancer: conceptual and assessment issues. Psychosomatics. 2002;43(4):259–81.

Hollen PJ, Gralla RJ, Liepa AM, Symanowski JT, Rusthoven JJ. Adapting the lung cancer symptom scale (LCSS) to mesothelioma: using the LCSS-Meso conceptual model for validation. Cancer. 2004;101(3):587–97.

Homsi J, Walsh D, Nelson K. Important drugs for cough in advanced cancer. Support Care Cancer. 2001;9:565–74.

Jim H, Pustejovsky J, Park C, Danhauer S, Sherman A, et al. Religion, spirituality, and physical health in cancer patients: a meta-analysis. Cancer. 2015;121(21):3760–8.

Kao SC, Vardy J, Harvie R, et al. Health-related quality of life and inflammatory markers in malignant pleural mesothelioma. Support Care Cancer. 2013;21(3):697–705.

Lingerfelt BM, et al. Nebulized lidocaine for intractable cough near the end of life. J Support Oncol. 2007;7:301–2.

Mercadante S, Degiovanni D, Casuccio A. Symptoms burden in mesothelioma patients admitted to home palliative care. Curr Med Res Opin. 2016;32(12):1985–8.

National Cancer Institute. Caring for the caregiver. 2014. https://www.cancer.gov/publications/patient-education/caring-for-the-caregiver. Accessed 30 Oct 2017.

Pearson E, Morris M, McKinstry C. Cancer-related fatigue: appraising evidence-based guidelines for screening, assessment and management. Support Care Cancer. 2016;24(9):3935–42.

Psallidas I, Yousuf A, Talwar A, et al. Assessment of patient-reported outcome measures in pleural interventions. BMJ Open Respir Res. 2017;4(1):e000171.

Puspawati NLPD, Sitorus R, Herawati T. Hand-held fan airflow stimulation relieves dyspnea in lung Cancer patients. Asia Pac J Oncol Nurs. 2017;4(2):162–7.

Quist M, Adamsen L, Rørth M, Laursen JH, Christensen K, Langer S. The impact of a multidimensional exercise intervention on physical and functional capacity, anxiety, and depression in patients with advanced-stage lung cancer undergoing chemotherapy. Integr Cancer Ther. 2015;14(4):341–9.

Ryan N, Birring S, Gibson P. Gabapentin for refractory chronic cough: a randomised, double-blind, placebo-controlled trial. Lancet. 2012;380(9853):1583–9.

Smith TJ, Temin S, Alesi ER, et al. J Clin Oncol. 2012;30:880–7.

Temel J, Greer J, Muzikansky A, Gallagher E, Admane S, et al. Early palliative care for patients with metastatic non-small-cell lung cancer. N Engl J Med. 2010;363:733–42.

Wiskemann J, Hummler S, Diepold C, Keil M, Abel U, et al. POSITIVE study: physical exercise program in non-operable lung cancer patients undergoing palliative treatment. BMC Cancer. 2016;16:499.

World Health Organization. WHO definition of palliative care. 2017. http://www.who.int/cancer/palliative/definition/en/. Accessed 31 Oct 2017.

Yennurajalingam S, Frisbee-Hume S, Palmer J, Delgado-Guay M, Bull J, Bruera E. Reduction of cancer-related fatigue with dexamethasone: a double-blind, randomized, placebo-controlled trial in patients with advanced cancer. J Clin Oncol. 2013;31(25):3076–82.

Jadmin L. Mostel and Gleneara E. Bates-Pappas

1 Part I: Difficult Conversation and Healthy Boundaries with Patients During Treatment

1.1 Talking to Patients and Their Loved Ones During Treatment: How to Engage in Supportive Decision-Making with Patients

Throughout the treatment process, it is important that patients and families are included in discussions surrounding the treatment plan and future outcomes. Medical jargon is confusing, and patients can easily feel they have little voice when undergoing treatment. With mesothelioma, there are many important keywords that need to be defined and can make a world of differences to the patient when engaging in treatment conversations. It is important for medical professionals to understand the power they have when discussing treatment with patients and their families. Using language that allows for a dialogue around treatment options may reduce treatment regret among patients and their families.

Supportive decision-making, also known as shared decision-making (SDM), is an imperative part of a patient's treatment plan and supports the idea of patient-centered care. Instead of patients being informed of the treatment that they will undergo, this paradigm promotes collaboration between practitioners and patients (Durand et al. 2014). Under this model, practitioners give patients all of their options, weigh the pros and cons concerning quality of life and treatment efficacy,

J. L. Mostel (✉)
Johns Hopkins Bloomberg School of Public Health, Baltimore, MD, USA

G. E. Bates-Pappas
City University of New York Graduate Center, New York, NY, USA
e-mail: gbates@gradcenter.cuny.edu

© Springer Nature Switzerland AG 2019
M. Hesdorffer, G. E. Bates-Pappas (eds.), *Caring for Patients with Mesothelioma: Principles and Guidelines*,
https://doi.org/10.1007/978-3-319-96244-3_14

and work together with the patient to find the best solution for their needs. Clinicians work with patients to identify patient's goals, develop realistic plans, and highlight parts of the plan that patients can manage on their own in an effort to empower them (McCorkle et al. 2011). One review suggests that using the SDM model improves outcomes in disadvantaged groups, such as groups with low socioeconomic status. Using SDM is imperative when treating mesothelioma patients, one reason being that mesothelioma characteristically affects individuals of low socioeconomic status, and can effectively navigate the challenges of consent forms, medication regimens, and discussing treatment options with practitioners (Durand et al. 2014). SDM helps patients and families take back some semblance of control over their disease, reduces decisional conflict, and increases knowledge concerning the disease (Durand et al. 2014).

Using the SDM paradigm frequently involves altering the language in which medical information is conveyed. There is not a standard SDM protocol, for SDM interventions must be customized for each individual patient. For example, in order to effectively engage in SDM practices, language must be stripped down to what the patient and family can understand, medical jargon must be appropriately used, and a simpler presentation of information may be needed (Durand et al. 2014). When used correctly, practitioners can use SDM as a powerful tool to empower their patients to take ownership of their own treatment and regain decision-making abilities for their own health (Durand et al. 2014).

1.2   Talking to Patients and Their Loved Ones During Treatment: After Disease Progression

As disease progresses, it is important that patients are given the opportunity to participate in meaningful discussions regarding future treatment and care (Parry et al. 2014). With mesothelioma's high mortality rate, medical professionals should be aware of disease progression and introduce conversations about advance care planning when appropriate. These conversations can be challenging and uncomfortable to facilitate and, more so, difficult to ascertain when it is appropriate to introduce these topics to patients and their loved ones (Parry et al. 2014). Practitioners may be faced with an overwhelming reluctance from patients to engage in these conversations, and that is okay; however, these conversations must be introduced to give patients the ability to decide their willingness to participate before disease progression becomes too advanced.

There are a variety of communicative routes to engage in these difficult conversations with patients and their loved ones. For example, if looking to gently inquire if the patient is willing to discuss advance care planning, using an indirect approach could be an option (Parry et al. 2014). Using euphemisms, referring to mesothelioma as "it," and hinting at future disease outcomes are all examples of indirect language, deflecting some of the emotional toll and creating a scenario where the practitioner may judge the patient's reaction to understand if the conversation should continue (Parry et al. 2014). If looking to stay more on topic without as many options to deflect difficult topics, practitioners could use a hypothetical approach (Parry et al. 2014). In this approach, asking hypothetical scenarios, such as "say that your mesothelioma continues to metastasize into other body parts. Who will help you make decision during this time?" can produce more direct answers from patients that stay on the topic of end-of-life care/planning (Parry et al. 2014).

1.3   Talking to Patients and Their Loved Ones During Treatment: About Transitioning to Hospice Care

Transitioning a patient to hospice care can be a challenging time for the practitioners, patient, and family. Family members may doubt their decision, perhaps inquiring if a last-shot at aggressive treatment is appropriate, or wonder if in-home hospice would be more advantageous than a hospice care facility. One study aimed to examine the role of PCPs in this transition and found that most take a psychosocial support approach, focusing on educating, supporting, and reassuring patients and families (Shalev et al. 2017). As patients and families navigate the transition to hospice, it is important that the role of each practitioner is made clear to manage expectations of families (Shalev et al. 2017).

2   Part II: Life After Active Treatment (Survivorship)

2.1   Transiting Back to Primary Care Team

The transition back to a patient's PCP team posttreatment can be challenging for the patient and family, primarily because of ambiguity about expectations. This unique phase is termed survivorship, and issues related to short-term care are lessened and are replaced with questions surrounding follow-up care and management of effects of treatment (Grunfeld and Earle 2010). Tasks within the survivorship phase may include follow-up visits, understanding signs of mesothelioma recurrence, managing the effects of treatment, reengaging with pre-diagnosis routines, and managing psychological issues that resulted from diagnosis and treatment (McCorkle et al. 2011). Patients may not be aware which of their providers (PCP, oncologist, and other medical clinicians) are responsible for these tasks, and, as a result, patients entering their posttreatment phase should be given an individualized survivorship care plan (SCP) from their oncologist to facilitate this transition (Blanch-Hartigan et al. 2014). Like supportive/shared decision-making (SDM, discussed in another chapter), patients must be included in forming this SCP to enhance patient empowerment, engagement, and adherence to medical recommendations (Blanch-Hartigan et al. 2014).

2.2   Reducing Feelings of Abandonment After Treatment

There are many transitions that the patient navigates posttreatment, but the most prominent include transitioning to maintenance scans/follow-ups and transitioning to PCP and/or local oncologist (Bates et al. 2017). These transitions can prove psychologically challenging to the patient when departing from their oncologist's constant care into the care of a PCP (Bates et al. 2017). The patient may feel abandoned of medical care and fear of posttreatment navigation without supervision (Bates et al. 2017). Having open discussions at the beginning of their transition with the patient about their individualized SCP can help, and it will be beneficial to include the PCP within these conversations (Blanch-Hartigan et al. 2014). This will lessen any conflicting advice between oncologist and PCP, will help in care coordination, and will make ambiguous instructions more lucid (Blanch-Hartigan et al. 2014). Being aware of a patient's potential heightened feeling of abandonment can aid in the presentation of SCP language and future interaction with the patient.

2.3   Helping Patients Manage Physical Change After Treatment

The physical changes for patients after treatment can be challenging to navigate, in part due to discomfort but also due to the physiological effects brought forth by these new bodily challenges.

(a) *Fatigue* is a common side effect of cancer treatment and may continue to affect a patient many years after treatment (Bower 2014). The intensity of fatigue felt by cancer survivors can be more severe than fatigue felt from sleep deprivation or overexertion (Bower 2014). When related to cancer and cancer treatment, fatigue can develop in physical, mental, and emotional ways that impact concentration, motivation, and day-to-day engagement (Bower 2014). Although there is not a ubiquitous standard for treating fatigue, there are a number of options for patients to utilize, such as exercise, psychosocial interventions, meditation or yoga, and pharmacologic treatments (Bower 2014).

(b) Cognitive issues, such as *memory and concentration* impairments, are frequently reported as side effects among patients undergoing chemotherapy and/or radiation treatment (Janelsins et al. 2014). Cognitive impairment can affect a patient's quality of life, can influence adherence to treatment, and may be temporary or permanent (Janelsins et al. 2014). Some ways to improve the effects of memory and concentration impairments include cognitive behavioral therapy approaches and physical activity (Janelsins et al. 2014).

(c) *Biologic change* (*menopause*). Female cancer patients have unique biological responses to chemotherapeutic treatment. In some cases chemotherapy can cause menopause to occur. This can be practically challenging and/or upsetting for women diagnosed within their childbearing years. As the rate of survival continues to increase, providing female patients with appropriate information on how to cope with biological changes after active treatment could possibly reduce feels of anxiety and depression as they navigate their new normal.

(d) *Intimacy after treatment* can be a challenging subject to navigate. Patients may feel ashamed to discuss intimacy topics and also may not know what kinds of questions to ask. Erectile difficulties, bodily pain, and decreased sexual desire may be a few challenges patients experience after undergoing cancer treatment (Ussher et al. 2013). One way to combat the effects of intimacy challenges include renegotiate sex and to incorporate other forms of intimacy such as cuddling, massages, or kissing (Ussher et al. 2013). When engaging in sexual intercourse, the use of lubricant can combat any vaginal dryness.

(e) *Changes in body image.* Physical changes after treatment can be hard for patients to accept. The most common physical changes patients will experience are hair loss; fatigue; skin dryness; swelling of the face, legs, and arms; weight loss; weight gain; scars from surgery; skin discoloration from irradiation; and bowel and bladder changes (Bates et al. 2016). Patients who undergo surgical treatment and radiotherapy may have visible scars. Explaining to patients the physical changes they may experience after treatment can help them prepare for life after active treatment, thus allowing them to feel a sense of ownership over their body post active treatment.

References

Bates G, Taub RN, West H. Intimacy, body image, and cancer. JAMA Oncol. 2016;2(12):1667. https://doi.org/10.1001/jamaoncol.2016.1196.

Bates GE, Mostel JL, Hesdorffer M. Mesothelioma survivorship: challenges in delivering quality care. Expert Rev Qual Life Cancer Care. 2017;2(3):177–80.

Blanch-Hartigan D, et al. Provision and discussion of survivorship care plans among cancer survivors: results of a nationally representative survey of oncologists and primary care physicians. J Clin Oncol. 2014;32(15):1578–85.

Bower JE. Cancer-related fatigue—mechanisms, risk factors, and treatments. Nat Rev Clin Oncol. 2014;11(10):597–609.

Durand M-A, et al. Do interventions designed to support shared decision-making reduce health inequalities? A systematic review and meta-analysis. PLoS One. 2014;9(4):e94670.

Grunfeld E, Earle CC. The interface between primary and oncology specialty care: treatment through survivorship. J Natl Cancer Inst Monogr. 2010;2010(40):25–30.

Janelsins MC, et al. Prevalence, mechanisms, and management of cancer-related cognitive impairment. Int Rev Psychiatry. 2014;26(1):102–13.

McCorkle R, et al. Self-management: enabling and empowering patients living with cancer as a chronic illness. CA Cancer J Clin. 2011;61(1):50–62.

Parry R, Land V, Seymour J. How to communicate with patients about future illness progression and end of life: a systematic review. BMJ Support Palliat Care. 2014;4(4):331–41.

Shalev A, et al. Examining the role of primary care physicians and challenges faced when their patients transition to home hospice care. Am J Hosp Palliat Med. 2017; https://doi.org/10.1177/1049909117734845.

Ussher JM, et al. Renegotiating sex and intimacy after cancer: resisting the coital imperative. Cancer Nurs. 2013;36(6):454–62.

End-of-Life Care

15

Karlynn BrintzenhofeSzoc and Louisa Daratsos

1 Introduction

Mesothelioma is a complex disease that does not have a predictable path from pre-diagnosis to death. An additional aspect of the complexity to those with mesothelioma is the legal- and compensation-related issues (Moore et al. 2010). Mesothelioma is a rare cancer that is most often the result of exposure to asbestos. The time from exposure to the development of cancer ranges from 20 to 40 years (Linton et al. 2014; Taioli et al. 2015; NCCN 2017a). Even though there is no known cure for mesothelioma, there are guidelines for the treatment of malignant pleural mesothelioma developed by the National Comprehensive Cancer Network (NCCN 2017a). The treatment guidelines, for both clinicians and patients, are based on the stage of the disease and include supportive and palliative care (Meyerhoff et al. 2015; NCCN 2016, 2017a).

Currently, the outcome of a diagnosis of mesothelioma is death. As noted in much of the literature, life expectancy of a person diagnosed with mesothelioma is based on multiple factors (Meyerhoff et al. 2015; Musk et al. 2011; Taioli et al. 2015). Death is not the outcome most people who are involved with this disease want. Those involved include the person with the disease, family members who provide direct care, family and friends who care for and about the person with the disease, and members of the healthcare team that provides medical, psychosocial, and spiritual care. Dying and death are not topics that come up in conversation with ease in our society. The conversations about death and dying usually start when someone is diagnosed with a life-limiting disease or is told that the person with a

K. BrintzenhofeSzoc (✉)
University of Cincinnati, Cincinnati, OH, USA
e-mail: brintzkn@ucmail.uc.edu

L. Daratsos
VA NY Harbor Healthcare System, Brooklyn, NY, USA

© Springer Nature Switzerland AG 2019
M. Hesdorffer, G. E. Bates-Pappas (eds.), *Caring for Patients with Mesothelioma: Principles and Guidelines*,
https://doi.org/10.1007/978-3-319-96244-3_15

disease has days to weeks or weeks to months to live. The topic continues to be taboo due to fear that talking about it will make it happen sooner, and the conversation about death and dying brings up a lot of emotions for most involved. These emotions are positive and negative and often both at the same time. Often, both the person with the disease that will lead to death and all others involved don't want to talk about death as it might upset the other. At the core of the fear to talk about, think about, and plan for death is that death is one of the rare experiences that no one really knows what happens as it starts, progresses, and, finally, occurs.

As discussed in Chap. 18, *Palliative Care*, including palliative care providers as members of the healthcare team, the discussion of death and dying will more likely occur. The conversations with palliative care start with the identification of goals of care from the person with the disease and the family perspectives. The palliative care team focuses not only on the medical treatment course but also on the quality of life, goal setting, pain management, symptom management, and psychosocial-spiritual sexual issues. In these conversations, the topic of death and dying is often initiated. Thus, those persons with mesothelioma, caregivers, and carers will have had the experience of talking about death and dying with few negative outcomes. This may result in more comfort in talking about the end of life as it nears which meets the request for more information about the trajectory of the disease (Hughes and Arber 2008; Moore et al. 2010).

The goal of this chapter is to cover what is known about how people respond to an upcoming death, the actual dying process, and after the death (see Fig. 15.1). So as not to overlap with the previous chapter on palliative care, the focus will be on the last 2 weeks of life. The chapter will provide guidance on what patients, caregivers, and those who care can do that might be helpful and what might not be helpful,

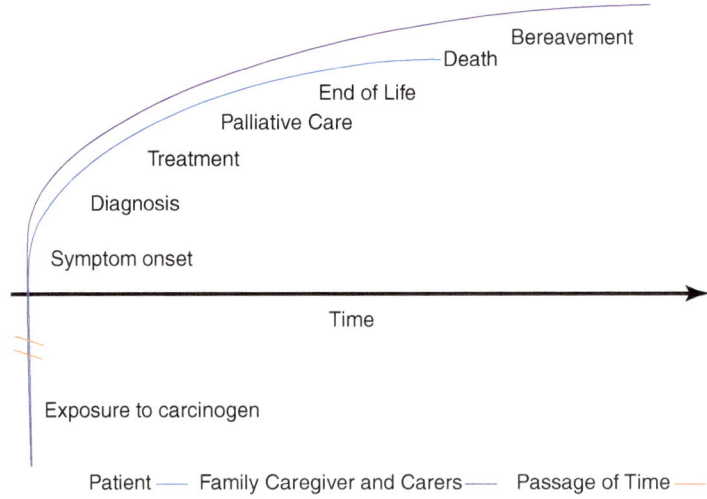

Fig. 15.1 The mesothelioma trajectory

including how to find information. The concrete tasks that can be done before death will be discussed as well as those that must occur after the death are addressed.

As mentioned previously, mesothelioma is a complex disease and manifests with physical symptoms, emotional symptoms, and social issues. As the disease progress and the symptoms become worse, there is a direct relationship with declining functional ability of the person with the disease. This leads to a greater need for basic help from family caregivers and other carers to help the patients have their needs met. Further, these symptoms and issues are reported to be more burdensome to those with mesothelioma, family caregivers, and other carers than in other diseases. Some of this additional burden may be due to the small number of people with mesothelioma, family members, and carers being in the same healthcare setting at the same time. This will likely change over time as the incidence of mesothelioma is expected to continue to grow. Being a patient or family member of this rare disease in a setting where there are few others can exacerbate the symptoms and problems due to isolation, lack of support, and lack of specialized services. Being that the vast majority of people diagnosed with mesothelioma were exposed at work can add yet another layer of complexity (Moore et al. 2010; van Zandwijk et al. 2013).

2   End-of-Life Overview

At some point during the treatment of mesothelioma, a patient and family may be told that treatment options might be exhausted. The American Cancer Society (ACS, 2016) website offers a patient education handout, "If Treatment of Malignant Mesothelioma Stops Working," which can be a very helpful resource to help patients, families, and carers determine the most appropriate next steps for the months to weeks ahead.

Many patients and families will be shocked to learn that their treatment has stopped working and that there may be limited options to continue treatment. As ACS writes, "…[A]t some point, you need to consider that treatment is not likely to improve your health or change your outcome or survival." The handout suggests patients, families, and the treatment team have a discussion about the risks and benefits of potential treatments. The objective of such conversations is to have patients and families reach an understanding that any potential treatment options may pose harm and may not arrest the progression of mesothelioma nor lessen its symptoms. Some patients may appreciate this news since the symptoms and treatment of mesothelioma have so radically changed their lives and the lives of their loved ones. Even patients and caregivers who report positive relationships with their treatment teams often do not take active roles in questioning how long should the treatment phase last. While visiting the clinic, taking treatments and occasional hospitalizations became analogous to other careers for patients and their caregivers, there is now an opportunity to assess what matters most in life and to try to create opportunities to achieve goals and to make meaningful memories with family and friends.

It is important to recognize that even if doctors say there is no treatment to contain the cancer, there are many treatments to reduce uncomfortable symptoms. At this point, the patient and family may be introduced to the palliative care team. This is an interdisciplinary team usually consisting of at least a physician, nurse or nurse practitioner, social worker, and chaplain. Larger teams often have psychologists, pharmacists, rehabilitation therapists, and even complementary medicine practitioners such as Reiki therapists. "Palliate" comes from the Latin word meaning comfort, and the palliative care team's goal is to help patients improve their quality of life. These teams do this by assessing patients and families' biopsychosocial functioning and helping patients and families identify their definition of quality of life for them to maintain functioning and even attain goals as much as possible. An example of palliative care's work at this stage of a person's life with mesothelioma would be this:

Mr. and Mrs. A are 1 month shy of their 60th anniversary. At Mr. A.'s last medical oncology appointment, he was told that his CT scan showed progression of his disease and it was unlikely he could tolerate another cycle of chemotherapy. He and his wife were able to meet the palliative care team the same day he was in the clinic. When the palliative care team social worker asked the couple what mattered to them most, they each said they knew Mr. A did not have much longer to live. The couple decided to give themselves an anniversary party with their closest family and friends present. They decided they would give their children and their respective families a sum of money to come home for the weekend celebration. Mr. A had been expressing to his wife that the weekly 9 am visits to the clinic were exhausting him. He was glad he could now be free to spend the next week at home to gather his strength for the party. The following week, Mrs. A came to the medical center to show the staff pictures of the gathering. She shared that the couple had long ago planned to spend this anniversary on a cruise, but they were grateful for the information about her husband's grave condition so that they could make alternative but very meaningful plans to celebrate the life they built together.

This case illustrates what life without active treatment at the end of life can offer. In the days before the A.'s party, Mr. A. was able to direct his attention to resting instead of thinking about all the tasks associated with getting to his next clinic appointment. He was able to wake up on his own schedule, not worry about arranging for someone to help him out of the house and driving him to the medical center, etc. The party showed him how it is possible to look toward the future with hopeful anticipation instead of the worry he often felt before coming to the medical center.

Hospice care is a specific kind of palliative care. It is a program, most often brought to the patient's home, which focuses caring for the patient when life expectancy is likely to be 6 months or less and patients are receiving symptom management and not active therapy. Like palliative care teams, hospice teams usually include a physician, nurse, social worker, and chaplain. Often, hospice programs offer home healthcare for several hours a week and a 24-hour number to call if the patient is experiencing troublesome symptoms during nonbusiness hours. Hospice programs also allow for durable medical equipment to be placed in the home such as a hospital bed and wheelchair. For people over the age of 65 who have Medicare, hospice can postpone or avoid admission to a nursing home because the range of services it offers.

The National Cancer Institute's (2015) PDQ Last Days of Life (Patient Version) states that when patients, caregivers, and carers plan for end-of-life care, patients and their loved ones are better able to make the decisions that must be made at critical moments. There are many books and resources to help patients and families through the final days starting with the hospice program's information packet and asking the hospice team for recommendations given your particular situation.

3   Symptoms of Advancing Mesothelioma

As people with cancer enter the end of life, they may experience symptoms that are calling cards of the beginning of the dying process. A wide variety of symptoms occur regardless of the type of cancer, but those discussed here are specific to mesothelioma. The symptoms can range from being an irritant to very distressing for the person with mesothelioma who is approaching death and the family caregivers and others who care. Most of the symptoms that people with mesothelioma experienced before the initial diagnosis are the same ones that identify the beginning of the end of life. Hughes and Arber (2008) report that people with mesothelioma and caregivers wanted more information about the trajectory of the disease. Thus, being aware that the progression of symptoms is a sign of the end of life is important for people with mesothelioma, caregivers, and other carers to understanding the process. Knowing this information may decrease fears and anxiety about the changing symptoms. Further, it may answer the following question: How do we know that we are coming close to the end of life? Some of the symptoms can be minimized with the help of healthcare providers as well as things family members and others who care can do simply.

Common symptoms experienced by persons with mesothelioma that when they deteriorate or worsen can identify the beginning of the end of life: dyspnea, dysphagia, fatigue, weight loss, insomnia, and a cough (van Zandwjik 2013).

Dyspnea (pronounced dysp ne a) is shortness of breath. Dyspnea can be the result of a pleural effusion, fluid buildup between the lung and the wall of the chest. It can also be the result of the lining around the lung, which is where mesothelioma most often occurs and thickens. This thickening constrains the lung from fully expanding. Having lungs that no longer fully expand can cause chest pain, a feeling of tightness in the chest, and difficulty breathing or labored breathing. Dyspnea is also caused by anxiety. According to Guirimand et al. (2015) and Kamal et al. (2012), dyspnea is one of the common symptoms identified by people with advanced disease near the end of their life, starting between 4 and 6 days before death.

Fatigue (pronounced fa teg) is feeling extremely tired that is not relieved by rest. According to the NCCN, cancer-related fatigue is defined as "distressing, persistent, subjective sense of physical, emotional and/or cognitive tiredness or exhaustion … not proportional to activity and that interferes with usual functioning". Between 76% and 99% of both people with cancer and those receiving palliative care report fatigue as a difficult symptom (Kirshbaum et al. 2013).

Dysphagia (dis fa gia) means difficulty swallowing. Dysphagia can be the result of the disease putting pressure on the lungs as well as from having a dry mouth. Usually, it is difficult to swallow food, but it can be both food and liquids. Dysphagia can feel like the food is stuck in the throat, chest, or behind the breastbone and may result in gagging or coughing. This symptom can result in extreme weight loss and dehydration. If the food or liquid is going down the airway rather than the esophagus, the result could be aspiration pneumonia or other respiratory problems.

Weight loss or anorexia (pronounced an a rex i a) is a common symptom of mesothelioma. Weight loss can be the result of some of the symptoms mentioned already, dyspnea and dysphagia. It can also be the result of the spread of the cancer itself. Also, as the disease progresses, the person with mesothelioma may no longer be hungry or thirsty. This can be scary as it might seem that they are giving up or the family caregiver and other carers may get frustrated feeling that their offer of food is a rejection.

Can you as a family member help with someone who is living with end-stage mesothelioma? We say this is a very broad question, but yes, whether you are someone's blood relative or family member of creation, there is so much you can do for your loved one. The first thing you can do is listen to the fears and concerns of your loved one and be prepared to act on requests which you can fulfill and be clear about what you cannot do. For example, you can screen calls and visitors for times when your loved one is asking for quiet time or cook someone's favorite meal. You cannot, on the other hand, have superhuman powers to tend to all of your loved one's physical, emotional, and spiritual needs. You may have other people who depend upon you, you may have financial responsibilities, and you may have your own health needs to pay attention to. In short, you have to have a realistic assessment of what you can and cannot do. When you come to a task which you cannot do, that is the time to ask others in your family or social circle to pitch in or discuss your need for external support with someone whom you trust.

For most patients and families, the gateway to getting external support is a hospice program. Hospice programs are not only an interdisciplinary team of specialists who assist with the last months of life, but they are also able to refer you to other specialists and sources of assistance. Because they specialize in the end-of-life experience, the professionals who work in hospice programs know the types of problems family such as yours endure when a loved one is dying of mesothelioma. Hospices frequently have volunteers who can perform a wide variety of tasks from friendly visiting to dog walking, to handyman chores, etc. Similarly, hospice counselors can refer families to free or low-cost attorneys, find other sources of home care and assist with funeral planning, etc.

4   Common Emotions

Van Zandwijk et al. (2013) cite a study published by The British Lung Foundation (BLF) entitled *Survey of mesothelioma patients and their carers*. They collected data from people diagnosed with mesothelioma and their caregivers. One finding was that both those with mesothelioma and their caregivers had different experiences of the same emotions. The emotions and the percentage who endorsed most or some of the time by each group are as follows:

- Anger. Forty-six percent of patients and 89% of caregivers experienced anger most or some of the time. Anxiety. Sixty-eight percent and 84% of patients and caregivers, respectively, dealt with anxiety.
- Depression. Depression was reported by 72% and 80% of patients and caregivers, respectively. Isolation. The experience of isolation was 41% and 89%, respectively.
- Fear. Seventy-three percent of those with mesothelioma and 66% of caregivers experienced fear. In a small study from Australia, over 94% of patients were fearful of dying, and 43% experienced this fear every day (Dooley et al. 2010).
- Peace and acceptance: Seventy-one percent of those with mesothelioma reported being at peace and accepting this situation in comparison to 23% of the carers.

Given the percent of the patient and caregiver participants who completed this survey had some level of experience with the same emotions, some were higher for one than the other. As noted by Buchholz (2017), the informal caregivers and other carers have similar emotional reactions to the trajectory of the disease as the person with the disease.

5   The Dying Process

As someone is dying, the loss of appetite and no longer being thirsty are common (Lynn et al. 2011; Quill and Byock 2000). This can be distressing for caregivers and carers as one way to show love is to feed someone. At the end of life, the appetite decreases as the body is focusing on shutting down. It is more comfortable for the person dying only to drink if they ask for it. Being dehydrated decreases potential problems that could be uncomfortable for the dying person. One example is that being dehydrated results in urinating less, which can decrease the chance for the development of bed sores and less skin breakdown (Lynn et al. 2011).

6   Signs of Dying

Along the dying trajectory for anyone, there are specific things that start happening that are signs of impending death. These include slipping in and out of consciousness and becoming confused and having difficulty communicating. They may be drowsy, sleep more, and at times be unresponsive. They may be less interested in interactions with others. Unfortunately, one of the signs of dying is an increasing difficulty in managing pain and involuntary sounds and body movements.

As death approaches, the person extremities will be cool, and the parts of the body touching the bed or chair will have a purplish color. Breathing will be uneven, sometimes it will be rapid, and other times it will stop for a couple of seconds. These signs are usually observed up to 2 days before death. The closer one is to death the more likely the breathing starts being noisy. This is the result of the relaxing of the muscles in the throat. The noise is the saliva and other fluids that collect in the throat not being swallowed as before. Though it might be upsetting to the caregivers and carers, it is not causing the person who is dying discomfort. This sign of dying is called the "death rattle" and has been reported to be present in about half of people as they are dying. If the sound is upsetting to those who chose to be with the person, you might try to reposition the person in bed.

7   How to Know the Person Is Dead

One might think that it would be straightforward to know when someone is dead; this is not always true. Since one of the processes of dying is interrupted breathing, you might think a dying person is done breathing, and then they take another breath. You can assure someone is dead when they are no longer breathing. So, you may have to wait a bit to see that no more breathes are taken. There will be no pulse once a person dies.

In death all the muscles relax; this can result in either the bowel or the bladder emptying once the sphincter muscles release. If the person has not been eating much in the days before the death, it is less likely that they will defecate. It is also less likely for the bladder to empty if the person has not been drinking much or getting fluids intravenously.

If you have hospice providing care at the end of life, the hospice nurse will give you information on how to know when the person who is dying is dead. They will ask you to call them when you think the person is dead. If you are worried, scared, or not sure, please do call the hospice, and they will talk with you and help you figure out what has, is, and will happen. If you are involved with a hospice, do not be shy about calling them for help, guidance, and support.

8   Dying in the Hospital Versus at Home

Families caring for a person with mesothelioma can find it difficult to keep their family member at home as it becomes more difficult to manage the symptoms of advanced disease and think the person needs to be in the hospital to manage end-of-life symptoms and pain. As life with mesothelioma includes the thickening of the lining of the lungs which results in breathing becoming very difficult, it makes sense that the person who is dying and the family want to be in a hospital in the hopes it will be easier for all.

The discussion about where the person with mesothelioma wants to be when they die is extraordinarily important to have before the process starts. If the dying person wants to die at home, it is important to be associated with hospice before the dying process starts. Hospice services provide hands-on care for the person who is dying as well as a plethora of services and support to all involved. They are available for the person who is dying, the family, and other carers. Hospice staff have an amazing amount of experience with people dying at home and can help everyone providing care for a person with mesothelioma. They will provide education on all aspects of what to expect and how to respond to the changes that will likely occur, offer 24-hour access to nursing support, and come to the house if necessary. Hospice services include a physician, nurses, social worker, chaplains, and volunteers.

If the person with mesothelioma does not want to die in their home or the household is not able to accommodate a dying person, it is important to have this discussion with the healthcare providers. The most common alternative to dying at one's own home or the home of a caregiver is to have the person admitted to a nursing home, preferably a nursing home associated with a hospice program.

Often the person who is dying of mesothelioma wants to die at their home or the home of a loved one. This is acceptable to family caregivers and other carers until the symptoms are difficult to manage and it is difficult to accept that the dying person really wants to experience this at home. This is often when the person is taken to the emergency department or 911 is called. If 911 is called, the Emergency Medical Service (EMS) personnel will do everything to keep the person alive unless the dying person has completed a specific state document expressing medical procedures he/she does not want to be done if they are anywhere except a hospital. All communites are required by law to have the EMS pesonnel start resuscitation unless there is a signed form that is the mandoatory format, color, and is placed as specified by the jurisdiction.

This document has a variety of titles depending upon your locality:

- Do-Not-Resuscitate (DNR) Comfort Care
- Emergency Medical Services Do-Not-Resuscitate (DNR) Order
- Medical Orders for Life-Sustaining Treatments (MOLSTP)
- Physician Orders for Life-Sustaining Treatment (POLST)
- Physician Orders for Scope of Treatment (POST)
- Out-of-Hospital Do-Not-Resuscitate Declaration and Order

The person with mesothelioma or a family caregiver can start the conversation with either the physician or hospice team about obtaining an Out-of-Hospital DNR form. Some states have requirements for the color of the paper this document is to be printed on, where it is to be displayed, and if a bracelet or a necklace is required. The purpose of the document states that the treating physician has determined you are either terminally ill or extremely old and frail and that resuscitation, also known as CPR, would not be in your best interest or what you desire. The form may include a section on exactly what types of treatment you do want, such as comfort care and alleviation of pain. The document must be signed by a physician.

9   What Needs to Occur Right After the Death

In the United States, if your family member dies at home from mesothelioma, you call the healthcare provider who was providing care. This might be a hospice, a primary care provider, an oncologist, or a home health agency. The provider will notify the necessary organizations on your behalf. At some point after the death, the family needs to call the funeral home they plan to use to transport the body from the place of death. The funeral home is responsible for obtaining the death certificate.

In England and Wales, upon the death of someone with mesothelioma, the first person to call is the coroner. The coroner may or may not conduct an autopsy or just collect specimens. This is followed by an inquest to make the determination if the death was caused by mesothelioma, an occupational disease. A final death certificate cannot be released until after the inquest. In Northern Ireland, a coroner must be notified of the death, but an inquest is not mandated. The coroner usually only communicates with the provider who cared for the person to make a determination if the disease was occupationally related. In Scotland, the procurator fiscal (a legal officer who functions as a coroner) has to be notified by the provider. The procurator fiscal will then make a determination of whether an autopsy is necessary or not (British Lung Foundation 2017).

Depending on the wishes of the person who died or what the carers wish, a funeral may be organized with the body present in a coffin, or it could be a memorial service with the body not present if the person wanted to be cremated, it could be a memorial service, with the urn present. Sometimes there is no formal recognition of the death, or it occurs months after the death. This ritual is based on the family tradition, culture, or religious beliefs. Again, this time immediately after death is a bit easier if the decision about the final ritual is determined before the death.

10   Bereavement

Bereavement generally occurs after death. Typically, we think of the first several weeks after death as being the most intense, since the survivors have to arrange a burial and tend to some administrative tasks while, at the same time, adjusting to the loss of one's loved one. Social workers and chaplains in hospitals, nursing homes, and hospice programs can assist in helping families access burial and survivor benefits. There is no process of bereavement that every person, even within the same family, will experience. Hospice programs have bereavement counselors and see the bereaved individuals regardless of where and how a person died. Other sources of bereavement assistance include places of worship, hospitals, cancer treatment centers, and senior centers. In addition, there are telephone and internet support groups such as those offered by the Mesothelioma Applied Research Foundation and Cancer Care.

Finally, as mesothelioma is most often the result of occupational exposure to asbestos, many patients and their families may decide to file a claim for compensation. See the addendum on end-life-care and the legal process for more information.

Helpful Resources for Veterans:

- For example, the Department of Veterans Affairs administers the National Cemetery Administration which has jurisdiction over the 135 veterans cemeteries in the United States and in some instances can offer survivors a monthly income support (https://www.benefits.va.gov and https://www.cem.va.gov). Also, many states have veterans cemeteries of their own.

Helpful resources for patient and their families:

- The Mesothelioma Applied Research Foundation
  http://www.curemeso.org
- CancerCare
  https://www.cancercare.org/

Addendum: End-Life-Care and the Legal Process

While the discussion on the legal process may not be germane to the direct care of mesothelioma patients due to the high mortality, elucidating the legal process as it relates to end-of-life care may be an important resource for patients and their families, because financial and legal matters may be important to maintaining quality of life for the patient and his family.

The information presented below should not be interpreted as legal advice. Healthcare professional should exercise caution when discussing the legal process with patients and their families.

Legal Process

As mesothelioma is most often the result of occupational exposure to asbestos, filing a claim for compensation is a common course of action. There is an abundance of law firms around the world who claim to focus specifically on working with people with mesothelioma. Be thoughtful about how you select your legal assistance. When filing a claim against a previous employer where the exposure took place, it doesn't matter if the company knew they were putting employees at risk or not.

With the extended time between the exposure to asbestos and the diagnosis of mesothelioma, statutes of limitations have been revised to take this into account. The statutes of limitations are rules related to how long a person has before they must file a claim. In most cases, the time starts with exposure or when the injury took place. In the case of mesothelioma, the statute of limitations, which differs by state and the type of legal claim, the time to file ranges from 1 to 4 years from diagnosis (Hartley and Hesdorffer 2017).

There are three main routes to file a claim for the exposure that resulted in mesothelioma. The first is through a bankruptcy trust, the second is litigation, and, finally, if you are a veteran and you think your exposure was during your service, you would file veterans claim. A bankruptcy trust is a fund the companies where exposure to asbestos was known to have occurred were required to set up before they either close or claim bankruptcy to cover future legal claims. Litigation is when a lawsuit is filed with the intention of appearing in court. In many cases, these lawsuits can be settled out of court. A veteran who thinks they were exposed to asbestos while on active duty will file a claim for disability compensation through the Veterans Benefits Administration (https://www.benefits.va.gov/benefits/). You will also want to contact the VA Environmental Health Coordinator. You can find your local coordinator at https://www.publichealth.va.gov/exposures/asbestos/index.asp. There are two types of claims: personal injury and wrongful death.

When the person diagnosed with mesothelioma files a claim, it is a personal injury claim, within the statute of limitations for mesothelioma in the state you are filing. The claim can be filed to cover medical expenses, lost income (past, present, and future), and psychical and emotional pain. If the person with mesothelioma filed a claim after they were diagnosed and before they died, once the claim is settled, it becomes a part of the estate. This means that the executor of the estate will continue working with the lawyer the person with mesothelioma was working with to finalize the claim. There will likely be changes in what is covered once the person with mesothelioma dies. Since there will be no additional medical costs and the emotional distress does not continue beyond the death, the amount of the settlement may be impacted. Surviving family members can contact their local government office for state-specific information regarding legal proceedings and compensation (Hartley and Hesdorffer 2017).

References

American Cancer Society. If treatment of malignant mesothelioma stops working. 2016. Available at: https://www.cancer.org/cancer/malignant-mesothelioma/after-treatment/no-longer-working.html. Accessed 1 Dec 2017.
British Lung Foundation. End of life with mesothelioma. 2017. Accessed 20 Nov 2017.
Buchholz WM. The Patient's experience of malignant mesothelioma. In: Testa J, editor. Asbestos and mesothelioma. Cham: Springer; 2017. p. 381–407.
Dooley JJ, Wilson JP, Anderson VA. Stress and depression of facing death: Investigation of psychological symptoms in patients with mesothelioma. Aust J Psychol. 2010;62(3):160–8.
Guirimand F, Sahut d'izarn M, Laporte L, Francillard M, Richard J, Aegerter P. Sequential occurrence of dyspnea at the end of life in palliative care, according to the underlying cancer. Cancer Med. 2015;4(4):532–9.
Hartley K, Hesdorffer M. Challenges facing mesothelioma patients and their families: medical/legal intersections. In: Testa J, editor. Asbestos and mesothelioma. Cham: Springer; 2017. p. 359–81.
Hughes N, Arber A. The lived experience of patients with pleural mesothelioma. Int J Palliat Nurs. 2008;14(2):66–71.
Ionvno J. Mesothelioma statute of limitations. 2017. Accessed 10 Nov 2017.
Kamal AH, Maguire JM, Wheeler JL, Currow DC, Abernethy AP. Dyspnea review for the palliative care professional: treatment goals and therapeutic options. J Palliat Med. 2012;15(1):16–114.

Kirshbaum MN, Olson K, Pongthavornkamol K, Graffigna G. Understanding the meaning of fatigue at the end of life: an ethnoscience approach. Eur J Oncol Nurs. 2013;17(2):146.

Linton A, Pavlakis N, O'connell R, Soeberg M, Kao S, Clarke S, et al. Factors associated with survival in a large series of patients with malignant pleural mesothelioma in New South Wales. Br J Cancer. 2014;111(9):1860–9.

Lynn J, Harrold J, Schuster JL. Handbook for mortals: Guidance for people facing serious illness. 2nd ed. New York: Oxford University Press; 2011.

Meyerhoff RR, Yang CJ, Speicher PJ, Gulack BC, Hartwig MG, D'Amico TA, et al. Impact of mesothelioma histologic subtype on outcomes in the surveillance, epidemiology, and end results database. J Surg Res. 2015;196(1):23.

Moore S, Darlison L, Tod AM. Living with mesothelioma. A literature review. Eur J Cancer Care. 2010;19(4):458.

Musk AW, Olsen N, Alfonso H, Reid A, Mina R, Franklin P, et al. Predicting survival in malignant mesothelioma. Eur Respir J. 2011;38(6):1420–4.

National Cancer Institute. Planning the transition to end-of-life care in advanced cancer. 2015. Accessed 18 Nov 2017.

National Comprehensive Cancer Network. Malignant pleural mesothelioma guideline for patients. 2016. Available at: https://www.nccn.org/patients/guidelines/mpm/files/assets/basic-html/page-1.html

National Comprehensive Cancer Network. Malignant pleural mesothelioma. 2017a. Accessed 7 Nov 2017.

National Comprehensive Cancer Network. Cancer-related fatigue. 2017b. Accessed 18 Nov 2017.

Quill TE, Byock IR, for the ACP-ASIM End-of-Life Care Consensus Panel. Responding to Intractable Terminal Suffering: The Role of Terminal Sedation and Voluntary Refusal of Food and Fluids. Ann Intern Med. 132:408–414. https://doi.org/10.7326/0003-4819-132-5-200003070-00012.

Taioli E, Wolf AS, Camacho-Rivera M, Kaufman A, Lee D, Nicastri D, et al. Determinants of survival in malignant pleural mesothelioma: a surveillance, epidemiology, and end results (SEER) study of 14,228 patients. POLS One. 2015;10(12):e0145039.

van Zandwijk N, Clarke C, Henderson D, Musk AW, Fong K, Nowak A, et al. Guidelines for the diagnosis and treatment of malignant pleural mesothelioma. J Thorac Dis. 2013;5(6):E254.

Public Health Impact of Asbestos Worldwide

Public Health Impact of Asbestos
Worldwide: What Is the Current Public
Health Impact?

16

Jadmin L. Mostel, Gleneara E. Bates-Pappas,
and Gregory Pappas

1   History of Asbestos

The use of asbestos dates back to ancient times when it was used as wick material for oil lamps (Darcey and Alleman 2004). As asbestos' highly resistant properties came to light, it was subsequently woven into cloth, combined with clay in 2500 BC to create greater material strength, and, to this day, is still used as a fortifying agent in paint, concrete, and cement (Darcey and Alleman 2004). However, currently, public health issues dominate the conversations surrounding asbestos, and asbestos use is permitted in products such as roofing, millboard, automatic transmission components, disc brake pads, brake linings, cement products, and more (Darcey and Alleman 2004).

Commercial use of asbestos was banned in Germany since 1993, in Sweden since 1982, and in Italy since 1992 (3, 4, and 7). While Canada has yet to ban asbestos, asbestos mining has been halted since 2012, with plans to ban all asbestos by 2018. The United States remains one of the major industrialized countries that has yet to ban all asbestos production and use (8).

J. L. Mostel (✉)
Johns Hopkins Bloomberg School of Public Health, Baltimore, MD, USA
e-mail: jmostel@curemeso.org

G. E. Bates-Pappas
City University of New York Graduate Center, New York, NY, USA
e-mail: gbates@gradcenter.cuny.edu

G. Pappas
Department of Kinesiology and Applied Physiology, Rutgers University,
New Brunswick, NJ, USA
e-mail: gbates@gradcenter.cuny.edu

© Springer Nature Switzerland AG 2019
M. Hesdorffer, G. E. Bates-Pappas (eds.), *Caring for Patients with Mesothelioma: Principles and Guidelines*,
https://doi.org/10.1007/978-3-319-96244-3_16

1.1   Why Has Asbestos Been Slow to Ban?

Asbestos continues to be used because of its advantageous properties – such as good electrical resistance, tensile strength, sound insulation, heat insulation, and resistance to chemical and biological mediums, to name a few – and is low cost to produce (Hwang and Park 2016). In fact, it is these economic advantages that largely contribute to its ubiquitous application. Because asbestos is mined, rather than being a manufactured material, it is not closely monitored by producers or consumers and remains accessible for industrial exploitation in many countries (Darcey and Alleman 2004). As a natural product, there are little manufacturing and development costs, keeping it an affordable and accessible substance (Darcey and Alleman 2004). Because of these attractive properties, asbestos has been slow to ban in many countries; it is difficult to find an alternative substance of similar efficacy with a comparable low economic impact. As asbestos use has diminished in traditional capacities such as shipbuilding and home construction, some talc powder products were recently found to be contaminated with asbestos in Korea (Hwang and Park 2016).

1.2   What's Next After an Asbestos Ban?

A study conducted in Sweden examined recent deaths attributed to mesothelioma in the context of the country's asbestos ban in 1982. Although asbestos has been removed from the Swedish market for over 35 years, a declivity in the number of mesothelioma cases each year has not been clearly documented (Plato et al. 2016). While this may be attributed to the long latency period of mesothelioma, many individuals still experience non-occupational exposure to asbestos through DIY construction, which will continue to expose individuals to asbestos for the indefinite future. As a result, an asbestos ban does not negate the need for educational resources for respiratory protection for fiber inhalation and the dangers of handling asbestos materials.

Developed countries have a responsibility to ban asbestos for developing countries. Developing countries will likely continue to lack the resources for this education and lack the correct respiratory protection for handling asbestos materials. The responsibility of global health falls to those that have the power to make positive change: a global ban in the mining and exportation of asbestos rests at the decisions of developed countries.

2   What Is the Current Public Health Impact?

2.1   Non-occupational Asbestos Exposure

Much of asbestos literature documents the incidence of occupational-related exposure. However, non-occupational asbestos exposure has increasingly become a prominent issue in the mesothelioma community. Throughout the 1900s until the 1960s, many homes built in the United States used insulating materials that contained asbestos. These older homes are now often undergoing renovations, creating a new avenue of potential asbestos exposure. With the latency period of mesothelioma to be 20–50 years, and without proper precautions taken during home renovation projects, cases of individuals with mesothelioma due to DIY home renovations are beginning to emerge.

Studies conducted in Australia have suggested this trend in malignant mesothelioma (MM) cases due to non-occupational-related asbestos exposure is on the rise. One study conducted in Australia suggests that MM cases due to non-occupational exposure accounts for 8.4% of men and 35.7% of women diagnosed (Olsen et al. 2011). Olsen et al. also suggest a shorter latency period for MM due to non-occupational asbestos exposure. This could be due to a variety of factors, such as shorter follow-up periods and inability to recall exposure dates (Olsen et al. 2011). With this, it is likely that an increase in non-occupational mesothelioma cases will have an acclivity in diagnosis (Olsen et al. 2011). Another study conducted in Australia suggests the lack of adequate safety precautions for respiratory protection during DIY projects can lead to increases in non-occupational asbestos exposure and likely an increase in mesothelioma cases (Park et al. 2013). Asbestos dust may be released as home renovators continue to DIY renovate their houses, and without proper respiratory protection, this asbestos dust could be easily respired.

Schools are one area of concern for non-occupational secondhand exposure as many were built with asbestos-containing surface materials. As maintenance and/or renovations of schools occur, asbestos fibers may be released into the air (Darcey and Alleman 2004). Some studies examining asbestos abatement in schools have shown that there was little change in the air levels of asbestos fibers before and after asbestos removal, thus calling into question the health risks vs. benefits of asbestos abatement (Darcey and Alleman 2004). A study performed by the EPA indicated that while asbestos fibers did escape during the process of encapsulation and abatement, encapsulation did seem to result in a net reduction in asbestos fiber levels (Darcey and Alleman 2004). This suggests that instead of asbestos abatement, asbestos encapsulation may be the better option to take preventative measures to combat fiber inhalation (Darcey and Alleman 2004).

A second, albeit much less common route of non-occupational asbestos exposure, is through environmental exposure. Asbestos is a naturally occurring mineral, and environmental exposure can result from weathering and erosion of rocks containing asbestos, therefore releasing asbestos fibers into the air, and/or the weathering of road surfaces built with asbestos materials. (Darcey and Alleman 2004) Areas in the United States that have high concentration of source rock *and* high population density include eastern Pennsylvania, southwestern Connecticut, southeastern New York, Los Angeles, and San Francisco; these areas could indicate more critical points for environmental exposure to asbestos (Darcey and Alleman 2004).

There is a dearth in literature documenting non-occupational asbestos exposure in the United States. However, as these older homes continue to be renovated and other DIY projects are performed to the structure of the house and a rise in non-occupational mesothelioma cases is expected, it is essential that renovators are educated on proper safety procedures when handling asbestos materials and the risks involved.

2.2   Occupational Exposure

Occupations with high levels of asbestos exposure are strongly associated with the high rates of mesothelioma. Studies from various countries demonstrate mesothelioma diagnosis trends in high-exposure occupations such as industry, construction, factory, and shipyard workers. Historically, asbestos was a widely used material across industries because of its useful qualities in insulating, reduction of fire risk, and corrosion resistance (Darcey and Alleman 2004). As asbestos is cheap to mine and produce, it was widely used in many common household products such as clothes, fireproofing materials, vehicle brakes, and construction materials (Darcey and Alleman 2004).

With mesothelioma so strongly linked to occupation, there is also a geographical trend associated with occupational exposure. Mesothelioma rates tend to be higher in regions with a history of asbestos-using occupations or production sites, such as factories, shipyards, railways, or construction yards. Italy was a prominent asbestos user from approximately 1950 until its ban in 1992, with peak production and use around 1976–1980. A 2015 study in Italy sought to identify and characterize territorial clusters of malignant mesothelioma using the Italian National Mesothelioma Registry (ReNaM). Results identified 32 clusters of MM cases, primarily in northern Italy, the site of asbestos-containing manufacturing plants and shipyards (Corfiati et al. 2014). Many studies support the strong link between mesothelioma and occupation: A 2005 study using the British mesothelioma registry found the highest rates of mesothelioma deaths in men were associated with regions containing shipyards and other asbestos-containing occupations, and a 2014 Canadian study found mesothelioma rates highest in the regions with the highest reported occupational asbestos exposure (McElvenny et al. 2005; Pefoyo et al. 2014).

Many countries have implemented safety measures to reduce occupational exposure risk and/or have banned asbestos use and production. One study in Italy found that the rate of pleural mesothelioma diagnosis declined from 2005 to 2010 (D'Agostin et al. 2017). The authors suggest this could be the positive effects of asbestos exposure workplace safety measures implemented in Friuli Venezia Giulia in 1975, although more research is needed to confirm this trend (D'Agostin et al. 2017). Similar studies examining mesothelioma incidence have been performed in France. A 2009 study found a slight declivity in mesothelioma rates in males from 2000 to 2003 (Le Stang et al. 2009). The authors also speculate this could be related to work safety regulations put in place since 1977 (Le Stang et al. 2009). Despite some positive effects demonstrated in declines of mesothelioma diagnosis, many asbestos bans, such as those in Sweden and Canada, have not supported a significant decrease in mesothelioma diagnosis to date (Plato et al. 2016; Pefoyo et al. 2014).

Occupational asbestos exposure and mesothelioma diagnosis historically tend to be more prevalent in men than women, presumably due to men working in high asbestos exposure occupations. Mesothelioma diagnosis in women, seemingly on the rise, could be due to a number of factors, including para-occupational exposure in which workers unknowingly bring home asbestos fibers on their clothes or other work materials. Family members are exposed to these asbestos fibers through laundry or other forms of contact (Noonan 2017; Goswami et al. 2013). Although women are generally thought to be exposed to asbestos para-occupationally, occupational exposure in women may be due to the textile industry, schools, or offices. Additionally, a rise in mesothelioma rates in women could be due to more accurate diagnosis.

3   Summary and Future

Despite its long history of adverse health effects, asbestos-containing products are still used all over the world. Efforts to ban, limit, or reduce exposure to asbestos across many countries have started to come into place. While there has been a seismic shift in attitudes, regarding asbestos lead by grass-roots organizations, there continue to be challenges in banning the use of asbestos. Industry continues to lobby for the "controlled use of asbestos" arguing that asbestos can be used safely with minimal risk to workers (Kazan-Allen 2012). However, history has shown that despite regulations and legislation, the safe sue of asbestos has proven to be impossible. Despite the scientific evidence quantifying the social cost of the use of asbestos, industry and government officials have yet to develop regulations and policies that truly protect unsuspecting populations from the risk of asbestos exposure (Kazan-Allen 2011).

References

Corfiati M, et al. Epidemiological patterns of asbestos exposure and spatial clusters of incident cases of malignant mesothelioma from the Italian national registry. BMC Cancer. 2014;15:286.

D'Agostin F, De Michieli P, Chermaz C, Negro C. Pleural and peritoneal mesotheliomas in the Friuli Venezia Giulia register: data analysis from 1995 to 2015 in Northeastern Italy. J Thorac Dis. 2017;9:1032–45.

Darcey DJ, Alleman T. Occupational and environmental exposure to asbestos. In: Pathology of asbestos-associated diseases. New York: Springer; 2004. p. 17–33.

Goswami E, et al. Domestic asbestos exposure: a review of epidemiologic and exposure data. Int J Environ Res Public Health. 2013;10(11):5629–70.

Hwang SH, Park WM. Evaluation of asbestos-containing products and released fibers in home appliances. J Air Waste Manag Assoc. 2016;66(9):922–9.

Kazan-Allen, L. Ban asbestos phenomenon: the winds of change. New Sol, 2012;21(4):629–36. https://doi.org/10.2190/NS.21.4.j.

Le Stang N, et al. Evolution of pleural cancers and malignant pleural mesothelioma incidence in France between 1980 and 2005. Int J Cancer. 2009;126(1):232–8.

McElvenny DM, Darnton AJ, Price MJ, Hodgson JT. Mesothelioma mortality in Great Britain from 1968 to 2001. Occup Med. 2005;55:79–87.

Noonan CW. Environmental asbestos exposure and risk of mesothelioma. Ann Transl Med. 2017;5(11):234.

Olsen N, et al. Increasing incidence of malignant mesothelioma after exposure to asbestos during home maintenance and renovation. Med J Aust. 2011;195:271.

Park E, Yates D, Hyland R, Johnson A. Asbestos exposure during home renovation in New South Wales. Med J Aust. 2013;199(6):410–3.

Pefoyo AJK, et al. Exploring the usefulness of occupational exposure registries for surveillance: the case of the Ontario Asbestos Workers Registry (1986–2012). J Occup Environ Med. 2014;56:1100–10.

Plato N, et al. Occupation and mesothelioma in Sweden: updated incidence in men and women in the 27 years after the asbestos ban. Epidemiol Health. 2016;38:e2016039.

Part V

The Future of Mesothelioma Research

Aaron Mansfield, Dennis Wigle, and Tobias Peikert

1 Introduction to Clinical Research Studies in Mesothelioma

Clinical trials are research studies in humans. They are designed to find out if certain treatments are safe and effective—for example, whether a new or existing drug is more effective in treating mesothelioma compared to the current standard therapy. While most clinical trials may involve new drugs or new ways of giving patients those drugs—such as combinations of medications—they are also investigating new surgical and radiation treatments, medical devices, vaccines, symptom management strategies, diagnostic tests and biomarkers for early detection, diagnosis and prediction of disease outcomes, and therapeutic responses. In order to be marketed in the United States, devices, drugs, and medical tests must pass strict regulatory conditions set by the Food and Drug Administration (FDA). Based on estimates by the National Institutes of Health, there are approximately 250,000 clinical trials in progress worldwide. These clinical trials range across the entire spectrum of medicine.

Clinical research studies in oncology represent the leading edge for advances in diagnostic testing and therapeutic innovations for patients with mesothelioma and other cancers. These trials are most commonly available at large academic medical centers and are led by investigators with expertise in mesothelioma. The purpose of these research studies is to investigate new diagnostic tests, procedures, or treatment strategies to improve the standard of care. These studies

A. Mansfield (✉) · D. Wigle (✉) · T. Peikert (✉)
Mayo Clinic, Rochester, MN, USA
e-mail: Mansfield.Aaron@mayo.edu; Wigle.Dennis@mayo.edu; Peikert.Tobias@mayo.edu

© Springer Nature Switzerland AG 2019
M. Hesdorffer, G. E. Bates-Pappas (eds.), *Caring for Patients with Mesothelioma: Principles and Guidelines*,
https://doi.org/10.1007/978-3-319-96244-3_17

frequently compare new diagnostic tests, therapeutic procedures, or drug treatments to the current standard of care in order to determine if there are advantages with the new approach. Without research studies doctors and their patients have no way to systematically understand whether the benefits of new tests, devices, procedures, or drugs outweigh their risks and improve patient care. Consequently, clinical research also represents the key component for the regulatory approval and ultimately insurance coverage decisions for new diagnostic tests, devices, and drugs.

Patients facing a new diagnosis of malignant mesothelioma are frequently overwhelmed by the diagnosis and struggle to understand the information about the prognosis and therapeutic options of this deadly disease. Many patients and their caregivers frequently do not have prior exposure to clinical trials and their associated terminology.

Participation in a clinical trial may not be the right fit for every patient. Even if patients are willing to consider receiving a promising but unproven type of treatment or to contribute to advance the understanding, diagnosis, and management of mesothelioma, there are always advantages and disadvantages to consider before making the decision to enter a trial. Herein we will try to provide you the resources to help with this decision.

Clinical trials are typically designed to answer specific questions about safety and efficacy. Based on the stages of development, there are many possible clinical trial designs that can be used to assess safety and efficacy. The technical terms used to describe these trials and their designs can make it challenging for patients and their families to make a fully informed decision whether or not to participate in clinical research (Tables 17.1 and 17.2). Furthermore, common misperceptions of patients being used as "guinea pigs" are partially based of previous unethical trials conducted in the twentieth century fuel concerns by patients and families over participation in current clinical trials. Fortunately, over the last few decades, clinical research has become highly regulated and include extensive protections for patients. In this chapter, we will review the basic

Table 17.1 Common clinical trial designs

Type of clinical trial	Goals or definitions
Phase 1	Determine the safety of a new drug or combination of drugs
Phase 2	To detect a preliminary signal of efficacy of a new drug or combination of drugs once safety has been establish
Phase 3	To definitively determine the efficacy of a new drug or combination of drugs
Basket trial	A trial that includes patients with one of multiple types of cancers with a common biomarker
Umbrella trial	A trial that assigns treatment patients with one type of cancer to one of many treatments based on the presence of a biomarker

Table 17.2 Meaning of common clinical trial terms

Term	Definition
Randomization	Process by which participants are assigned to a treatment
Blinding	Process of preventing participants and study staff from being aware of which treatment is being administered, often with the use of a placebo
Placebo	An inactive substance that is designed to look like the treatment it is being compared to
Crossover	Process by which participants receiving standard of care treatment may receive the experimental treatment after their tumors grow
Biomarker	A substance that can be measured or detected such as a DNA mutation or protein that is used to select or assign a treatment

designs and components of clinical trials specifically as they relate to the unique and multidisciplinary care for patients with mesothelioma.

2   The Traditional Phases of Clinical Trials and Drug Development

2.1   Phase 1 Clinical Trials

Most people consider clinical trials in the context of a new treatment strategy (new drugs, devices, or surgical interventions). A new treatment is sometimes brought forward for testing in patients often after many years of laboratory work, and various laboratory models have been tested to determine that a drug may be effective in a particular setting such as mesothelioma. These models are also used to test the potential safety of these interventions in patients. If an intervention being tested has never been approved for other purposes in human patients, its safety in humans needs to be established, and that is typically done through a phase 1 clinical trial. Other times, novel combinations of drugs are being tested requiring the establishment of safety and dosing parameters. The traditional phase 1 clinical trial with a single anticancer agent will test escalating doses of this agent and monitor patients for safety in what is called a 3 + 3 cohort expansion design. If the first group of patients tolerates the initial dose of a drug well, the dose is then escalated and tested in a second group. Alternatively, if patients experience side effects that are thought to be related to the drug, more patients may be asked to participate at the current dose level, or the dose may be reduced for the next group of patients. Based on the nature of the drug being tested, there could be many dose levels that are explored. Also, based on the emerging signals from these clinical trials, the design may be modified to add additional cohorts of patients to help determine the safety and efficacy of the new drug (Ivy et al. 2010). The ultimate goal of the traditional phase 1 clinical trial is to identify the highest safe dose of a novel drug that can be tested for efficacy in a larger clinical trial (LoRusso et al. 2010).

An improved understanding of tumor biology and the development of more efficient clinical trial designs have resulted in changes to the classic phase 1 clinical trial. For example, although safety is always at the forefront of phase 1 clinical trials, blood and tumor tissue-based biomarkers may be used to select the recommended phase 2 dose of a drug rather than the maximum tolerated dose. In other words, the dose of the drug may be selected based on its biological effect rather than the highest dose of a drug that patients can tolerate. Similarly, continual reassessment methods are used in phase 1 clinical trials to select the dose of a drug for the next patient based on the side effects observed in all patients previously treated in the clinical trial (Paoletti et al. 2017). Regardless of the design, phase 1 clinical trials often require frequent visits with the medical team for safety monitoring, additional blood work, and sometimes tumor biopsies that otherwise would not be performed during standard therapy outside of a clinical trial. Also, because of concerns about potential side effects of the drugs/interventions being tested, additional medical tests such as ophthalmologic or cardiac examinations are often required to monitor for safety. Most patients who are invited to participate in phase 1 clinical trials have often received and stopped benefitting from prior therapies. As is the case for most clinical trials, patients who participate in phase 1 clinical trials must have a good performance status, have not suffered other significant medical complications, and have no severely abnormal laboratory results.

2.2   Phase 2 Clinical Trials

Once the safety of a new drug or a treatment strategy has been established, phase 2 clinical trials are traditionally performed to estimate the effect of the intervention on the disease such as mesothelioma. There are many variations of phase 2 clinical trials which reflect the diverse goals of these trials (Seymour et al. 2010). Sometimes these trials are performed to broadly explore anticancer activity of the drug in many tumor types; other times these are performed to determine if the intervention should be investigated in a larger, randomized phase 3 clinical trial in a particular disease. Accordingly, some phase 2 clinical trials enroll all patients at the same dose of the drug and monitor outcomes to be compared with historical controls, meaning that all patients in the study receive the investigational therapy. In contrast, other phase 2 clinical trials will randomize patients to receive an experimental therapy, one of the multiple experimental therapies, or standard of care therapy. When phase 2 clinical trials randomize patients to one of two treatments, "crossover" (switching over) to the experimental treatment may be allowed if there is progression of disease with the standard of care. Although placebo controls (sham treatments) are more commonly used in phase 3 clinical trials, sometimes this strategy is also used in phase 2 studies to blind patients and the treating medical team to whether a patient is receiving an experimental drug or standard of care. For example, sometimes all patients in a trial will receive the standard of care therapy, but half will also receive an experimental drug, and the other half will receive a placebo. The experimental drug and placebo can be designed to look the same so that patients and physicians are not aware of which one is which. Pure placebo groups in the absence of any active therapy are rare in aggressive diseases such as mesothelioma. Given the development of many molecular targeted therapies and advances in the development of biomarkers potentially predicting treatment responses, phase 2 clinical trials now more commonly select patients based on the presence of a biomarker or monitor changes in biomarkers before, during, and after a treatment. Also, based on the safety signal that emerged in prior phase 1 clinical trials or other trials with the drug under development, additional safety monitoring may be required such as with echocardiograms or ophthalmological exams. There are many ways to determine if a drug is efficacious in phase 2 clinical trials, but there is some controversy as to which is most appropriate to use. The shrinkge of tumor or the lack of progression of disease as determined through radiologic imaging can be used to determine efficacy. The ultimate goal of these studies is to identify new and improved therapies that potentially will result in improved survival time with good quality of life.

2.3   Phase 3 Clinical Trials

Once the safety of the drug has been established and there is a preliminary signal of efficacy, phase 3 clinical trials are conducted to definitively test whether a treatment should become standard of care. Accordingly, phase 3 clinical trials typically randomize patients to receive a new treatment or the current standard of care. In some trial designs, all patients receive the standard of care, but one group of patients will receive a drug that is added to the standard regimen. The current standard of care for the systemic treatment of mesothelioma is based on a phase 3 clinical trial that randomized patients to receive cisplatin or a combination of cisplatin and pemetrexed (Vogelzang et al. 2003). More recently, a trial in France randomized patients to receive the standard of care cisplatin and pemetrexed or the combination of cisplatin and pemetrexed with bevacizumab (Zalcman et al. 2016). The addition of bevacizumab to cisplatin and pemetrexed improved survival and has been incorporated into the National Comprehensive Cancer Network guidelines (Ettinger et al. 2016). Given the strict eligibility criteria for this clinical trial and the lack of submission for approval of this regimen by the US Food and Drug Administration, some have questioned the applicability of the cisplatin, pemetrexed, and bevacizumab regimen to a wider population of patients (Levin and Dowell 2017). Accordingly, the use of this three-drug regimen has not been completely adopted, and some clinical trials do not include it as the standard of care comparator.

Blinding is a critical component of clinical trials that prevents patients, physicians, and other study personnel from knowing which treatment a participant is receiving. This is important because knowledge of which treatment a participant is receiving may influence how investigators assess responses and outcomes or influence the supportive care they provide. For example, in a clinical trial that is not blinded, an investigator might be inclined to look for more adverse events in the group of patients not receiving the experimental therapy. Similarly, an investigator might be more inclined to attribute a symptom to a treatment that may have occurred anyway when a study is not blinded. Blinding minimizes these influences and improves the quality of the information obtained from the clinical trial. In terms of systemic therapies, blinding may include the use of a placebo. A placebo is an inactive agent that is designed to be indistinguishable from the experimental therapy. In terms of surgeries or medical procedures, a sham procedure in which the intervention is not performed is akin to a placebo in a drug trial; however, this may preclude blinding of some of the study personnel. The use of a placebo or sham procedure alone is appropriate in some medical situations for which there is no standard of care. For patients with mesothelioma, there is no standard of care maintenance therapy after cisplatin and pemetrexed. Accordingly, an ongoing clinical trial as of December 2017 randomizes patients to receive a new drug, nintedanib, or a placebo after initial treatment with cisplatin and pemetrexed to determine if nintedanib is superior to no treatment in this setting (Scagliotti et al. 2017). In this study both investigators and participants are blinded to whether someone is receiving a nintedanib or a placebo.

Some clinical trials that randomize participants to one of two treatments allow crossover to the experimental arm after participants experience disease progression with the standard of care. Crossover can provide a mechanism for most participants to receive an experimental therapy and improve enthusiasm for participation, but its use may complicate the interpretation of trial outcomes (Prasad 2013). Blinding of treatments, as discussed previously, would preclude crossover unless there is unblinding of the treatment received.

The federal Food and Drug Administration (FDA) provided additional information to patients about clinical trials (https://www.fda.gov/ForPatients/ClinicalTrials/default.htm).

3   Novel Clinical Trial Designs: Basket and Umbrella Studies

Biomedical research is rapidly advancing with novel technologies. Most cancers like mesothelioma are thought to be caused by changes or mutations in DNA. DNA sequencing techniques allow the identification of mutations that might be susceptible to targeted therapies that have been designed to block these changes. Although some mutations may be specific to a single type of cancer, other mutations may be present in many types of cancer. In addition to DNA mutations, cancer cells may aberrantly express proteins that can be targeted with various therapies. Both DNA mutations and aberrantly expressed proteins can be considered biomarkers. Given that most novel therapeutics are designed to target a specific biomarker, the clinical trial landscape has changed significantly to incorporate biomarkers into the selection of participants for treatment (Renfro and Sargent 2017; Verma et al. 2017; West 2017; Woodcock and LaVange 2017; Simon 2017). One example of a biomarker-based clinical trial is an umbrella trial. In an umbrella trial, patients with a single type of cancer such as mesothelioma are screened for the presence of biomarkers.

Treatment may then be assigned to a therapy that targets the specific biomarker that was identified. Another example of a biomarker-based clinical trial is a basket trial. A basket trial typically allows the screening of many cancers or disease subtypes for a single biomarker, and assignment is made to a targeted therapy if this biomarker is present. An example of a basket trial is KEYNOTE-28 (NCT02054806) which screened patients with one of many cancer types for the immune checkpoint programmed cell death 1 ligand 1 (PD-L1, aka B7-H1 and CD274). The expression of PD-L1 has been associated with a poor prognosis in mesothelioma (Mansfield et al. 2014), and drugs have been developed to limit the immunosuppressive effects of PD-L1 (Mansfield 2017). For example, in KEYNOTE-28 patients with mesothelioma that expressed PD-L1 were assigned to treatment with pembrolizumab which was shown to have some promising activity in this setting (Alley et al. 2017).

Biomarkers have been incorporated into the design of clinical trials that do not qualify as basket or umbrella studies. Mesothelin is another biomarker that is commonly expressed by mesotheliomas and can be targeted (Hassan et al. 2016). Some recent clinical trials have screened patients' tumors for the presence of mesothelin to select participants to receive therapy that targets mesothelin. This biomarker-screening design excludes patients whose tumors lack a biomarker and are therefore unlikely to benefit from targeting this biomarker. These biomarker selection trials are increasingly common with DNA sequencing and other technologies.

4 Expanded Access and Off-Label Use

Unfortunately, current standard of care therapies available to treat mesothelioma eventually fail in most cases, and patients and their families are often interested in trying other therapies. In this situation we strongly encourage them to consider participation in available clinical trials and to consider local consensus guidelines for treatment of mesothelioma, for example, National Comprehensive Cancer Network (NCCN, https://www.nccn.org/professionals/physician_gls/default.aspx) and the American Society of Clinical Oncology (ASCO) (Hedy et al. 2018). Regardless, questions of "compassionate use" and "off-label use" frequently arise in clinic. When a drug is not approved by the FDA for any indication, expanded access (sometimes called "compassionate use") could be considered. In order to pursue expanded access in the United States, a physician has to submit form FDA 3926 to the FDA to obtain an Investigational New Drug (IND) number (Department of Health and Human Services Food and Drug Administration). Submitting an IND application requires support from the pharmaceutical company that makes the drug of interest and their commitment to provide the drug (Caplan et al. 2016). Despite popular conception, the FDA actually rapidly approves the majority of expanded access requests that are supported by a manufacturer. The drug companies are not under legal obligation to do this. Once an IND number has been assigned by the FDA, the physician has to obtain approval by their local institutional review board to prescribe this compassionate use medication. Expanded access represents a significant burden on physicians due to the many hours required to complete paperwork, to submit an IRB proposal, and to comply with the monitoring and regulatory requirements of what is essentially a single patient clinical trial. Also given the unknown risks of non-FDA approved medications to the patient, expanded access should only be considered if there is a strong biologic rationale such as the presence of a mutation targeted by a novel therapeutic and prior demonstration that an agent may be safe to administer. This justification to pursue expanded access is often lacking. In other cases, the promising activity of a drug may lead to many requests for single patient expanded access INDs. In this situation, pharmaceutical companies may create an expanded access protocol which has the goal of making a novel therapeutic available to patients likely to benefit from it.

When a drug is approved by the FDA for an indication other than mesothelioma, some patients or family members request off-label use of that drug. Even though precision medicine or the use of DNA sequencing to select targeted therapies has advanced treatments for non-small cell lung cancer and other cancers, treating variants of undetermined significance with off-label therapies has had limited applicability and benefit at some major academic centers (Bryce et al. 2017). Similar to requests for expanded access, the use of off-label drugs often is not justified. Prescription of off-label drugs is often complicated by payment issues. If a health insurance company or health system is not willing to cover the costs of an off-label therapy, a patient would have to pay out of pocket for these treatments. Given the escalating costs of therapies, this is not feasible for most people. In this context the description used for these therapies may matter. There have been recent efforts by physicians and the FDA to replace the term "off-label" use with physician-directed therapy which highlights that this is not the random use of an unapproved medication but rather based on a strong and plausible biological rationale (Position Statement by the American Academy of Orthopedic Surgeons, https://www.aaos. org/uploadedFiles/PreProduction/About/Opinion_Statements/position/1177%20 Physician%20Directed%20Use%20of%20Medical%20Products.pdf). When might expanded access or off-label use be appropriate? There are many factors that a physician considers when recommending expanded access or off-label use for patients who have exhausted other options. One setting that might be appropriate is for a patient who does not meet the eligibility criteria for a clinical trial because of a minor issue, or when the experimental therapy has demonstrated a strong signal of efficacy against tumors with a biomarker that is also present in this patient's tumor. Some success stories have been published with this approach (Mansfield et al. 2016). The safety of the drug in question, its reported efficacy, insurance coverage, and patient eligibility and geographical access to ongoing clinical trials testing the agent should all be considered to determine if physician-guided "off-label" use is appropriate (Mailankody and Prasad 2016).

5   Multimodality Therapy Studies in Mesothelioma

The routine clinical use of aggressive multimodality therapy represented by the sequential use of surgery, chemotherapy and radiation therapy in mesothelioma remains controversial. The use of this approach varies largely across the world. In the

United States, different approaches to multimodality therapy are offered to mesothelioma patients across the country. There is a lack of consensus regarding the patient selection, staging procedures, and the sequencing of the components of a multimodality treatment plan for mesothelioma. In our hands, multimodality therapy is typically considered in patients with early-stage epithelioid tumors confided to a unilateral pleural space in the absence of lymph node or systemic metastasis. The goal for the surgical intervention is to remove all visible tumors with the least invasive approach. There are several previous and ongoing trials investigating multimodality therapy for mesothelioma in the United States (Verma et al. 2017; Batirel et al. 2016; Bovolato et al. 2014; Burt et al. 2014; Cao et al. 2014; Flores et al. 2008; Friedberg et al. 2017; Marulli et al. 2017; Schwartz et al. 2017; Shaikh et al. 2017; Taioli et al. 2015). Most of these studies have been relatively small single institution studies. Investigators in Britain completed the Mesothelioma and Radical Surgery (MARS) study, which compared combination therapy including surgery (extrapleural pneumonectomy), postoperative radiotherapy, and chemotherapy with chemotherapy alone (Treasure et al. 2011). Unfortunately, the study was stopped early due to decreased survival and worse quality of life in the aggressively treated patients (Treasure et al. 2011). The follow-up Mesothelioma and Radical Surgery 2 (MARS-2) study is investigating a less aggressive lung-sparing surgical approach of pleurectomy and decortication (Trialists and Lim 2017). This study has surpassed the first futility endpoint and continues to recruit patients in the United Kingdom. However there are many remaining questions which include patient selection, the contribution of the individual therapeutic modalities and their sequencing, the type of surgical procedure used, and the delivery modality of radiation therapy. Ideally we need additional randomized studies comparing various multimodality therapeutic protocols such as neoadjuvant radiotherapy followed by extrapleural pneumonectomy and pleurectomy decortication followed by intensity-modulated radiation therapy (IMRT) or the direct comparison of the use of different intraoperative therapies such as heated chemotherapy, photodynamic therapy, and povidone (Friedberg et al. 2017; Shaikh et al. 2017; Chan et al. 2017; de Perrot et al. 2016; Rimner et al. 2016). In this context we would like to strongly encourage patients to consider participation in multimodality therapy studies for mesothelioma if they are interested in this treatment approach and are considered candidates by their treating physician.

The window of opportunity studies represent a subgroup of surgical studies for mesothelioma. These studies typically involve the neoadjuvant (prior to surgery) administration of a drug, vaccine, or other interventions (radiation or freezing) prior to a surgical intervention. This approach typically provides invaluable data regarding the effects of the tested intervention on the tumor since tissue sample from before and after the intervention can be analyzed.

6 Cell Therapy Studies

Cell therapy is a very exciting area in cancer research. While bone marrow transplantation has been used for many hematologic malignancies for a number of years, more specific interventions such as chimeric antigen receptor T-cell (CAR T-cell) therapy have become more popular as a cancer therapy recently. While there has been considerable success and now FDA approval of CAR T-cells in hematological malignancies, clinical studies of CAR T-cells in solid tumors including mesothelioma are still ongoing. These studies involve the isolation of the patients' T-cells and their retargeting to the tumor by expression of a chimeric T-cell receptor, representing an antibody fragment that binds to a tumor-specific surface protein. In the case of mesothelioma, the most commonly targeted antigen is mesothelin. While there is considerable overlap between the clinical trial design for other therapeutic interventions and cell therapy, there are a number of differences which allow for an accelerated regulatory approval process for effective cell therapeutic products.

7 Non-therapeutic Research Studies

There are also a number of mesothelioma research studies that are not primarily focused on the investigation of new therapies for the disease. These studies primarily try to better understand mesothelioma and to facilitate its early detection and diagnosis. In contrast to therapeutic clinical trials, these studies have less potential benefits for the individual participating patient but may impact future patients by developing new biomarkers and diagnostic techniques and discovering novel potential therapeutic strategies. These studies commonly involve the collection of clinical information, questionnaire data, blood and tumor tissue or the application of new imaging or other diagnostic tests. While these studies are less likely to impact the clinical disease course of the participating patients, they are typically associated with only "minimal" risks and provide extremely valuable information for future patients. A very successful example for this type of research study is the National Mesothelioma Virtual Tissue Bank (NMVB) (https://www.mesotissue.org/). The NMVB database represents a collection of well-annotated and de-identified blood, tissue, and pleural fluid specimens donated by mesothelioma patients across several large referral centers in the United States. This unique collection of clinical information and biospecimens is accessible to mesothelioma researchers at no cost and has supported a large number of successful research projects. It currently includes >1500 annotated cases and >1800 biospecimens. It is important to recognize that some of these highly valuable tumor specimens would otherwise be considered surgical waste and be discarded after the biopsy or surgical procedure.

8 How Do I Find a Clinical Trial and Decide If It Is Right for Me?

Finding a clinical trial for mesothelioma that suits the particular needs of a specific patient requires significant research. It is typically best to start by discussing your interest in clinical research with your treating physician first. This discussion should provide you with a good understanding of the clinical trial opportunities that are available in your local area. There are also a number of online resources. However given the legal implications of a diagnosis of mesothelioma, patients should be careful about online resources that use links and descriptions of clinical trials to recruit patients as clients for law firms. Therefore we would like to highlight some comprehensive unbiased resources. It is always a good idea to start by searching the NIH's www.ClinicalTrials.gov website for mesothelioma studies. This is one of the largest databases for both privately and publicly funded clinical trials. The search strategy can be focused on a particular disease such as mesothelioma and a specific geographical area. Another excellent resource is the Mesothelioma Applied Research Foundation (MARF, www.curemeso.org). They provide patient support regarding the selection of clinical trials over the phone, online, and during regional and national meetings. In addition patients can also research the websites of large mesothelioma programs such as Mayo Clinic; MD Anderson Cancer Center, New York University, the University of Pennsylvania, Memorial Sloan Kettering Cancer Center, the National Cancer Institute, Princess Margaret Cancer Center, the University of Western Australia, etc. Given that most clinical trials require regular follow-up visits at the site of the clinical study, patients need to consider geographic proximity and the impact of travel when making a decision about specific clinical studies.

How do I find out if I qualify for a clinical trial? Most clinical trials have rigorous inclusion and exclusion criteria to identify appropriate participants. Clinical trial participation typically includes a screening visit and frequently some additional testing to determine if a patient is a candidate for a particular study. Important factors for mesothelioma include the histological disease type (epithelioid, biphasic, or sarcomatoid), disease stage (surgical versus non-surgical), performance status, and the presence of other medical problems including a history of other cancers. A recent diagnosis of another malignancy with the exception of non-melanoma skin cancer and few selected other indolent cancers typically represents an exclusion criterion for most therapeutic clinical trials. The presence of measurable disease, tumor that can be reliably measured on an imaging study, is usually also required. The main reason for establishing and reinforcing strict eligibility criteria is to make trials as safe as possible for participants and to ensure that the study yields consistent and scientifically valid results for the investigators.

Who is in charge of my medical care in a clinical trial? Every clinical mesothelioma study has a principal investigator, usually a physician and mesothelioma expert. For multicenter studies there is an overall study principal investigator and a site-specific principal investigator. These are supported by a research team made up of other physicians, study nurses, and study coordinators. Your research team will monitor your progress throughout the research study and will also communicate with your usual clinical team. It is possible that some of the prior and ongoing treatments are not compatible with participation in a specific clinical trial. Consequently sometimes there will be adjustments to ongoing treatments.

Mesothelioma clinical trials are paid (funded) by multiple different sources, including the government, e.g., the National Institute of Health and the Department of Defense, pharmaceutical companies, and foundations. Research funds typically pay for the research-related interventions and therapies as well as all research-related testing. These charges are not submitted to insurance companies. However all standard of care testing including safety monitoring and standard interval follow-up imaging are considered standard of care and are billed to insurance companies. These charges are subject to plan coverage and co-payments according to the specific health insurance policy.

Participation in clinical research is completely voluntary. Specifically if patients decide not to participate in clinical research, they should otherwise be offered standard of care or best supportive care. Furthermore patients can always change their mind and discontinue any clinical study at any time without having to provide a specific reason for that decision.

While patients with mesothelioma are enrolled into clinical trials, they will be carefully monitored for any potential side effects. Standardized systems such as the National Cancer Institute's (NCI) Common Terminology Criteria for Adverse Events (CTCAE, https://ctep.cancer.gov/protocoldevelopment/electronic_applications/ctc.htm) and the new patient-reported outcome companion tool (PRO-CTCAE, https://healthcaredelivery.cancer.gov/pro-ctcae/) are typically used to report symptomatic adverse events (AE) in mesothelioma trials. This task is routinely performed by the study investigators and other study personnel supervised by the investigator. The responses to the development of these side effects are specified in the study protocol. Severe side effects may result in the discontinuation of the study treatment.

In mesothelioma clinical trials, treatment response can be monitored clinically, based on patient symptoms and by imaging studies. For mesothelioma imaging mostly focuses computed tomography at intervals ranging between 4 and 12 weeks. Since mesothelioma does not typically represent a spherical three-dimensional tumor but a rather complex space occupying lesion involving the pleural lining standard three-dimensional size, measurements are not effective to monitor disease progression. Most studies use the modified RECIST criteria for mesothelioma (Byrne and Nowak 2004). The measurement represents the sum of up to six perpendicular measurements of the tumor thickness at three different levels within the chest where each measurement is perpendicular to a known anatomic structure. Based on these measurements, patients are classified as complete response (all tumor disappeared), partial response (>30% decrease in the measurement), stable disease, or disease progression (>20% increase in tumor measurement or development of new lesions). Study treatments are typically stopped if there is disease progression. These response criteria were originally designed for chemotherapy-based studies. Since chemotherapeutic drugs typically directly kill tumor cells, disease response is typically paralleled by a decrease in tumor size as measure by RECIST. However other therapeutic approaches such as immunotherapy, cancer cell death occurs indirectly. In this context the immunotherapy such as the immune checkpoint inhibitor activates immune cells, which subsequently infiltrate the tumor to kill the cancer cells. The associated tumor inflammation can lead to the transient enlargement of the tumor. This phenomenon is called "pseudo-progression." Pseudo-progression should not be associated with a clinical deterioration of the patient. With the increased utilization of immunotherapy in clinical trials, new immune-related response criteria (irRC) have been developed and are now being used in mesothelioma studies using immunotherapy (Wolchok et al. 2009).

While radiological and/or clinical disease progression represents the most common determinants for the continuation or discontinuation of study treatment progression-free survival, patient-reported quality of life outcomes and overall survival represent much more important variables in determining the effectiveness of study treatments. However, overall survival is fortunately not a short-term outcome, and collection of survival outcome data requires long-term follow-up. Fortunately in mesothelioma measurements of disease progression, using the modified RECIST criteria appears to correlate with the overall survival highlighting the importance of these measurements (Mansfield et al. 2017). This being said better radiological techniques allowing the volumetric tumor assessment are needed to improve the diagnostic performance of the modified RECIST criteria for mesothelioma (Gill et al. 2012; Rusch et al. 2016).

What happens to patients if their disease progresses? For most patients whose disease progresses, the clinical trial is finished. However depending on the clinical trial design, there may be the option to cross over to another treatment arm. Alternatively patients could consider participation in another clinical trial or other clinical treatment options.

If patients have not experienced progression of disease at the end of the study, treatments might be able to be continued through expanded access, off-label use, or by the pharmaceutical company. However patients need to understand that drug companies are under no obligation to continue to provide the investigational drug to patients after the termination of the study. Examples for potentially helpful questions to the study staff of a clinical trial are shown in Table 17.3.

In summary clinical research including therapeutic clinical trials is essential for improving the medical care of patients with mesothelioma. Given that mesothelioma is a relatively rare disease, medical advances in the early detection, diagnosis, staging, and treatment of this often devastating disease largely rely on the motivation, altruism, and selflessness of mesothelioma patients who are willing to participate in these studies. Additional, studies investigating and comparing different multimodality treatments and window of opportunity studies are needed. The medical community needs to optimize the geographic availability, referral network, and the pre-screening process for study eligibility to minimize any existing hurdles for patients with mesothelioma to participate in clinical trials.

Table 17.3   Patient questions regarding clinical trials

What are important questions to ask the researchers prior to joining a clinical trial?
What is the goal of this research study and who is funding it?
If this is a treatment trial, are all patients receiving active therapy or is there a control (placebo) group?
How much is known about how this treatment works in mesothelioma patients?
How many patients are already in the study and what has been the experience of these patients to date?
How long does it take to determine if I am a candidate for the study and what additional tests are required?
What are the potential side effects, and how will those be addressed if they come up?
How will this trial affect any of the other treatments, medications, and supplements I am currently receiving?

References

Department of Health and Human Services Food and Drug Administration. Individual patient expanded access investigational new drug application (IND).

Alley EW, et al. Clinical safety and activity of pembrolizumab in patients with malignant pleural mesothelioma (KEYNOTE-028): preliminary results from a non-randomised, open-label, phase 1b trial. Lancet Oncol. 2017;18:623–30. https://doi.org/10.1016/S1470-2045(17)30169-9.

Batirel HF, et al. Adoption of pleurectomy and decortication for malignant mesothelioma leads to similar survival as extrapleural pneumonectomy. J Thorac Cardiovasc Surg. 2016;151:478–84. https://doi.org/10.1016/j.jtcvs.2015.09.121.

Bovolato P, et al. Does surgery improve survival of patients with malignant pleural mesothelioma?: a multicenter retrospective analysis of 1365 consecutive patients. J Thorac Oncol. 2014;9:390–6. https://doi.org/10.1097/JTO.0000000000000064.

Bryce AH, et al. Experience with precision genomics and tumor board, indicates frequent target identification, but barriers to delivery. Oncotarget. 2017;8:27145–54. https://doi.org/10.18632/oncotarget.16057.

Burt BM, et al. Malignant pleural mesothelioma and the Society of Thoracic Surgeons Database: an analysis of surgical morbidity and mortality. J Thorac Cardiovasc Surg. 2014;148:30–5. https://doi.org/10.1016/j.jtcvs.2014.03.011.

Byrne M. J., Nowak A. K., Modified RECIST criteria for assessment of response in malignant pleural mesothelioma. Ann Oncol. 2004;15:257–60. https://doi.org/10.1093/annonc/mdh059.

Cao C, et al. A systematic review and meta-analysis of surgical treatments for malignant pleural mesothelioma. Lung Cancer. 2014;83:240–5. https://doi.org/10.1016/j.lungcan.2013.11.026.

Caplan AL, Bateman-House A, Waldstreicher J. Compassionate use: a modest proposal. Am Soc Clin Oncol Educ Book. 2016;35:e2–4. https://doi.org/10.14694/EDBK_156130.

Chan WH, Sugarbaker DJ, Burt BM. Intraoperative adjuncts for malignant pleural mesothelioma. Transl Lung Cancer Res. 2017;6:285–94. https://doi.org/10.21037/tlcr.2017.05.04.

de Perrot M, et al. Accelerated hemithoracic radiation followed by extrapleural pneumonectomy for malignant pleural mesothelioma. J Thorac Cardiovasc Surg. 2016;151:468–73. https://doi.org/10.1016/j.jtcvs.2015.09.129.

Ettinger DS, et al. NCCN guidelines insights: malignant pleural mesothelioma, version 3.2016. J Natl Compr Cancer Netw. 2016;14:825–36.

Flores RM, et al. Extrapleural pneumonectomy versus pleurectomy/decortication in the surgical management of malignant pleural mesothelioma: results in 663 patients. J Thorac Cardiovasc Surg. 2008;135:620–6, 626 e621–623. https://doi.org/10.1016/j.jtcvs.2007.10.054.

Friedberg JS, et al. Extended pleurectomy-decortication-based treatment for advanced stage epithelial mesothelioma yielding a median survival of nearly three years. Ann Thorac Surg. 2017;103:912–9. https://doi.org/10.1016/j.athoracsur.2016.08.071.

Gill RR, et al. Epithelial malignant pleural mesothelioma after extrapleural pneumonectomy: stratification of survival with CT-derived tumor volume. AJR Am J Roentgenol. 2012;198:359–63. https://doi.org/10.2214/AJR.11.7015.

Hassan R, et al. Mesothelin immunotherapy for cancer: ready for prime time? J Clin Oncol. 2016;34:4171–9. https://doi.org/10.1200/JCO.2016.68.3672.

Hedy L, Kindler NI, Armato SG III, Bueno R, Hesdorffer M, Jahan T, Jones CM, Miettinen M, Pass H, Rimner A, Rusch V, Sterman D, Thomas A, Hassan R. Treatment of malignant pleural mesothelioma: American Society of Clinical Oncology Clinical Practice Guideline. J Clin Oncol. 2018;36(13):1343–73.

Ivy SP, Siu LL, Garrett-Mayer E, Rubinstein L. Approaches to phase 1 clinical trial design focused on safety, efficiency, and selected patient populations: a report from the clinical trial design task force of the national cancer institute investigational drug steering committee. Clin Cancer Res. 2010;16:1726–36. https://doi.org/10.1158/1078-0432.CCR-09-1961.

Levin PA, Dowell JE. Spotlight on bevacizumab and its potential in the treatment of malignant pleural mesothelioma: the evidence to date. Onco Targets Ther. 2017;10:2057–66. https://doi.org/10.2147/OTT.S113598.

LoRusso PM, Boerner SA, Seymour L. An overview of the optimal planning, design, and conduct of phase I studies of new therapeutics. Clin Cancer Res. 2010;16:1710–8. https://doi.org/10.1158/1078-0432.CCR-09-1993.

Mailankody S, Prasad V. Thinking systematically about the off-label use of cancer drugs and combinations for patients who have exhausted proven therapies. Oncologist. 2016;21:1031–2. https://doi.org/10.1634/theoncologist.2016-0086.

Mansfield AS. Immune checkpoint inhibition in malignant mesothelioma: does it have a future? Lung Cancer. 2017;105:49–51. https://doi.org/10.1016/j.lungcan.2017.01.004.

Mansfield AS, et al. B7-H1 expression in malignant pleural mesothelioma is associated with sarcomatoid histology and poor prognosis. J Thorac Oncol. 2014;9:1036–40. https://doi.org/10.1097/JTO.0000000000000177.

Mansfield AS, et al. Chromoplectic TPM3-ALK rearrangement in a patient with inflammatory myofibroblastic tumor who responded to ceritinib after progression on crizotinib. Ann Oncol. 2016;27:2111–7. https://doi.org/10.1093/annonc/mdw405.

Mansfield A, Peikert T, Vogelzang N, Symanowski J. Effects of tumor burden reduction on survival in epithelioid pleural mesothelioma. J Thorac Oncol. 2017;12

Mansfield A, Peikert T, Vogelzang N, Symanowski J. Effects of tumor burden reduction on survival in epithelioid pleural mesothelioma. Mayo Clin Proc. 2018;93(8):1026–33. https://doi.org/10.1016/j.mayocp.2018.01.032. Epub 2018 May 24

Marulli G, et al. Pleurectomy-decortication in malignant pleural mesothelioma: are different surgical techniques associated with different outcomes? Results from a multicentre study. Eur J Cardiothorac Surg. 2017;52:63–9. https://doi.org/10.1093/ejcts/ezx079.

Paoletti X, Drubay D, Collette L. Dose-finding methods: moving away from the 3 + 3 to include richer outcomes. Clin Cancer Res. 2017;23:3977–9. https://doi.org/10.1158/1078-0432.CCR-17-1306.

Prasad V. Double-crossed: why crossover in clinical trials may be distorting medical science. J Natl Compr Cancer Netw. 2013;11:625–7.

Renfro LA, Sargent DJ. Statistical controversies in clinical research: basket trials, umbrella trials, and other master protocols: a review and examples. Ann Oncol. 2017;28:34–43. https://doi.org/10.1093/annonc/mdw413.

Rimner A, et al. Phase II study of hemithoracic intensity-modulated pleural radiation therapy (IMPRINT) as part of lung-sparing multimodality therapy in patients with malignant pleural mesothelioma. J Clin Oncol. 2016;34:2761–8. https://doi.org/10.1200/JCO.2016.67.2675.

Rusch VW, et al. A multicenter study of volumetric computed tomography for staging malignant pleural mesothelioma. Ann Thorac Surg. 2016;102:1059–66. https://doi.org/10.1016/j.athoracsur.2016.06.069.

Scagliotti GV, et al. LUME-Meso: design and rationale of the phase III part of a placebo-controlled study of nintedanib and pemetrexed/cisplatin followed by maintenance nintedanib in patients with unresectable malignant pleural mesothelioma. Clin Lung Cancer. 2017;18:589–93. https://doi.org/10.1016/j.cllc.2017.03.010.

Schwartz RM, Watson A, Wolf A, Flores R, Taioli E. The impact of surgical approach on quality of life for pleural malignant mesothelioma. Ann Transl Med. 2017;5:230. https://doi.org/10.21037/atm.2017.03.41.

Seymour L, et al. The design of phase II clinical trials testing cancer therapeutics: consensus recommendations from the clinical trial design task force of the national cancer institute investigational drug steering committee. Clin Cancer Res. 2010;16:1764–9. https://doi.org/10.1158/1078-0432.CCR-09-3287.

Shaikh F, et al. Improved outcomes with modern lung-sparing trimodality therapy in patients with malignant pleural mesothelioma. J Thorac Oncol. 2017;12:993–1000. https://doi.org/10.1016/j.jtho.2017.02.026.

Simon R. Critical review of umbrella, basket, and platform designs for oncology clinical trials. Clin Pharmacol Ther. 2017;102:934–41. https://doi.org/10.1002/cpt.814.

Taioli E, Wolf AS, Flores RM. Meta-analysis of survival after pleurectomy decortication versus extrapleural pneumonectomy in mesothelioma. Ann Thorac Surg. 2015;99:472–80. https://doi.org/10.1016/j.athoracsur.2014.09.056.

Treasure T, et al. Extra-pleural pneumonectomy versus no extra-pleural pneumonectomy for patients with malignant pleural mesothelioma: clinical outcomes of the Mesothelioma and Radical Surgery (MARS) randomised feasibility study. Lancet Oncol. 2011;12:763–72. https://doi.org/10.1016/s1470-2045(11)70149-8.

Trialists M, Lim E. Surgical selection in pleurectomy decortication for mesothelioma – an overview from screening and selection from MARS 2 pilot. J Thorac Oncol. 2017;12:S1748.

Verma V, et al. National cancer database report on pneumonectomy versus lung-sparing surgery for malignant pleural mesothelioma. J Thorac Oncol. 2017;12:1704–14. https://doi.org/10.1016/j.jtho.2017.08.012.

Vogelzang NJ, et al. Phase III study of pemetrexed in combination with cisplatin versus cisplatin alone in patients with malignant pleural mesothelioma. J Clin Oncol. 2003;21:2636–44. https://doi.org/10.1200/JCO.2003.11.136.

West HJ. Novel precision medicine trial designs: umbrellas and baskets. JAMA Oncol. 2017;3:423. https://doi.org/10.1001/jamaoncol.2016.5299.

Wolchok JD, et al. Guidelines for the evaluation of immune therapy activity in solid tumors: immune-related response criteria. Clin Cancer Res. 2009;15:7412–20. https://doi.org/10.1158/1078-0432.CCR-09-1624.

Woodcock J, LaVange LM. Master protocols to study multiple therapies, multiple diseases, or both. N Engl J Med. 2017;377:62–70. https://doi.org/10.1056/NEJMra1510062.

Zalcman G, et al. Bevacizumab for newly diagnosed pleural mesothelioma in the Mesothelioma Avastin Cisplatin Pemetrexed Study (MAPS): a randomised, controlled, open-label, phase 3 trial. Lancet. 2016;387:1405–14. https://doi.org/10.1016/S0140-6736(15)01238-6.

The Future of Mesothelioma Research: Basic Science Research

18

Vanessa S. Fear, Alistair M. Cook, and Scott A. Fisher

1   Introduction

Much of our current understanding of the causes, biological mechanisms, risk factors, and potential treatments for mesothelioma are derived not from the clinic, but from basic research that involves a mixture of in vitro work using cell lines grown in the lab and in vivo experiments where treatments are explored in a variety of animal models of mesothelioma (predominantly mice). This section gives an overview of the cutting-edge preclinical research currently being performed in the field. Pre–clinical models are discussed in the context of conventional therapies, followed by new and emerging treatments.

2   Pre–clinical Models

Clinical studies of mesothelioma are somewhat limited by the low numbers of patients presenting at any one location. Therefore, establishment of cell lines and disease-representative animal models has been important for our understanding of the development, biology, and progression of this aggressive disease. Key aspects include isolation of human tumour cell lines and development of asbestos-derived mesothelioma cell lines from mice, plus the establishment of models of solid tumours, orthotopic models of local and metastatic disease, and long-term asbestos exposure. Each model has specific advantages and limitations as discussed below.

V. S. Fear (✉) · A. M. Cook · S. A. Fisher
National Centre for Asbestos Related Diseases, The University of Western Australia, School of Biomedical Sciences, Perth, WA, Australia
e-mail: Vanessa.Fear@telethonkids.org.au; alistair.cook@uwa.edu.au; scott.fisher@uwa.edu.au

© Springer Nature Switzerland AG 2019
M. Hesdorffer, G. E. Bates-Pappas (eds.), *Caring for Patients with Mesothelioma: Principles and Guidelines*,
https://doi.org/10.1007/978-3-319-96244-3_18

2.1   Mesothelioma Cell Lines

In early studies, human malignant mesothelioma cell lines were used extensively to study drug susceptibility, cytokine production, and response of immune effector cells in vitro. Furthermore, these cell lines helped define various phenotypic and genetic characteristics of human tumours, e.g. epithelioid or sarcomatoid (Table 18.1).

Human cell lines provided information regarding the resistance of mesothelioma to cytotoxic drugs such as actinomycin D, cisplatin, etoposide, methotrexate, 5'flu-orouracil, mitomycin C, and vinblastine. Further human cell line studies determined the response of mesothelioma cells to cytokines including TNFα, IFNγ, and IFNα, indicating reduced proliferation of some cell lines. Later notable immunology studies included stimulation of cytotoxic T cells or natural killer (NK) cells with cytokines to stimulate tumour cell killing. This led to the notion that immunotherapeutic approaches to mesothelioma may be more effective in vivo rather than assayed by direct anti-tumour activity on cell lines.

Cell monolayer cultures are easy to handle and suitable for large-scale drug testing, but drug sensitivity in vitro often does not translate to the clinic. A potential limitation of research using human cell lines is that continued long-term culturing may result in highly selected clonal tumour cell populations that only partially represent the original tumour.

To overcome such issues, recent research has focused on the use of 3D spheroid cultures, which more closely mimic solid tumours (Schunselaar et al. 2016). Mesothelioma is particularly resistant to chemotherapy, an outcome not always accurately reflected when using in vitro monolayer cultures. Conversely, 3D spheroid cultures have shown chemotherapy resistance profiles similar to that observed in patients. However, the use of 3D cultures is still limited by the intrinsic complications associated with quantifying cell survival.

Table 18.1 Mesothelioma cell lines

Cell lines	Phenotype/source	Species	References
NO-36	Pleural effusion	Human	Manning et al. (1991)
JU-77	Pleural effusion	Human	
LO-68	Pleural effusion	Human	
ONE-58	Pleural effusion	Human	
DeHI28(M)	Pleural effusion	Human	
REN MM cell line	Primary tumour	Human	Taguchi et al. (1993)
AB1, AB2, AB12, AB13, AB22	Sarcomatoid	Mouse BALB/cArc (H-2^d)	Davis et al. (1992)
AC14, AC16, AC24, AC28, AC29, AC31, AC32, AC34, AC36	Sarcomatoid	Mouse CBA (H-2^k)	
AE17	Sarcomatoid	Mouse C57BL/6 (H-2^b)	Jackaman et al. (2003)
40	Highly invasive, metastatic	Mouse C57BL/6	Goodglick et al. (1997)

Other in vitro models include primary cell culture using single cells isolated from patients that are cultured for a short period of time. These cultures, often taken from pleural effusions, more closely represent the original tumour in cell complexity, cytology, and cellular biology. In some hands, primary tumour cultures have resistance to drug treatment mirroring the clinical setting (Schunselaar et al. 2016). However, establishing primary tissue cultures is often difficult, and in vitro resistance to drug treatment is extremely variable between patients.

2.2 Animal Models of Mesothelioma

The refractive nature of malignant pleural mesothelioma to aggressive trimodal treatment (surgery, chemotherapy, and/or radiation) has patient survival at only 1–2 years depending on stage and histology at time of diagnosis (Rusch et al. 2012). Accordingly, new treatment strategies are urgently required, and here we discuss current preclinical research efforts. Early studies in animal models assessed the carcinogenicity of different fibre types, with identification of asbestos fibre exposure leading to mesothelioma. Other animal models include xenograft models with human tissue, orthotopic models at the site of mesothelioma formation, solid tumour models, and genetic predisposition models. Preclinical mesothelioma models are listed in Table 18.2.

Table 18.2 Features of preclinical models and their application

Model	Applications	Tumour mimic	Time	Benefits	Disadvantages
Cell line models					
Monolayer	Large-scale drug testing	Low	Short	High throughput	Lack of immune system, poor translation
Spheroids		Yes	Long	Mimics tumour response	Technically demanding and difficult to quantitate
Tumour primary tissue culture					
Monolayer	Drug sensitivity	Low	Short	Patient tumour cells	Lack of immune system, poor translation
3D spheroids	Drug testing	Yes	Long	Mimics tumour	Technically demanding and difficult to quantitate
Tumour biopsy	Drug testing	Yes	Long	Mimics tumour; stromal cells	
Asbestos-induced models					
Intraperitoneal	Disease development	Yes	Long	Technically easy	20–30% incidence; tumour hard to measure; peritoneal mesothelioma represents 10–20% of patient disease
Intrapleural	Disease development	Yes	Long	Local invasion; ascites development; aetiology	Technically difficult; long latency; development of adenocarcinoma/lung cancer; difficult to measure

(continued)

Table 18.2 (continued)

Model	Applications	Tumour mimic	Time	Benefits	Disadvantages
Xenograft models					
	Drug testing	Yes	Long	Human cells used	No immune system; irrelevant anatomical site
Mouse orthotopic models					
Intrapleural	Drug testing; tumour development	Yes	Short	Anatomically relevant site	High level of technical expertise; risk of complications; difficult to measure
Mouse solid tumour models					
	Drug testing	Yes	Short	Immune system; high throughput	Irrelevant anatomical site/ microenvironment
Genetic predisposition mouse models					
NF2+/− KO	Disease development	Yes	Mid	Ascites; tumour dissemination and invasion; use of asbestos	Artificial bias in the gene setting; only 85% of mice develop disease; cannot measure tumour directly
P53+/− KO	Disease development	Yes	Long	Local tissue invasion and lymph node metastases; use of asbestos	Not all mice develop disease; not a key gene for mesothelioma; formation of spontaneous tumours
NF2,P53, p16^{Ink4a}/p19^{Arf} KO	Disease development	Yes	Short	Inducible P53 expression	Mesothelioma induced without asbestos; high tumour incidence (80–100%) but not all mesothelioma
MexTAg (SV40 large T antigen)	Asbestos-induced disease development	Yes	Mid to long	Asbestos-induced ascites; tumour dissemination and invasion	SV40 TAg phenocopies p16 loss leading to high incidence (85–100%) of mesothelioma after asbestos exposure. Little to no spontaneous non-mesothelioma tumours in absence or presence of asbestos

2.3   Asbestos Exposure Models

Using animal models to study human cancer is a widely accepted strategy that can yield answers that would not otherwise be achievable. Mesothelioma has been reported in many different animals including rodents, dogs, horses, goats, and even tigers, indicating that all mammals with pleura or peritonea are susceptible to environmental asbestos exposure (Cleo Robinson et al. 2014).

   Disease pathology stems from inhalation of long, thin asbestos fibres (3 μm–5 μm, aspect ratio >1:3) that penetrate deep into the lung and enter the pleural space. Subsequently, a continuous inflammatory cycle of pleural irritation, DNA damage, and repair leads to mutations in mesothelial cells leading to the onset of disease. Inflammatory cytokines, including transforming growth factor-β, (TGF-β), platelet-derived growth factor (PDGF), and vascular endothelial growth factor (VEGF), promote proliferation and angiogenesis. Phagocytosis of asbestos fibres leads to release of oxygen free radicals inducing DNA mutations, and fibre penetration of mesothelial cells interferes with mitosis. Not all individuals exposed to asbestos develop mesothelioma, suggesting host genetics may predispose some individuals to disease. Rodents, particularly mice, from different genetic backgrounds have been exposed to asbestos fibres and monitored for development of mesothelioma. Strikingly, asbestos-induced mesothelioma in mice recapitulates the human disease with regard to disease latency, growth of tumour on the mesothelium, histopathology, and chromosomal abnormalities (see Sect. 2.5 below). Many murine cell lines have since been developed from asbestos-exposed mice (Table 18.1) and have contributed significantly to our current understanding of mesothelioma biology.

2.4   Inhalation Models

Although inhalation studies are more representative of human exposure, their use is limited by a number of factors. Firstly, it is often difficult to regulate the number of asbestos fibres inhaled. Additionally, there is a high asbestos exposure risk to research staff and the immediate study environment. As such, inhalation studies often require specialised equipment and facilities at a cost that is often prohibitive to many research labs. Conversely, instillation of asbestos fibres via intraperitoneal (i.p.), intrapleural (i.pl), or intratracheal (i.tr) injection is more common as it is cost-effective and easily performed with minimal training. Both models are equally important, and it is the hypothesis being tested that should dictate which type of model is ultimately used. When investigating the potential carcinogenicity of airborne particles on human health, an inhalation study is warranted. However, when investigating biological processes that occur once disease is induced, injection models are no less useful; how the disease is induced is not the primary concern, but what happens biologically afterwards is.

2.5   Injection Models

Following exposure of mice to asbestos fibres (crocidolite) via intraperitoneal injection, tumours resembling mesothelioma develop in the peritoneal cavity after 24 weeks in a29/Sv mice and C57BL/6 mice, 29 weeks in BALB/c mice, and 56 weeks in CBA mice (Davis et al. 1992). These models closely resemble the onset of human disease in terms of disease incidence (20–30% of exposed mice) and histological and morphological features, with the notable exception that unlike human mesothelioma, most mouse-derived mesotheliomas are sarcomatoid, with very little epithelioid or biphasic subtypes observed (Robinson et al. 2006). Nonetheless, these models have significantly aided our understanding of the mechanisms leading to onset of mesothelioma. Although many mouse exposure models recapitulate human mesothelioma, the low disease incidence (20–30% of exposed mice), and long latency period lag time to disease onset, is prolonged (0.5–2 years); asbestos exposure models are therefore inappropriate for many investigations such as molecular tumourigenesis and drug testing.

2.6   Xenograft Models

Xenograft models of mesothelioma involve the transplantation of human solid tumours or tumour cell lines into mice and are useful for investigating drug toxicity and the molecular mechanisms of tumour growth.

Xenograft models most commonly implant human mesothelioma cell lines into mice that are immune-compromised (i.e. lack an intact immune system) in order to avoid a foreign tissue response. These include mice strains such as the hairless 'nude' mouse (lack T cells), severe combined immunodeficient (SCID) mice (lack T and B cells), and recombination-activating gene (RAG) knockout mice (lack adaptive immune cells) and are often used for drug targeting of oncogenic pathways.

Other xenograft models transplant intact tumour pieces into immune-compromised mice. The advantage of these models is that the structure and integrity of the tumour is maintained, in particular the stromal compartment. Accordingly, the biological and clinical behaviour of tumour growth in the mice seems to correlate well with that observed in patients. A major disadvantage of xenograft models is that the lack of an intact immune system impacts on both tumour growth parameters and/or drug treatment response. Therefore, whilst xenograft models provide a valuable tool for assessment of targeted drug treatment of oncogenic pathways (Cleo Robinson et al. 2014), they are not suitable for investigation of immune-based treatments, such as chemoimmunotherapy.

2.7   Subcutaneous Models

Various murine tumour models have been developed in which tumour cells are injected directly under the skin where they develop as subcutaneous solid tumours. The advantage of these models is the visualisation of tumour growth and response to therapy. Additionally, tumours develop in the context of vasculature, connective, and lymphatic tissues allowing drug metabolism in situ to be assessed with consideration of drug pharmacokinetics, tumour accessibility, tumour biology, and the contribution of the immune system.

Mesothelioma tumours grown subcutaneously retain many morphological features of disease and can be validated by histology. The tumour size is easily measured and therefore response to drug treatment is easily assessed over time. As tumour growth is rapid in these models, they provide a relatively high throughput mouse model for the assessment of novel therapeutics.

The disadvantage of the subcutaneous model is that tumours develop at an anatomically irrelevant site and that rapid tumour growth may preclude normal stromal development or limit the efficacy of anti-tumour immune responses. As such, there can be significant differences in treatment responses between subcutaneous and orthotopic tumour models. In addition, the majority of murine-derived mesotheliomas used in subcutaneous models display the sarcomatoid phenotype and not the epithelioid phenotype that is more common in human mesothelioma. Therefore, the suitability of the subcutaneous mouse tumours model has been questioned for relevance in the disease setting. Despite this, many therapies that are currently in the clinic for many cancer types, including chemotherapy and immunotherapy, were developed using subcutaneous mouse models (Cleo Robinson et al. 2014).

The benefits of the subcutaneous model lie in the simplicity of the method, the ability to monitor tumour growth over time, and the presence of an immune cell response to tumour growth. Some of the issues regarding translation of findings in these solid tumour models are addressed by testing treatment in a number of different subcutaneous mesothelioma models, to confirm efficacy of treatment interventions.

2.8   Orthotopic Models

Orthotopic models have been developed for pleural and intraperitoneal mesothelioma. These models represent a more human-like disease model, since tumours develop in an anatomically relevant site and are often more invasive relative to subcutaneous tumour models.

Orthotopic mesothelioma models mimic human disease closely, in that tumour cells grow along the serosal surfaces, form nodules in the peritoneum, develop metastases, and in some cases form ascitic fluid. Importantly, tumours develop in the context of the host tissue, and tumour growth is subject to relevant host factors such as the immune system, vasculature, metabolites, and microenvironment.

A high level of technical expertise is required for the intrapleural orthotopic model due to risk associated with intrapleural injections such as hemothorax and pneumothorax (Cleo Robinson et al. 2014). For this reason, intraperitoneal models of mesothelioma are more commonly used as they conserve the same biological features of disease as the intrapleural model but are easier to perform, even by less skilled personnel.

A potential disadvantage of the orthotopic model is the inability to directly monitor tumour growth. This can be overcome by the use of small animal imaging techniques where growth of cancer cells expressing a fluorescent reporter protein, or the luciferin gene that converts substrate to emit light, can be measured. Additionally, the development of small animal imaging platforms that mimic clinical disease detection such as PET-CT and MRI and the utilisation of radio-nucleotide tracers are becoming more readily available.

2.9   Genetic Predisposition Models

Mesothelioma is a disease of genetic loss, often characterised by the deletion of the tumour suppressor genes *CDKN2A*, encoding the proteins p16^{INK4a} and p14^{Arf} (p19^{Arf} in mice), *NF2*, *BAP1*, and to a lesser extent *p53*. Accordingly, mouse models have been developed in which these genes, either individually or in combination, are no longer expressed, i.e. the genes have been 'knocked out' (KO models). Mice in which a single copy of *NF2* or *p53* have been deleted (heterozygous KO mice) display increased incidence of mesothelioma (up to 80% of mice) and a shorter disease latency following asbestos exposure. Importantly, both *NF2* and *p53* heterozygous mice develop other types of highly metastatic lesions (Cleo Robinson et al. 2014) and other spontaneous cancers, such as lymphomas, sarcomas, and adenocarcinomas. It is also notable that these mouse models don't require exposure to asbestos for disease development and become complicated by spontaneous occurrence of many non-mesothelioma tumours. Whilst a disadvantage of these models is the induction of mesothelioma in the absence of asbestos exposure, they have still been instrumental in elucidating the molecular mechanisms that lead to mesothelioma following asbestos exposure.

2.10   MexTAg Mice

Our lab developed the MexTAg transgenic mouse model of mesothelioma in which mesothelial cells have been engineered to express the oncogenic SV40 virus large T antigen (SV40 TAg) (Robinson et al. 2006). Whilst SV40 does not play a causative role in human mesothelioma, we utilise the oncogenic potential of TAg as a disease accelerator, producing a mouse model in which mesothelioma development is predictable, uniform, and reproducible, but only *after asbestos exposure*. MexTAg mice have higher disease incidence (up to 100%), develop mesothelioma with similar pathology, and show comparable treatment responses to human mesothelioma (Robinson et al. 2006, 2011,). Importantly, MexTAg mice are less likely to develop unrelated tumours compared to wild-type mice or the heterozygous or conditional mesothelioma knockout mouse models mentioned above. Expression analysis comparing MexTAg and wild-type mesotheliomas with their counterpart normal mesothelial cells demonstrates highly homologous gene expression profiles that suggest the TAg transgene does not affect the overall mechanism of mesothelioma development, but rather it phenocopies p16 loss – leading to increased disease incidence in these mice after asbestos exposure (Robinson et al. 2015). Thus, the MexTAg model is a functional equivalent of the deletion of tumour suppressor genes such as *CDKN2A* (*p16^{INK4a}/p14^{Arf}*), *NF2*, *BAP1*, or *p53* that characterise human mesothelioma.

The reproducibility and high incidence of disease in asbestos-exposed MexTAg mice make this model ideal for disease prevention studies as well as assessing the potential carcinogenicity of minerals and materials that share asbestos-like characteristics such as long carbon nanotubes and non-asbestiform elongated mineral particles (Table 18.2).

3   Conventional Therapies

3.1   Surgery

The benefits of surgery in pleural mesothelioma are hotly debated (Opitz and Weder 2017). Factors taken into consideration when recommending patients for surgery include disease stage and histology. Patients with less bulky tumours are often treated with pleurectomy/decortication (P/D) surgery, whilst high-risk patients undergo the more radical extrapleural pneumonectomy (EPP). The IASLC database, however, indicates an OS benefit of 40 months for EPP and 23 months after P/D. This is further complicated by 30-day mortality rates at 2–5% after EPP surgery. This is unsurprising as many patients selected for EPP are already high risk, and the procedure has a relative risk for technical complications including haemorrhage, empyema, failure at reconstruction of the diaphragms or pericardium, atrial fibrillation, and acute respiratory distress syndrome (ARDS).

Given the low frequency of MM patients suitable for surgical resection, some centres are now trialing neoadjuvant chemotherapy or radiotherapy to patients (see below).

3.2   Chemotherapy

Current studies indicate that neoadjuvant chemotherapy prior to surgery is feasible; however it is yet to be determined if there is an associated survival benefit.

Historically, chemotherapy has been considered immunosuppressive via depletion of immune cells sensitive to treatment. The action of chemotherapy was thought to occur primarily by inhibition of tumour cell division. More recently there has been overwhelming evidence of the positive effects of chemotherapy on anti-tumour immune responses. These immune benefits include stimulation of immunogenic tumour cell death, tumour antigen presentation, depletion of suppressive cells, and stimulation of anti-tumour T cell immune responses. Types of chemotherapy for use in mesothelioma, their target, and immunomodulatory properties are listed in Table 18.3.

3.2.1   Immunogenic Tumour Cell Death

Under normal physiological conditions, cells die in a manner that does not provoke an immune response (i.e. non-immunogenic), avoiding immune reactivity to self-proteins. Some chemotherapies, however, are able to kill cells in an immunogenic manner. Here, chemotherapy may promote tumour antigen uptake by dendritic cells whilst inducing activation of those DC through release of alarmin proteins. Additionally, chemotherapy can induce recruitment and maturation of dendritic cells that ultimately induces an anti-tumour immune response (Aston et al. 2014).

3.2.2   Dendritic Cell Cross-Presentation

Mature dendritic cells can uptake and display tumour-derived peptides on MHC class I molecules to CD8 T cells in a process known as cross-presentation.

Table 18.3 Chemotherapy, class, immunomodulation, and current disease treatment

Name	Trade name	Alternate name	Use	Class
Bleomycin	Blenoxane[R]	Bleomycin sulphate	Lymphoma; solid tumours; squamous cell carcinoma, melanoma, sarcoma; malignant pleural effusion	Anti-tumour antibiotic
Cisplatin	Platinol[R]	CDDP	Mesothelioma; solid tumours; lung cancer, lymphoma, sarcoma, multiple myeloma, and melanoma	Platinum compound
Cyclophosphamide	Cytotaxan[R], Neosar[R]	Cytophosphane	Non-Hodgkin's lymphoma; breast cancer; neuroblastoma, sarcoma, small cell lung cancer, blood cancers	Alkylating agent
Docetaxel	Taxotere[R]	Docefrez	Small cell lung cancer; breast cancer; solid tumour, sarcoma	Antimicrotubule agent
Doxorubicin	Adriamycin[R], Rubex[R]	Doxil, Caelyx, Myocet	Solid tumours; haematopoietic malignancy	Anthracycline antibiotic
Etoposide	Toposar[R], VePesid[R]	VP-16, etoposide phosphate	Solid tumours; lymphomas, neuroblastoma	Topoisomerase inhibitor
5'Fluorouracil	Adrucil[R]	Fluorouracil, 5-FU	Solid tumours, skin cancer	Antimetabolite
Gemcitabine	Gemzar[R]	Gemcitabine hydrochloride	NSCLC and solid tumours; metastatic breast cancer; sarcoma	Antimetabolite
Irinotecan	Camptosar[R]	Camptothecan-11	Metastatic colon or renal cancer	Topoisomerase inhibitor
Methotrexate	Otrexup[TM], Rasuvo[R], Rheumatrex[R], Trexall[TM]	Amethopterin, Methotrexate sodium	Non-Hodgkin's lymphoma, acute lymphoblastic leukaemia, sarcoma, solid tumour	Antimetabolite
Mitomycin C	Mutamycin[R]	MTC	Adenocarcinoma, solid tumour incl. NSCLC	Anti-tumour antibiotic
Paclitaxel	Taxol[R], Onxal[R]	NSC 125973, Paxene	Solid tumours	Antimicrotubule agent
Pemetrexed	Alimta[R]	Disodium pemetrexed	Mesothelioma; metastatic or advanced NSCLC	Antimetabolite
Vinblastine	Velban[R], Alkaban-AQ[R]	Vinblastine sulphate, vincaleukoblastine	Solid tumours incl. NSCLC, soft tissue sarcoma, choriocarcinoma	Plant alkaloid
Vinorelbine	Navelbine[R]	Vinorelbine tartrate, 5'-nor-anhydrovinblastine	NSCLC, solid tumour, Hodgkin's lymphoma	Plant alkaloid

NSCLC non-small cell lung cancer

Gemcitabine, a chemotherapy used in thoracic cancer, enhances dendritic cell cross-presentation, leading to activation of tumour-specific CD8 T cells in murine mesothelioma (Nowak et al. 2003a). Chemo-modulation of dendritic cells has also been demonstrated with low-dose paclitaxel, doxorubicin, mitomycin C, methotrexate, and vincristine (Aston et al. 2014).

3.2.3 Depletion of Immune Suppressive Cells

Tumour cells secrete IL-10 and TGFβ to enhance the suppressive immune function of Treg cells and myeloid-derived suppressor cells (MDSCs). In a murine mesothelioma model, tumour eradication after low-dose cyclophosphamide is achieved, in part, due to depletion of suppressive Treg cells (Aston et al. 2014). Other chemotherapeutics such as gemcitabine and 5'fluorouracil (5'FU) deplete MDSCs and augment lung tumour regression (Aston et al. 2014). Conversely, gemcitabine and 5'FU chemotherapy may blunt the anti-tumour response by activating the NOD-like receptor protein (NLRP) inflammasome and release of the immunosuppressive cytokine IL1-β. This example highlights the need for careful delineation of mechanism of action of chemotherapeutic drugs to better inform decisions associated with combination therapy.

3.2.4 Enhancing Cytotoxic T Lymphocyte Activity

Cytotoxic T lymphocytes (CTLs) secrete the protease granzyme B to kill tumour cells. Paclitaxel, cisplatin, and doxorubicin increase tumour cell permeability, sensitising tumour cells to CTL killing (Ramakrishnan et al. 2010), whilst other platinum-based chemotherapies promote anti-tumour immunity by enhancing DC-mediated CTL activation (Lesterhuis et al. 2011). Additionally, in vitro studies using cisplatin have shown downregulation of T cell inhibitory ligands PD-L1 and PD-L2 on both tumour cells and DCs, thus enhancing T cell recognition in vitro.

3.3 Radiotherapy

Clinical MM has traditionally been considered radiotherapy resistant, despite in vitro studies showing mesothelioma cell lines to be sensitive to doses as little as 2 grays (Gy). Epithelial mesothelioma subtypes appear more susceptible to irradiation than sarcomatoid cell lines (Sharabi et al. 2015). More recently the development of new radiation therapy techniques such as intensity-modulated radiation therapy (IMRT), which allows delivery of high-dose radiotherapy to the hemithorax, has shown efficacy. In clinical trials IMRT after EPP led to a patient survival of 23.9–39.4 months (Perrot et al. 2017). Accordingly, IMRT adjuvant therapy has been introduced after P/D and EPP. Further studies are indicating that IMRT is a feasible option prior to surgery and may increase survival before EPP, as in the SMART protocol (Cho et al. 2014). Radiotherapy is also prophylactically used for biopsy tract metastases, which occur in around 20% of patients, but this is controversial and studies to date have been largely negative. A large randomised trial designed to definitively answer whether this procedure is beneficial is currently in progress (Bayman et al. 2016).

4   Emerging Therapies

Cutting-edge research into MM targets the immune system, oncogenes and their signaling pathways, early disease detection by biomarker identification, as well as novel studies including drug repositioning and combination treatment modalities. These topics are discussed below.

4.1   Immunotherapy

There is a strong immunological rationale for using immunotherapy to treat mesothelioma. Tumour biopsies with high levels of $CD8^+$ tumour-infiltrating lymphocytes (TILs) are positively correlated with tumour regression and improved survival. However, despite the infiltration of T effector (Teff) cells, tumours can escape elimination by the immune system through the involvement of T cell inhibitory molecules (CLTA-4 or PD-1, PD-L2), or the development of a suppressive tumour microenvironment (TME), characterised by high levels of Treg cells (Fisher et al. 2017) and suppressive cytokines such as TGF-β and IL-10.

New strategies for the treatment of cancer include therapies that target the immune system. The recognition of tumour by the immune system occurs in several stages (Figs. 18.1 and 18.2). Initially the immune system recognises tumour cells via direct presentation of tumour antigens in MHCI molecules on the tumour itself or via presentation of antigen on dendritic cells leading to activation of CD8 T cells in the lymph nodes. The activated CD8 T cells then traffic to the tumour site and are further presented with tumour antigen, via tumour cells or antigen-presenting cells. Following antigen exposure CD8 T cells then produce granzyme B and perforin in an anti-tumour cytotoxic response. However, at each stage of the immune process, there are checks in place to suppress or control the anti-tumour response. These checks to inhibit the immune response can be provided by tumour cells, antigen-presenting cells, immunosuppressive cells (i.e. Treg, MDSC), and/or the cytokine milieu.

Current emerging immunotherapy for treatment of mesothelioma includes immune checkpoint blockade (ICPB), CAR T cell therapy, T regulatory cell modulation, and neoantigen vaccination.

4.1.1   Immune Checkpoint Blockade

One of the most exciting recent advances in cancer therapy is immune checkpoint blockade (ICPB) where the therapy is focused on modulating the immune system rather than the tumour. Upon activation, immune cells express a variety of co-stimulatory and co-inhibitory molecules: molecular 'checkpoints' that dictate the amplitude and duration of the immune response (Steven et al. 2016). Inhibitory checkpoint molecules, such as cytotoxic T lymphocyte antigen (CTLA-4) and programmed cell death protein 1 (PD-1), are expressed on immune cells in order to protect host cells from prolonged inflammation and/or autoimmunity, acting as an 'off' signal for the immune system.

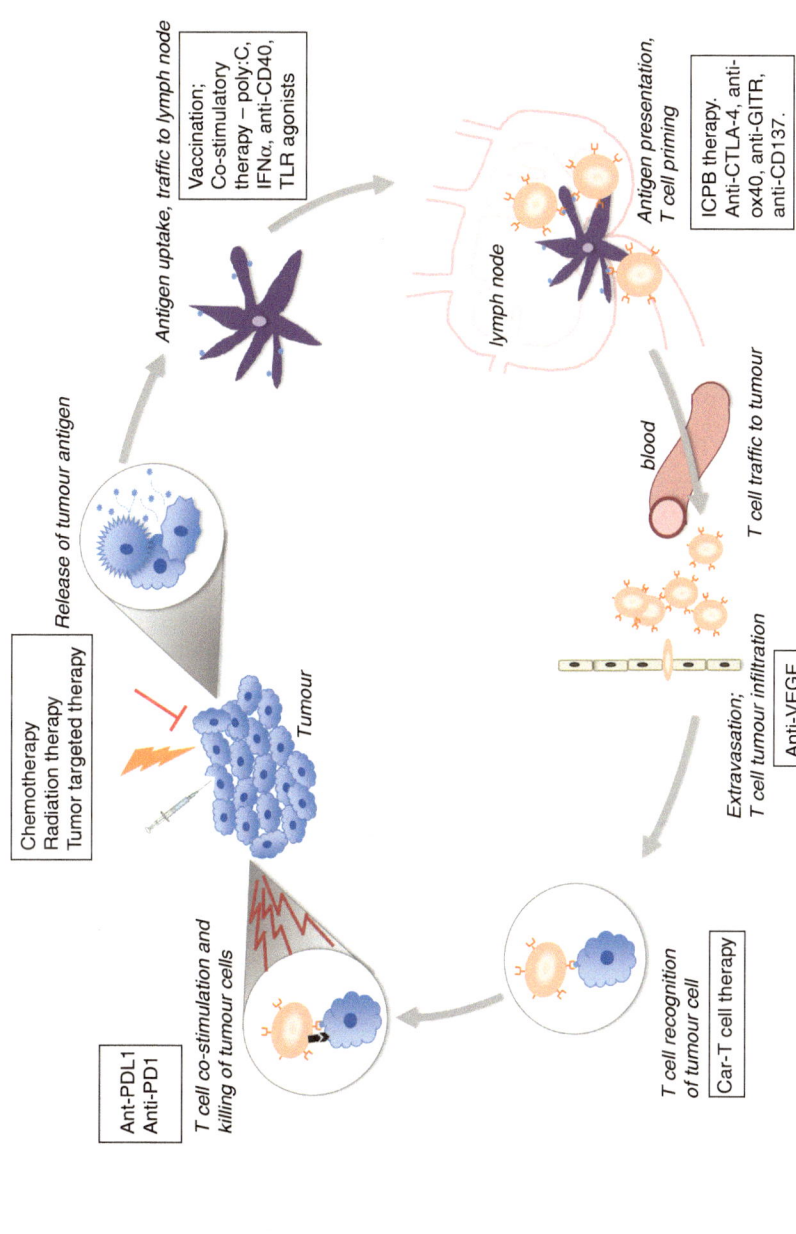

Fig. 18.1 Therapeutic intervention modulates anti-tumour immunity

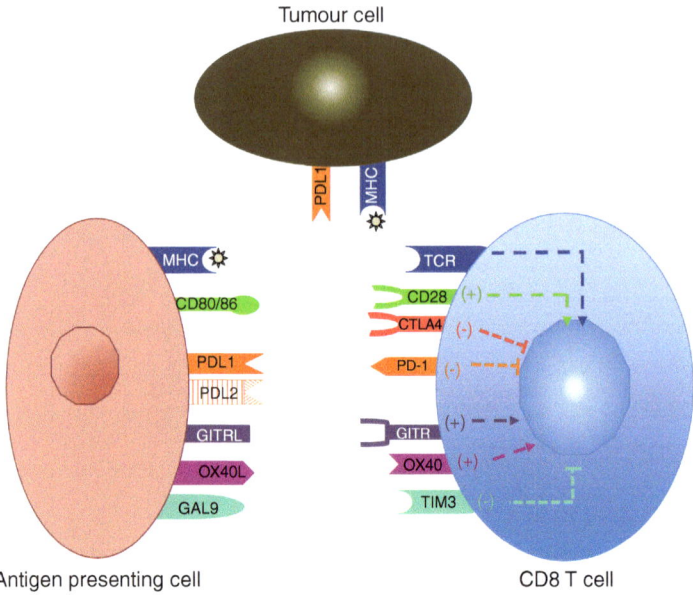

Fig. 18.2 Immune checkpoint receptors and their action on T cell activation

CTLA-4 opposes the co-stimulatory signals generated by CD28 during T cell activation, by disrupting binding of CD28 to its cognate ligands CD80/CD86. Binding of CTLA-4 to CD80/CD86 promotes Teff cell inhibition. In addition, CTLA-4 is constitutively expressed on immunosuppressive Treg cells. Targeted antibodies against CTLA-4 release the block on T cell activation and deplete T regulatory cells. In murine mesothelioma models, blockade of CTLA-4 using anti-CTLA-4 monoclonal antibodies delayed tumour growth.

PD-1 functions primarily in peripheral tissue to inhibit T cell activation, by binding to its cognate ligands programmed death ligand-1 (PD-L1) and programmed death ligand 2 (PD-L2), expressed on tumour and dendritic cells, respectively. Similar to CTLA-4, ligation of PD-1 inhibits T cell proliferation and secretion of effector cytokines. Limited preclinical information on PD-1 blockade is published in mesothelioma, but in combination with adjuvant therapies in other preclinical models, tumour growth is delayed.

Alternative new immune checkpoint targets, which include inhibitory receptor T cell immunoglobulin 3 (TIM-3), and stimulatory receptors OX40 and glucocorticoid-induced tumour necrosis factor receptor (TNFR)-related protein (GITR), are in the early stages of clinical development and may be alternative targets for ICPB therapy in mesothelioma. TIM-3 is an inhibitory molecule that mediates immune tolerance and along with PD-1 expression marks a dysfunctional population of CD8 T cells. Stimulatory OX40 and GITR promote the survival and proliferation of Teff cells and reduce the activity of immunosuppressive Treg cells.

Although ICPB shows promise for cancer therapy, only a small proportion of mesothelioma patients experience a durable response. Combined with the limited preclinical data on ICPB in mesothelioma, there is a clear need for increased preclinical research into the use of novel immune checkpoints or combination therapies.

4.1.2   CAR T Cell Therapy

T cell activation is a two-step process in which naïve T cells, via the T cell receptor (TCR), first recognise their cognate antigen in the context of a major histocompatibility complex (MHC). Once the TCR binds the MHC-antigen complex (signal 1), additional co-stimulatory signals, provided by CD3ζ and CD28 binding to CD80/CD86 (signal 2), are required to promote T cell activation. T cells that receive signal 1, but not signal 2, are considered anergic; they remain inactive and are non-functional.

A chimeric antigen receptor (CAR) combines the two-step activation process into a single activating receptor. A CAR incorporates the extracellular domain of the TCR specific to the tumour antigen with the intracellular activating domain of the CD3ζ cell receptor. To increase T cell activation in vivo, second- and third-generation CARs have been developed by fusing the CD3ζ-activating domain with additional co-stimulatory intracellular domains such as CD28 or 4-1BB (Zeltsman et al. 2017). Autologous T cells can then be transduced with a CAR construct to generate CAR T cells that can be fully activated upon binding to their cognate ligand.

To be useful as a cancer therapy, CAR T cells must recognise tumour-specific antigens. Initial studies assessing the efficacy of CAR T cells that recognise mesothelin, a protein that is overexpressed by mesothelioma but has low-level expression on normal mesothelial cells, indicated that although there was no off-target toxicity of mesothelin-specific CAR T cell therapy, there was no consistent clinical response (NCT02414269, NCT01583686, NCT02580747, NCT02159716, and NCT 01355965).

Nonetheless, preclinical studies have demonstrated the potential for effective CAR T cell therapy for mesothelioma. In an intrapleural mesothelioma mouse model, treatment with mesothelin-specific CAR T cells injected into the peritoneum induced potent, long-lasting anti-tumour immunity (Zeltsman et al. 2017).

Other targets for CAR T cells include components of the tumour-associated stroma, including fibroblast-activating protein (FAP) and vascular endothelial growth factor receptor 2 (VEGFR2). Preclinical studies demonstrate murine FAP-specific CAR T cells have efficacy in mice bearing subcutaneous mesothelioma with minimal toxicity (Zeltsman et al. 2017). A phase I clinical trial of human FAP-specific CAR T cells via intrapleural administration in mesothelioma patient has commenced (NCT01722149).

Alternative CAR T strategies in development for mesothelioma focus on co-expression of ErbB family members (EGFR, HER2, ErbB3, and ErbB4) in conjunction with chimeric cytokines receptors, which serve to promote IL-2-/IL-15-driven clonal expansion of CAR T cells in vivo (Zeltsman et al. 2017). Other candidates of interest for CAR T cell therapy include the oncofoetal cell surface glycoprotein (5 T4) and surface proteoglycan chondroitin sulphate proteoglycan 4 (CSPG4), which are known to be highly overexpressed in mesothelioma cell lines and biopsies.

Current strategies in murine models to enhance CAR T cell therapy are targeting suppression of soluble inhibitory signals (adenosine, TGFβ and PGE$_2$) and evasion of checkpoint inhibitors (such as PD-1) by addition of modified cell surface receptors to subvert their action.

4.1.3   Regulatory T Cell Modulation

Treg cells maintain peripheral tolerance and limit autoimmunity via crosstalk with antigen-presenting cells (APC) and Teff cells. In preclinical cancer models, depletion of Treg cells correlates with enhanced anti-tumour immunity. Indeed, we have shown that mesothelioma bearing BALB/c.FOXP3.dtr mice treated with diphtheria toxin (DTX) to systemically deplete Treg cells in a transient, dose dependent manner, leads to tumour clearance in 20–80% of mice (Fisher et al. 2017). Low dose-DTX mediated removal of Treg cells also enhanced the efficacy of tumour-specific vaccination. A major limitation to translating these data into the clinic is the ability to specifically target Treg cells in patients as there are no known reagents that specifically target Treg cells without affecting other Teff cell populations. We (Fear et al. 2018) and others (Marabelle et al. 2013) have shown that ICPB targeting OX40 and CTLA-4 (both highly expressed on Treg) has been successful in inducing tumour regression in mice, presumably by Treg depletion (Marabelle et al. 2013). However, Treg-specific immunotherapies have yet to be validated in the clinical setting.

4.1.4   Neoantigens and Vaccination

The host immune system is capable of recognising and targeting tumour cells. Numerous sources of tumour-associated antigens (TAAs) or neoantigens arise due to mutation of oncogenes and suppressor genes, oncofoetal proteins, oncogenic viruses, or overexpression of proteins. In order to stimulate an anti-tumour immune response, neoantigens must be present to T cells in the context of MHC molecules. To identify mutations, patient tumour samples are sequenced using next-generation sequencing (NGS) technology for aberrations compared to their normal cellular DNA. Mutation expression is confirmed by RNAseq, and MHC binding potential determine in silico. Finally, neoantigen peptide is compared to the normal (wild type; WT) peptide to identify tumour-specific T cell reactivity (Creaney et al. 2015).

The ability to identify tumour-specific neoantigens via NGS platforms has reinvigorated anti-cancer vaccination strategies. Patients can potentially be vaccinated with their own tumour-specific neoantigens (Chee et al. 2017), in a form of personalised medicine. Current vaccination strategies combine chemotherapy and/or immunotherapy treatment with peptide to stimulate anti-tumour immunity (Bakker et al. 2017).

4.2   Targeting Molecular Signaling Pathways, Oncogenes, and Tumour Suppressor Genes

4.2.1   Kinase Inhibitors

Dysregulation of cell surface receptor expression has been reported in mesothelioma. This includes EGFR overexpression; differential expression of PDGF subtypes; VEGF and VEGF-C constitutive activation of RTKs; and c-MET receptor autocrine loop/overexpression. These mutations induce downstream changes in a multitude of signaling pathways including Hippo, mTOR, MAPK, TP53, and PI3K/Akt.

EGF receptor pathway, PDGFR receptor pathway, VEGF pathway, and Notch receptor signal the phosphatidylinositol 3-kinase (PI3K/AKT) pathway and are frequently activated in mesothelioma (Ramos-Nino et al. 2006; Thellung et al. 2016). Activation of AKT triggers anti-apoptotic mechanisms, enhances NF-kB transcription, modulates angiogenesis, increases telomerase activity, potentiates tumour invasion, and inhibits cell cycle arrest (Ramos-Nino et al. 2006). Recent combination inhibitors against the PI3K and mTOR pathways mutual downstream signaling pathways have proven more effective than individual pathway targeting in human cell lines, and xenograft mouse models.

FAK, a non-receptor tyrosine kinase, belonging to signal pathways downstream of growth factor receptors and integrin-mediated cell adhesion (Thellung et al. 2016), is also overexpressed in mesothelioma. FAK signaling enhances cell survival, proliferation, migration, and tissue invasion. FAK-targeting pharmacological agents are currently being tested in the preclinical setting (Shapiro et al. 2014). Application of focal adhesion kinase (FAK) inhibitor, defactinib, demonstrated efficacy in NF-2-deficient tumours in vitro; however clinical trials were halted due to a lack of efficacy.

The c-MET receptor tyrosine kinase is often overexpressed in mesothelioma. Binding of the ligand receptor, hepatocyte growth factor (HGF), for this proto-oncogene enhanced cell proliferation, motility, and invasion, whilst promoting tumourigenesis and metastasis (Thellung et al. 2016). Notably combinatorial treatment with PI3K and c-Met RTK inhibitors has demonstrated increased efficacy in human mesothelioma cell line culture, resulting in G2-M arrest and apoptosis. Combination therapy in mouse models was also highly synergistic, reducing mesothelioma tumour growth.

Other drugs tested in the RTK space for mesothelioma treatment include EGFR inhibitors, BCR-Abl inhibitors, thalidomide, bortezomib, and vorinostat, all of which failed to improve patient outcome. Notably in each of these studies, a subgroup of patients appeared to benefit from treatment. Current studies are therefore underway to identify biomarkers for these treatment-sensitive subgroups.

4.2.2   Cancer Stem Cell Signaling

Cancer stem cells are commonly considered as the progenitor of tumour initiation, progression, recurrence, and resistance to treatment. This is because cancer stem cell progeny may be killed by chemotherapy or radiotherapy, whereas cancer stem cells are resistant. This therapy resistance may be attributed to the self-renewal capability of these cells and expression of stem-like intracellular signaling pathways. Activation of these stem-like pathways in mesothelioma patients associates with poor prognosis. Stem-like intracellular signaling mechanisms under investigation in mesothelioma include growth factor receptor pathways, Wnt signaling, Notch pathways, TGFβ, and Hippo and hedgehog pathway (Thellung et al. 2016).

The Wnt signaling pathway is involved in cell fate and proliferation in embryogenesis. Dysregulation of Wnt signaling by fizzled transmembrane receptors, is associated with tumourigenesis. Inhibition of Wnt signaling in mouse and human lung adenocarcinoma has been shown to inhibit tumour growth (Nusse and Clevers 2017).

4.2.3 Oncogenes and Tumour Suppressor Genes

Comprehensive genomic analysis of mesothelioma samples has found a landscape of mutated or altered tumour suppressor genes including BAP1, NF2, TP53, SETD2, and CDKN2A (Bueno et al. 2016). As loss of function genes, these cannot be targeted, and therefore downstream signaling molecules have been identified as potential therapeutic targets.

Chromatin is composed of DNA, RNA, and proteins. Histones form the basic protein structure of chromatin, where an octamer of histone subunits forms the nucleosome. DNA is wound around these nucleosome subunits to tightly pack DNA within the cell. Decondensation of the nucleosome is required for gene expression and involves epigenetic regulation including DNA methylation, as well as histone methylation, acetylation, and phosphorylation. Tumour suppressor genes can be regulated by epigenetic changes, leading to condensation of chromatin, and loss of heterozygosity. Histone acetyl transferases and deacetylases (HDACs) control DNA methylation and chromatin condensation. Early studies indicated a role for hypermethylation of CpG repeats in promoter regions of tumour suppressor genes in mesothelioma cell lines expressing SV40. Latter studies provide more convincing evidence for treatment of mesothelioma with histone deacetylase inhibitors (Paik and Krug 2010).

Treatment of mesothelioma cell lines with HDAC inhibitors (HDACi) leads to apoptosis. HDAC inhibitors tested include sodium butyrate, suberoylanilide hydroxamic acid, and depsipeptide that induce apoptosis via downregulation of the anti-apoptotic protein bcl-XL. In other studies, pan-HDAC inhibitor LBH589 or valproic acid treatment of mesothelioma cell lines induced apoptosis in a caspase-dependent manner, whilst valproic acid in combination with chemotherapy has now demonstrated increased efficacy in human epithelioid mesothelioma mouse xenograft models.

Clinical trials with the HDAC inhibitors belinostat (PXD101) and vorinostat are complete, however data has not yet been released. New pre-clinical studies, however, indicate increased efficacy of HDAC inhibitors in combination with chemotherapy. Further in a phase I clinical trial of five mesothelioma patients treated with vorinostat in combination with cisplatin and pemetrexed, 60% exhibited stable disease (Paik and Krug 2010).

The entire INK4a/ARF locus is deleted in greater than 70% of human mesothelioma cell lines. The INK4A/ARF locus encodes p16INK4a and p14ARF that regulate expression of the oncogene p53 and retinoblastoma protein (pRB) pathways, leading to G1 arrest and G0 arrest/apoptosis, respectively. Adenoviral p14ARF infection of human mesothelioma cell lines led to cell cycle arrest, growth inhibition, and apoptosis (Paik and Krug 2010). Further, p14ARF gene therapy restoration of p53 activity is being investigated as a tool to enhance the efficacy of radiation and chemotherapy treatment.

4.3 Biomarkers

The identification of biomarkers specific to mesothelioma is a useful tool for monitoring at-risk populations for early diagnosis and tumour response to therapy (Arnold and Maskell 2018). A good biomarker needs to be preferentially expressed at a relatively high level on mesothelioma cells and detected with high sensitivity and specificity. An ideal biomarker would be detectable in the serum of asbestos-exposed individuals at early stages of disease, prior to radiological confirmation of disease.

Candidate mesothelioma biomarkers include mesothelin, osteopontin, fibulin-3, and vascular endothelial growth factor (VEGF). Mesothelin is highly expressed on mesothelioma cells with low-level expression on some normal tissues (Robinson and Lake 2005). In mesothelioma patients, soluble mesothelin was detected in the blood with a sensitivity of 83% and specificity of 95%. As a predictive marker however, soluble mesothelin decreases to below an acceptable limit with only 75% of patients' serum positive at diagnosis, and patients with sarcomatoid phenotype have low or undetectable SM throughout disease. Importantly, after therapy decreased SM levels do correlate with surgical tumour debulking, response to therapy, or improved overall survival (Arnold and Maskell 2018).

Osteopontin (OPN) is a glycoprotein that mediates cell-cell interactions and is overexpressed on breast colon and lung malignancies. As a biomarker, OPN has low sensitivity (57%), and moderate specificity (81%), and therefore is not suitable for diagnostic testing. In addition OPN serial monitoring did not correlate with debulking surgery or response to chemotherapy. However, OPN has been demonstrated to have predictive potential of poor prognosis (Arnold and Maskell 2018).

Fibulin-3, thought to phosphorylate EGF, is reported in the serum of asbestos-exposed populations with a sensitivity of 87% and specificity of 89% and again falls below the level required for diagnostic testing. A number of studies indicate a correlation between high fibulin-3 serum levels at diagnosis and poor prognosis. VEGF similarly is elevated in mesothelioma with insufficient accuracy for a diagnostic test with 70.6% sensitivity and 88.1% specificity (Arnold and Maskell 2018).

The future of biomarker research is focused on identification of new biomarkers, validation of existing biomarkers or panels of biomarkers, and targeted biomarker research.

MicroRNA (miRNA) signatures have been identified in mesothelioma patients. These miRNA target mRNA after transcription and modulate translation. miRNAs are small non-coding RNA molecules that function as oncogenes or target tumour suppressor genes and are implicated in cell transformation. Identified markers of prognostic value include hsa-miR-29c*. In comparative studies on normal mesothelial and mesothelioma cells, there is upregulation of miR17-92 cluster. Other studies indicate downregulation of miR-126 in asbestos-exposed and mesothelioma patients; however 75% sensitivity and 54% specificity are too poor for diagnostic testing.

Hyaluronic acid is found in the blood and pleural effusions of patients with mesothelioma. New technology has allowed more accurate testing for hyaluronic acid. Recent studies indicate increased predictive value for combination testing of pleural fluid for hyaluronic acid and soluble mesothelin (Creaney et al. 2013) in diagnostic testing of mesothelioma. However the exact pathophysiology of these findings is uncertain and future optimisation is required.

Other studies have combined plasma mesothelin and microRNA miR-103a-3p detection. This sensitivity and specificity of mesothelioma patient testing increased from 74% and 89% to 95% and 81%, for mesothelin alone or combination testing, respectively. More recently studies show increased diagnostic significance for changes in the combination levels for miR-26, methylated thrombomodulin, and soluble mesothelin that are superior to current available screening tests (Santarelli et al. 2015).

New microRNA studies in mesothelioma are investigating the epigenetic methylation and inactivation of miRNA34/b/c. Active expression of miRNA34/b/c induces cell cycle arrest and inhibition of cell migration and invasion in both primary mesothelial cells and mesothelium cell lines. Further, xenograft mesothelioma studies have shown reduced tumour growth in adenovirus miRNA-34b/c-infected tumour cells. Other microRNAs such as oncogenic miR17 and miRNA-1 have also been targeted for modulation or re-expression to induce apoptosis in mesothelioma cells.

Finally, mesothelin has been investigated as an anti-tumour target using antibody therapy including anti-mesothelin immunotoxin SS1P and amatuximab (MORAb-009) or more recently the combination antibody-drug conjugate anetumab ravtansine (Thellung et al. 2016).

4.4 Novel Studies

4.4.1 Drug Repositioning

In the new technology age, many drugs are now being utilised off-target for disease treatment. This is possible as new DNA, RNA, and protein analysis can identify aberrant pathways in cancer cells, and then existing drugs can be used to interrupt these pathways and inhibit tumour cell growth (Thellung et al. 2016).

Metformin, used in type 2 diabetes, reduces tumour cell growth in many cancers. Whilst not tested in mesothelioma patients, mesothelioma cell treated with metformin had reduced intercellular communication a common structural feature in mesothelioma.

Disulfiram, a drug used to treat chronic alcoholism, has shown anti-tumour activity in humans, with suppressed proliferation in mesothelioma cells. Zoledronic acid, a nitrogen bisphosphonate, similarly arrests mesothelioma cells in S-phase. Estrogen receptor b (ERb) has been identified as tumour suppressor in mesothelioma. Treatment of mesothelioma in vitro and in vivo with the agonist KB9520 also had efficacy alone and increased sensitivity to cisplatin.

NSAIDs in the form of aspirin or Cox-2 selective inhibitors (celecoxib) have been investigated as a preventative for mesothelioma in that they may alleviate chronic inflammation after asbestos exposure. In mice there was significantly prolonged disease latency, but no change in rate of development or survival.

Itraconazole, an antifungal drug, has anti-tumour activity in mesothelioma at the level of angiogenesis and suppression of Hedgehog (Hh) signal transduction.

4.4.2 Viral and Gene Therapy

Viral therapy has been investigated as a therapy for mesothelioma (Pease and Kratzke 2017), with some success for non-replicating, conditional-replicating, and replication-competent viruses in preclinical models of mesothelioma.

Replication incompetent adenoviral vector expressing HSV-thymidine kinase suicide gene (Ad.HSV*tk)* rendered tumour cells susceptible to ganciclovir treatment both in vitro and in animal models (Pease and Kratzke 2017). Other adenovirus vectors expressing IFN-gamma also induced effective anti-tumour immunity, particularly with the addition of the expression of the co-stimulatory molecule CD40L (Friedlander et al. 2003).

In conditionally replicating adenoviruses, expression of viral protein is under the control of tumour-specific promoters. Accordingly, viral protein expression is limited to tumour cells and induced oncolysis in human mesothelioma cell lines.

Vaccinia viruses have been designed to infect tumour cells and stimulate and anti-tumour immune response. The replication-competent GLV-1 h68 virus successfully replicated and lysed multiple human mesothelioma cell lines in vitro. Importantly, this GLV-1 h68 virus reduced tumour burden and increases survival after intrapleural delivery in a murine model of mesothelioma (Belin et al. 2013).

4.4.3 Combination Treatment Modalities

The need for more effective treatment of mesothelioma and other solid tumours has led to exploration of combination modality treatments with ICPB, chemotherapy, radiation therapy, RTKs, anti-angiogenic drugs, and/or cytokine therapy.

Chemotherapy and ICPB

ICPB has met with limited success for mesothelioma, and new strategies are investigating combination treatment modalities for chemotherapy and ICPB. This is largely based on the somewhat recent findings of the immunomodulatory capacity of chemotherapy that may synergise with ICPB treatment.

The first study to demonstrate efficacy of combination chemotherapy and immunotherapy against mesothelioma was gemcitabine and anti-CD40 in a murine solid tumour model (Nowak et al. 2003b). More recent studies have combined anti-CTLA4 with the chemotherapies cisplatin, paclitaxel, etoposide, ixabepilone, and melphalan to demonstrate an additive effect of combination therapy (Aston et al. 2014). Interestingly, in these studies whilst little effect was observed for chemotherapy alone, a combination of therapy with CTLA-4 commonly induced 50% tumour regression.

PD-1/PD-L1 pathway blockade and low-dose cyclophosphamide also increased tumour immunity (Aston et al. 2014), potentially due to depletion of Treg cells, in solid tumour models. In other cancer models, efficacy of the combination PD-1/GITR with cisplatin and paclitaxel was greatly enhanced compared to monotherapy treatment (Aston et al. 2014). Combination chemotherapy with PD-1 pathway however is still in the early stages, and only a limited number of drug combinations have been tested in cancer models, and efficacy in mesothelioma is yet to be established.

ICPB and Radiotherapy

Increasing evidence from both clinical and preclinical settings suggests that radiotherapy may be a useful partner for ICPB, causing beneficial immune modulation and release of tumour-associated antigens but without the systemic toxicities associated with chemotherapy.

Mouse models of mesothelioma using hypo-fractionated dosing schedules, i.e. 15 Gy delivered over 3 fractions, were used to asses immunological response to radiotherapy. Two subcutaneous tumours, one on each flank, were used, with local radiotherapy to one tumour resulting in increased T cell infiltration to both tumours (Wu et al. 2015). When anti-CTLA-4 ICPB antibody was added following radiotherapy, tumour growth was delayed, and the presence of suppressive Treg cells was decreased with increased activated CD8 T cells in the spleen; expression of genes linked to immune activation in tumour was also upregulated (Wu et al. 2015). However, as in the clinic, tumour growth was not controlled in the majority of mice, and it may be that treatment scheduling was not optimal; for example, studies in other cancers have demonstrated that administration of anti-CTLA4 prior to radiotherapy may be more efficacious (Twyman-Saint Victor et al. 2015). Local radiotherapy has also been combined with anti-PD-1 and anti-PD-L1 ICPB antibodies in mouse mesothelioma, with both combinations currently showing to be less effective than radiotherapy plus anti-CTLA-4 (De La Maza et al. 2017).

Other Chemotherapy Combination Treatments

RTKs have a role in mesothelioma, and recent studies indicate that inhibition of the PI3K/AKT pathway enhances sensitivity to chemotherapeutic agents in preclinical studies. Other studies indicate the focal adhesion kinases and PD1 inhibitors may increase anti-tumour immunity (Schunselaar et al. 2016).

Neo-angiogenesis in cancer development provides nutrients to cancer cell proliferation and an avenue for metastasis. Mesothelioma cells secrete VEGF and have enhanced receptor expression to induce new vessel formation. High-level VEGF in patient serum is indicative of dismal mesothelioma prognosis. In combination the VEGF neutralising antibody, bevaciumab, with pemetrexed has shown efficacy in high-expression VEGF xenografts and is thought to control mesothelioma progression (Thellung et al. 2016).

5   Summary

A number of valuable mesothelioma models are available, each with their own advantages and shortcomings. Currently, mesothelioma mouse models must be selected on the attributes that best suit the specific research question. It is important that findings be replicated in multiple models to determine the reproducibility and robustness of results and increase the translatability of findings.

References

Arnold DT, Maskell NA. Biomarkers in mesothelioma. Ann Clin Biochem. 2018;55(1):49–58. https://doi.org/10.1177/0004563217741145.

Aston WJ, Fisher SA, Khong A, Mok C, Nowak AK, Lake RA, Joost Lesterhuis W. Combining chemotherapy and checkpoint blockade in thoracic cancer: how to proceed? Lung Cancer Manag. 2014;3(6):443–57.

Bakker E, Guazzelli A, Ashtiani F, Demonacos C, Krstic-Demonacos M, Mutti L. Immunotherapy advances for mesothelioma treatment. Expert Rev Anticancer Ther. 2017;17(9):799–814. https://doi.org/10.1080/14737140.2017.1358091.

Bayman N, Ardron D, Ashcroft L, Baldwin DR, Booton R, Darlison L, Edwards JG, Lang-Lazdunski L, Lester JF, Peake M, Rintoul RC, Snee M, Taylor P, Lunt C, Faivre-Finn C. Protocol for PIT: a phase III trial of prophylactic irradiation of tracts in patients with malignant pleural mesothelioma following invasive chest wall intervention. BMJ Open. 2016;6(1):e010589. https://doi.org/10.1136/bmjopen-2015-010589.

Belin LJ, Ady JW, Lewis C, Marano D, Gholami S, Mojica K, Eveno C, Longo V, Zanzonico PB, Chen NG, Szalay AA, Fong Y. An oncolytic vaccinia virus expressing the human sodium iodine symporter prolongs survival and facilitates SPECT/CT imaging in an orthotopic model of malignant pleural mesothelioma. Surgery. 2013;154(3):486–95. https://doi.org/10.1016/j.surg.2013.06.004.

Bueno R, Stawiski EW, Goldstein LD, Durinck S, De Rienzo A, Modrusan Z, Gnad F, Nguyen TT, Jaiswal BS, Chirieac LR, Sciaranghella D, Dao N, Gustafson CE, Munir KJ, Hackney JA, Chaudhuri A, Gupta R, Guillory J, Toy K, Ha C, Chen YJ, Stinson J, Chaudhuri S, Zhang N, Wu TD, Sugarbaker DJ, de Sauvage FJ, Richards WG, Seshagiri S. Comprehensive genomic analysis of malignant pleural mesothelioma identifies recurrent mutations, gene fusions and splicing alterations. Nat Genet. 2016;48(4):407–16. https://doi.org/10.1038/ng.3520.

Chee J, Robinson BW, Holt RA, Creaney J. Immunotherapy for lung malignancies: from gene sequencing to novel therapies. Chest. 2017;151(4):891–7. https://doi.org/10.1016/j.chest.2016.10.007.

Cho BC, Feld R, Leighl N, Opitz I, Anraku M, Tsao MS, Hwang DM, Hope A, de Perrot M. A feasibility study evaluating surgery for mesothelioma after radiation therapy: the "SMART" approach for resectable malignant pleural mesothelioma. J Thorac Oncol. 2014;9(3):397–402. https://doi.org/10.1097/JTO.0000000000000078.

Cleo Robinson JNS, Gary Lee YC, Lake RA, Joost Lesterhuis W. Mouse models of mesothelioma: strengths, limitations and clinical translation. Lung Cancer Manag. 2014;3(5). https://doi.org/10.2217/lmt.14.27.

Creaney J, Dick IM, Segal A, Musk AW, Robinson BW. Pleural effusion hyaluronic acid as a prognostic marker in pleural malignant mesothelioma. Lung Cancer. 2013;82(3):491–8. https://doi.org/10.1016/j.lungcan.2013.09.016.

Creaney J, Ma S, Sneddon SA, Tourigny MR, Dick IM, Leon JS, Khong A, Fisher SA, Lake RA, Lesterhuis WJ, Nowak AK, Leary S, Watson MW, Robinson BW. Strong spontaneous tumor neoantigen responses induced by a natural human carcinogen. Oncoimmunology. 2015;4(7):e1011492. https://doi.org/10.1080/2162402X.2015.1011492.

Davis MR, Manning LS, Whitaker D, Garlepp MJ, Robinson BW. Establishment of a murine model of malignant mesothelioma. Int J Cancer. 1992;52(6):881–6.

De La Maza L, Wu M, Wu L, Yun H, Zhao Y, Cattral M, McCart A, Cho BJ, de Perrot M. In situ vaccination after accelerated hypofractionated radiation and surgery in a mesothelioma mouse model. Clin Cancer Res. 2017;23(18):5502–13. https://doi.org/10.1158/1078-0432.CCR-17-0438.

Fear VS, Tilsed C, Chee J, Forbes CA, Casey T, Solin JN, Lansley SM, Joost Lesterhuis W, Dick IM, Nowak AK, Robinson BW, Lake RA, Fisher SA. Combination immune checkpoint blockade as an effective therapy for mesothelioma. Oncoimmunology. 2018;7(10):e1494111. https://doi.org/10.1080/2162402X.2018.1494111. eCollection 2018.

Fisher SA, Aston WJ, Chee J, Khong A, Cleaver AL, Solin JN, Ma S, Lesterhuis WJ, Dick I, Holt RA, Creaney J, Boon L, Robinson B, Lake RA. Transient Treg depletion enhances therapeutic anti-cancer vaccination. Immun Inflammation Dis. 2017;5(1):16–28. https://doi.org/10.1002/iid3.136.

Friedlander PL, Delaune CL, Abadie JM, Toups M, LaCour J, Marrero L, Zhong Q, Kolls JK. Efficacy of CD40 ligand gene therapy in malignant mesothelioma. Am J Respir Cell Mol Biol. 2003;29(3 Pt 1):321–30. https://doi.org/10.1165/rcmb.2002-0226OC.

Goodglick L, Vaslet CA, Messier NJ, Kane AB. Growth factor responses and protooncogene expression of murine mesothelial cell lines derived from asbestos-induced mesotheliomas. Toxicol Pathol. 1997;25(6):565–73.

Jackaman C, Bundell CS, Kinnear BF, Smith AM, Filion P, van Hagen D, Robinson BW, Nelson DJ. IL-2 intratumoral immunotherapy enhances CD8+ T cells that mediate destruction of tumor cells and tumor-associated vasculature: a novel mechanism for IL-2. J Immunol. 2003;171(10):5051–63.

Lesterhuis WJ, Punt CJ, Hato SV, Eleveld-Trancikova D, Jansen BJ, Nierkens S, Schreibelt G, de Boer A, Van Herpen CM, Kaanders JH, van Krieken JH, Adema GJ, Figdor CG, de Vries IJ. Platinum-based drugs disrupt STAT6-mediated suppression of immune responses against cancer in humans and mice. J Clin Invest. 2011;121(8):3100–8. https://doi.org/10.1172/JCI43656.

Manning L, Whitaker D, Murch AR, Garlepp MJ, Davis MR, Musk AW, Robinson BW. Establishment and characterization of five human malignant mesothelioma cell lines derived from pleural effusions. Int J Cancer. 1991;47(2):285–90.

Marabelle A, Kohrt H, Sagiv-Barfi I, Ajami B, Axtell RC, Zhou G, Rajapaksa R, Green MR, Torchia J, Brody J, Luong R, Rosenblum MD, Steinman L, Levitsky HI, Tse V, Levy R. Depleting tumor-specific Tregs at a single site eradicates disseminated tumors. J Clin Invest. 2013;123(6):2447–63. https://doi.org/10.1172/JCI64859.

Nowak AK, Lake RA, Marzo AL, Scott B, Heath WR, Collins EJ, Frelinger JA, Robinson BW. Induction of tumor cell apoptosis in vivo increases tumor antigen cross-presentation, cross-priming rather than cross-tolerizing host tumor-specific CD8 T cells. J Immunol. 2003a;170(10):4905–13.

Nowak AK, Robinson BW, Lake RA. Synergy between chemotherapy and immunotherapy in the treatment of established murine solid tumors. Cancer Res. 2003b;63(15):4490–6.

Nusse R, Clevers H. Wnt/beta-catenin Signaling, disease, and emerging therapeutic modalities. Cell. 2017;169(6):985–99. https://doi.org/10.1016/j.cell.2017.05.016.

Opitz I, Weder W. A nuanced view of extrapleural pneumonectomy for malignant pleural mesothelioma. Ann transl Med. 2017;5(11):237. https://doi.org/10.21037/atm.2017.03.88.

Paik PK, Krug LM. Histone deacetylase inhibitors in malignant pleural mesothelioma: preclinical rationale and clinical trials. J Thorac Oncol. 2010;5(2):275–9. https://doi.org/10.1097/JTO.0b013e3181c5e366.

Pease DF, Kratzke RA. Oncolytic viral therapy for mesothelioma. Front Oncol. 2017;7:179. https://doi.org/10.3389/fonc.2017.00179.

Perrot M, Wu L, Wu M, Cho BCJ. Radiotherapy for the treatment of malignant pleural mesothelioma. Lancet Oncol. 2017;18(9):e532–42. https://doi.org/10.1016/S1470-2045(17)30459-X.

Ramakrishnan R, Assudani D, Nagaraj S, Hunter T, Cho HI, Antonia S, Altiok S, Celis E, Gabrilovich DI. Chemotherapy enhances tumor cell susceptibility to CTL-mediated killing during cancer immunotherapy in mice. J Clin Invest. 2010;120(4):1111–24. https://doi.org/10.1172/JCI40269.

Ramos-Nino ME, Testa JR, Altomare DA, Pass HI, Carbone M, Bocchetta M, Mossman BT. Cellular and molecular parameters of mesothelioma. J Cell Biochem. 2006;98(4):723–34. https://doi.org/10.1002/jcb.20828.

Robinson BW, Lake RA. Advances in malignant mesothelioma. N Engl J Med. 2005;353(15):1591–603. https://doi.org/10.1056/NEJMra050152.

Robinson C, van Bruggen I, Segal A, Dunham M, Sherwood A, Koentgen F, Robinson BW, Lake RA. A novel SV40 TAg transgenic model of asbestos-induced mesothelioma: malignant transformation is dose dependent. Cancer Res. 2006;66(22):10786–94. https://doi.org/10.1158/0008-5472.CAN-05-4668.

Robinson C, Walsh A, Larma I, O'Halloran S, Nowak AK, Lake RA. MexTAg mice exposed to asbestos develop cancer that faithfully replicates key features of the pathogenesis of human mesothelioma. Eur J Cancer. 2011;47(1):151–61. https://doi.org/10.1016/j.ejca.2010.08.015.

Robinson C, Dick IM, Wise MJ, Holloway A, Diyagama D, Robinson BW, Creaney J, Lake RA. Consistent gene expression profiles in MexTAg transgenic mouse and wild type mouse asbestos-induced mesothelioma. BMC Cancer. 2015;15:983. https://doi.org/10.1186/s12885-015-1953-y.

Rusch VW, Giroux D, Kennedy C, Ruffini E, Cangir AK, Rice D, Pass H, Asamura H, Waller D, Edwards J, Weder W, Hoffmann H, van Meerbeeck JP, Committee IS. Initial analysis of the international association for the study of lung cancer mesothelioma database. J Thorac Oncol. 2012;7(11):1631–9. https://doi.org/10.1097/JTO.0b013e31826915f1.

Santarelli L, Staffolani S, Strafella E, Nocchi L, Manzella N, Grossi P, Bracci M, Pignotti E, Alleva R, Borghi B, Pompili C, Sabbatini A, Rubini C, Zuccatosta L, Bichisecchi E, Valentino M, Horwood K, Comar M, Bovenzi M, Dong LF, Neuzil J, Amati M, Tomasetti M. Combined circulating epigenetic markers to improve mesothelin performance in the diagnosis of malignant mesothelioma. Lung Cancer. 2015;90(3):457–64. https://doi.org/10.1016/j.lungcan.2015.09.021.

Schunselaar LM, Quispel-Janssen JM, Neefjes JJ, Baas P. A catalogue of treatment and technologies for malignant pleural mesothelioma. Expert Rev Anticancer Ther. 2016;16(4):455–63. https://doi.org/10.1586/14737140.2016.1162100.

Shapiro IM, Kolev VN, Vidal CM, Kadariya Y, Ring JE, Wright Q, Weaver DT, Menges C, Padval M, McClatchey AI, Xu Q, Testa JR, Pachter JA. Merlin deficiency predicts FAK inhibitor sensitivity: a synthetic lethal relationship. Sci Transl Med. 2014;6(237):237ra268. https://doi.org/10.1126/scitranslmed.3008639.

Sharabi AB, Lim M, DeWeese TL, Drake CG. Radiation and checkpoint blockade immunotherapy: radiosensitisation and potential mechanisms of synergy. Lancet Oncol. 2015;16(13):e498–509. https://doi.org/10.1016/S1470-2045(15)00007-8.

Steven A, Fisher SA, Robinson BW. Immunotherapy for lung cancer. Respirology. 2016;21(5):821–33. https://doi.org/10.1111/resp.12789.

Taguchi T, Jhanwar SC, Siegfried JM, Keller SM, Testa JR. Recurrent deletions of specific chromosomal sites in 1p, 3p, 6q, and 9p in human malignant mesothelioma. Cancer Res. 1993;53(18):4349–55.

Thellung S, Favoni RE, Wurth R, Nizzari M, Pattarozzi A, Daga A, Florio T, Barbieri F. Molecular pharmacology of malignant pleural mesothelioma: challenges and perspectives from preclinical and clinical studies. Curr Drug Targets. 2016;17(7):824–49.

Twyman-Saint Victor C, Rech AJ, Maity A, Rengan R, Pauken KE, Stelekati E, Benci JL, Xu B, Dada H, Odorizzi PM, Herati RS, Mansfield KD, Patsch D, Amaravadi RK, Schuchter LM, Ishwaran H, Mick R, Pryma DA, Xu X, Feldman MD, Gangadhar TC, Hahn SM, Wherry EJ, Vonderheide RH, Minn AJ. Radiation and dual checkpoint blockade activate non-redundant immune mechanisms in cancer. Nature. 2015;520(7547):373–7. https://doi.org/10.1038/nature14292.

Wu L, Wu MO, De la Maza L, Yun Z, Yu J, Zhao Y, Cho J, de Perrot M. Targeting the inhibitory receptor CTLA-4 on T cells increased abscopal effects in murine mesothelioma model. Oncotarget. 2015;6(14):12468–80. https://doi.org/10.18632/oncotarget.3487.

Zeltsman M, Dozier J, McGee E, Ngai D, Adusumilli PS. CAR T-cell therapy for lung cancer and malignant pleural mesothelioma. Transl Res. 2017;187:1–10. https://doi.org/10.1016/j.trsl.2017.04.004.

The Impact of the Internet on Mesothelioma Patients: The Good, the Bad, and the Ugly

19

Maja Belamaric and Mary Hesdorffer

At this point, it is hard for most of us to imagine a world where information isn't available to us at our fingertips. But the Internet, along with its ability to provide us with almost any knowledge we require in a matter of milliseconds, is a relatively new invention. Moreover, tools necessary to make the Internet actually useful are an even more recent occurrence. For perspective, Google, the most popular search engine, didn't exist before 1998 and wasn't quite helpful until the early 2000s when the company went public and underwent exponential improvements in its coverage as well as visibility (Wikipedia 2018). In terms of social media networks, it was 2006 when Facebook opened its product to the general public, though the network didn't gain much prominence until about 2010, when for the first time it reported 400 million users (Wikipedia 2017). As of September 2017, Facebook users have reached 2.07 billion monthly active users (Facebook 2017).

Just as it did for most Americans in general, the rise of the Internet has also had a huge impact on mesothelioma patients and on the ways in which they manage their cancer, learn about it, and cope with it. However, as patients and their families became more reliant on the stream of information readily available to them, Internet marketers have also became more ruthless in targeting this historically hard-to-find but incredibly valuable group.

1 The Dark Ages

Let's take a step back. Before the widespread availability of the Internet, a mesothelioma diagnosis generally meant the following:

M. Belamaric (✉) · M. Hesdorffer
Mesothelioma Applied Research Foundation, Alexandria, VA, USA
e-mail: mbelamaric@curemeso.org; mary@curemeso.org

© Springer Nature Switzerland AG 2019
M. Hesdorffer, G. E. Bates-Pappas (eds.), *Caring for Patients with Mesothelioma: Principles and Guidelines*,
https://doi.org/10.1007/978-3-319-96244-3_19

- The patient was told that they had a terminal illness; they had 6 months to live at most and only had enough time to get their affairs in order.
- The diagnosing physician wasn't able to offer patient-focused information about the disease.
- The diagnosing physician wasn't able to read about the disease beyond what information they had available in print, likely outdated.
- This was likely the diagnosing physician's first and only mesothelioma case throughout their career.

After receiving such grim news with no additional information attached, the patient had no way to learn more about their illness, find specialists, or find others facing a similar diagnosis.

2 The Good

Mesothelioma patients continue to face considerable challenges with their diagnosis – and will do so until the emergence of better treatments – something the Internet cannot directly improve. That said, because of communication tools available through the Internet, today's patients can immediately, on the first day of diagnosis, find information in the form of medical journal articles, articles written with the lay person in mind, clinical trial lists, and resources, and they can immediately begin the process of connecting with others facing the same diagnosis, undergoing similar treatments, and living... sometimes well past the elusive 5-year mark they're told they likely won't cross. For mesothelioma patients, connecting with the right resource can make all the difference between despair and hope.

According to the CDC report, most mesothelioma patients are 65 years old and above, a demographic seen as generally not very tech savvy. Even so, we have seen that this group is regardless able to reap the benefits of the information superhighway, often through their grown children's help. As this group continues to expand its use of technology, we also expect seeing them participating more in social media networks, particularly Facebook.

The way a patient usually finds online resources is fairly simple. It begins with a Google (or less often a different engine) search. After the shock of the diagnosis subsides, the patient or a close family member will search for the keyword "mesothelioma." The search will return pages upon pages of search results, some relevant, others less so. If the patient is lucky, they will find the website for the Mesothelioma Applied Research Foundation, the only legitimate nonprofit in the United States whose mission is to help patients and their families and to fund research to end mesothelioma. The reason they'll need luck to find this organization is because its website isn't listed until page three of Google search results. And this brings us to the bad and the ugly.

3   The Bad and the Ugly

Nearly overnight, patients went from complete darkness to suddenly having access to as much information as they could process, at seemingly little to no cost. However, as everything in life, nobody does anything for free, which begs the question: if the only nonprofit organization within the mesothelioma space isn't found until page 3 or lower of the Google search results, what are the websites that patients are actually finding? And even more importantly, why do such websites exist?

To properly explain this dynamic, it is very important to understand the value of mesothelioma patients to plaintiff attorneys. Mesothelioma is a cancer most often caused by exposure to asbestos, and as such it has profound legal and economic implications:

> Despite the lack of comprehensive, verifiable data, some will still ask for a view on an "average" recovery by a person with mesothelioma allegedly caused by asbestos. For current claimants (as opposed to past or future claimants), the subjective view of one author (K.H.) is that persons with well-documented asbestos exposures through occupational work with or around asbestos will on average obtain a total gross recovery (before expenses) in the range of $1.5–2.2 million, if represented by well-prepared plaintiff lawyers who can credibly take a case to trial against one or more defendants. Under that view, a net recovery for the person or family may run from $500,000 to $1.5 million, depending on the expenses of the case and the terms of a contingency fee agreement with a plaintiff's law firm. (Hartley and Hesdorffer 2017)

Almost instantly into the information revolution, those looking to profit from mesothelioma patients found ways to target them. And that's how a new business model was born (Fig. 19.1).

As the stakes rose, so did the investment into recruitment websites and search engine optimization. Suddenly, informational websites looking strikingly similar to nonprofit websites began flooding the web. Meanwhile, the keyword *mesothelioma*, and related keywords (such as *mesothelioma treatment* or *mesothelioma help*), became the epitome of outlandish Internet fads. While most industries were paying

Fig. 19.1 The business model of legal marketers

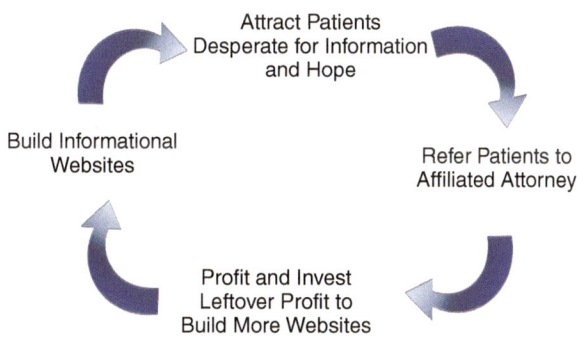

pennies per click for their keyword advertising, mesothelioma-related keyword clicks were exponentially rising first upward of $100, which seemed preposterous, and then by 2014 even higher than $300:

> Marketing of lawsuits to asbestos-exposed persons has become its own industry. Unfortunately, a result is that too many persons with cancer are lured to websites purporting to provide advocacy, expert advice, "support," and access to "top medical specialists." In our opinion, these assertions often are only barely true, and instead many of the websites are primarily about seeking out persons to become clients for some plaintiff law firms. This is not a complaint about the filing of lawsuits; they are often well-founded and much needed to provide economic resources to persons with cancer and/or their spouses or children. The complaint instead is that the client recruiting process too often diverts patients away from better sources of medical information and results in less than optimal medical care choices. For example, a patient may be diverted away from expert care fairly close to home and toward a doctor or medical center with which financial relationships have been developed. In some instances, this type of situation may needlessly delay care, and in some instances, it may decrease overall survival for a person with an aggressive mesothelioma. In other instances, persons may be discouraged from participating in clinical trials that need patient participation in order to advance research against this rare disease. (Hartley and Hesdorffer 2017)

Problems with this model abound and most notably include focus on client recruitment rather than providing objectively sound information and help. Such websites are marketing experts, not legal nor medical. They hire young, just-out-of-school marketers to help pump out as much content as they can, often styling it as clickbait. Therefore, factual accuracy is less important than obtaining clicks.

While the Internet may have been the most significant factor in the empowerment of mesothelioma patients, in the last decade, it has also become the easiest way to take advantage of them, mislead them, and provide them with false hope.

References

Facebook. Facebook reports third quarter 2017 results. 1 November 2017. https://investor.fb.com/investor-news/press-release-details/2017/Facebook-Reports-Third-Quarter-2017-Results/default.aspx. Accessed 15 Jan 2018.

Hartley K, Hesdorffer M. Challenges facing mesothelioma patients. In: Testa JR, editor. Asbestos and mesothelioma. Cham: Springer; 2017.

Wikipedia. History of Facebook. 19 December 2017. https://en.wikipedia.org/wiki/History_of_Facebook. Accessed 17 Jan 2018.

Wikipedia. History of Google. 12 January 2018. https://en.wikipedia.org/wiki/History_of_Google. Accessed 15 Jan 2018.

Raya Bodnarchuk

It turned out to be a gray and chilling day for the annual town yard sale. I was not feeling well but decided to join in for the usual camaraderie. My house is central, and my friends come to participate from this neighborhood and others. We line the street with our wares, so it is more like a street festival.

It was not usual for me to be tired, but I was coughing and my chest was heavy, and it felt like something was starting. I was worn out by the end of the day. My friend Dorothy, who is a doctor, had stayed behind and suggested that I see my doctor. He diagnosed bronchitis.

A few days later, I felt worse, so I went to the emergency room at Sibley Hospital. It was determined there that I had pneumonia, and I spent the next week on the fifth floor, attached to an IV drip, but with an unusual and magnificent view of the Potomac River. The view, the food, and the kindness of the workers and my friends got me through what turned out to be an unexpected and difficult week of the pulmonologist not quite being satisfied that pneumonia was the whole story. He ordered more tests, including a mediastinoscopy and bronchoscopy, and dug into my history. It was definitely the start of something.

I left Sibley with the pulmonologist hoping that the fluid, thought likely to be a part of the pneumonia, would subside. But he also recommended that I get a thoracoscopy (biopsy). I met with a couple of thoracic surgeons who could do this biopsy,

A practicing artist, specifically a sculptor, I was a fine art professor at the Corcoran College of Art and Design. I am now Professor Emeritus of Fine Art at the George Washington University.

R. Bodnarchuk (✉)
The Corcoran College of Art and Design, Washington, DC, USA

George Washington University, Washington, DC, USA

Rinehart School of Sculpture, Maryland Institute College of Art, Baltimore, MD, USA

Rhode Island School of Design, Sculpture, Providence, RI, USA

© Springer Nature Switzerland AG 2019
M. Hesdorffer, G. E. Bates-Pappas (eds.), *Caring for Patients with Mesothelioma: Principles and Guidelines*,
https://doi.org/10.1007/978-3-319-96244-3_20

and I ended up choosing one at Johns Hopkins. On July 19, 2012, I traveled to Baltimore where it was determined: I had pleural mesothelioma.

I was born into a family of artists. My father was a sculptor and my mother a painter and ceramicist and an art educator. Thus, I grew up surrounded by art and making things. And I grew up through art and making things, ultimately going to art school and graduate school in sculpture.

I had been teaching for 40 years when everything changed. I continued for 2 more years after the diagnosis, through chemotherapy and the frightening prognosis. The studio in which I taught was demanding, especially physically, given the environmental hazards. The loss of energy and stamina from the mesothelioma led to my having a different, less demanding teaching assignment.

Then I was turning 65, the institution was going under, and I had mesothelioma. That led to my stepping down and retiring from that job and life of 31 years. I had a farewell exhibition honoring my sculpture and two-dimensional work at the museum. I titled that show, "Letter to My Mother," in homage to my parents' contributions to my life in every way. I also revealed why I was leaving. Here is that letter:

LETTER TO MY MOTHER
February 24, 2014
Dear Mother,
Can you believe I am retiring from the Corcoran after teaching for 32 years! I feel I've been fortunate in so many ways – my colleagues were also my friends and my students always reminded me of what learning about art was like when I was their age. Though it comes down to doing my best work alone, I've also been surrounded and supported by people who experience the same struggles, share the same sense of enjoyment and celebrate the same accomplishments.

I appreciate so much what you and Daddy gave me. I didn't realize that I would be following in your footsteps. You were a great teacher for me and for all of your students, and I learned from your example that pursuing very simple ideas can lead to a fulfilling life's work. I believe that began when I was one-and-a-half and you gave me a shot glass of water and a little brush to paint on the refrigerator. Your encouragement and patience are unforgettable. You showed me what it means to be a great teacher. Daddy taught me how important tools and the knowledge of materials are. I sat right beside him as he worked and I made things in his footsteps. I learned many things that would have taken me twice as long to figure out by myself. You and Daddy made a rich and admirable life working side-by-side, and living with two wonderful artists gave me a view of the world of art from the very core.

You know my life changed two years ago when it was discovered that I have mesothelioma. I really didn't know what would happen with my aspirations. It was terrible. Everything was completely turned upside down.

Now I realize I have been freed to do more things with a renewed understanding of what is important and why. I thought about how long my life is going to last. I also wondered about what is going to happen to the work I've done and if I even would have the heart or the strength to continue working.

I think now I'm beginning to understand how incredibly simple the intertwining of art and life can be. I wish you could see my work and meet my colleagues and students right here in the gallery now. You know, my work has always been rooted in my personal experience and the things I hold dear. It's even more so presently. And it's not only about me – it's about the heritage you passed on to me and the progression and continuity of my work.

Looking ahead, I need to tell you how eager I am to cheer my students on into the future. I always wish them well and I hope they think of me.

I will miss my many students and will miss seeing my colleagues on a weekly basis. I loved working closely with Marie Ringwald, Rick Wall, Bill Suworoff and many more wonderful artists who were teachers, too. I will miss having the support of all the Corcoran staff and the guards at the college, the museum and the galleries. I wish you could have met them all.

Now I am looking forward to having time to myself and for my own work. Honestly, I think it will be as liberating as the change in my routine will be challenging.

I'll be missing you, Mom, and you will be happy to know that I am doing it. I won't ever stop.

Love, Raya

My life had changed quite a bit, and the treatments I had done at NIH made a huge difference in the disease. They stopped the pleural effusion from re-forming, and the tumors shrank and remained stable for the next 2 years. Without the full-time job, my art career could continue. I put my efforts into that—making and showing—and kept going. I have had to give up doing the larger works, which is a huge loss.

Since then, I have repeated the chemotherapy treatments two more times, 2 years between each time, and they did make a difference in keeping the cancer controlled. However, after the third round, I have not had positive results. Both the hope and the frightening aspects are a part of my life. I am always trying to figure out something better to do for myself. I try to do things in a positive way, with clarity, to keep living a productive life.

One part of that has been choosing NIH as my caregiving institution. Their care and attention to patients' well-being have made all the difference for me. NIH is a place of scientists and research doctors who are dedicated to finding a cure. However, I do not see an end to whatever medical treatments are required to keep the mesothelioma stable. I complement their work by taking care of myself through different health-promoting activities. These include acupuncture, yoga, exercise, proper nutrition, a rich social life, and counseling for the loss of good health. Recently, while enjoying good food with good friends on the other side of the Potomac River, looking back toward Sibley Hospital, I realized I have been living with the diagnosis of mesothelioma for 6 years.

1   Recommendations

I have been privileged to have such good care and respect from the medical professionals, and the scientists and researchers involved in my treatment. Though mesothelioma is considered rare, I have enjoyed meeting many fellow patients. I have some recommendations that could make mesothelioma treatment even better for all of us.

For Patients

- Research and hunt out the best doctor for oneself.
- Choose doctors who have experience with the mesothelioma you have (e.g., pleural, peritoneal, others).
- Interview doctors before making a decision.
- Get second opinions.
- Live your life, and do not become a total professional patient.
- Make you own decisions at every step.

For Medical Professionals

- Be kind.
- Be respectful.
- Respond to questions quickly (emails, phone calls).
- Be available to the patient.
- Avoid creating an impersonal atmosphere.
- Check in often enough so the patient does not feel frightened or forgotten.
- Take seriously even questions that may seem frivolous.
- Take seriously all reported side effects even if they seem insignificant or unusual.
- Schedule next appointments as soon as possible to reduce time for worry.

Correction to: Chemotherapy and Standard Treatment Options

Mary Hesdorffer and Gleneara E. Bates-Pappas

Correction to:
Chapter 5 in: M. Hesdorffer, G. E. Bates-Pappas (eds.),
Caring for Patients with Mesothelioma: Principles
and Guidelines, **https://doi.org/10.1007/978-3-319-96244-3_5**

The original version of the book was published in May 2019 without a key information about FDA approval for mesothelioma. The same has been included in this updated version.

The updated online version of this chapter can be found at
https://doi.org/10.1007/978-3-319-96244-3_5

© Springer Nature Switzerland AG 2019   C1
M. Hesdorffer, G. E. Bates-Pappas (eds.), *Caring for Patients*
with Mesothelioma: Principles and Guidelines,
https://doi.org/10.1007/978-3-319-96244-3_21

Helpful Resources

The Mesothelioma Applied Research Foundation
http://www.curemeso.org
Mesothelioma UK
https://www.mesothelioma.uk.com/
International Ban Asbestos Secretariat
http://ibasecretariat.org/index.htm
Bernie Banton Foundation
https://www.berniebanton.com.au/
National Cancer Institute: Comprehensive Cancer Information
https://www.cancer.gov/
International Association for the Study of Lung Cancer (IASLC)
https://www.iaslc.org/
International Mesothelioma Interest Group (IMIG)
https://imig.org/
The National Institute for Occupational Safety and Health (NIOSH)
https://www.cdc.gov/niosh/index.htm
National Organization for Rare Disorders
https://rarediseases.org/

© Springer Nature Switzerland AG 2019
M. Hesdorffer, G. E. Bates-Pappas (eds.), *Caring for Patients
with Mesothelioma: Principles and Guidelines*,
https://doi.org/10.1007/978-3-319-96244-3